CW00730146

Handbook of Family Planning
and Reproductive Health Care

For Churchill Livingstone

Commissioning Editor: Lucy Gardner
Copy Editor: Penelope Lyons
Project Manager: Nora Cameron
Design Direction: Sarah Cape
Pre-press Project Manager: Neil Dickson
Pre-press Desktop Operator: Kate Walshaw
Sales Promotion: Susan Jerdan-Taylor

Handbook of
Family Planning and
Reproductive Health Care

Edited by

Nancy Loudon OBE MB ChB FFFP
Vice-chairman, Health Education Board for Scotland,
Former Medical Co-ordinator, Family Planning and Well Woman Services,
Lothian Health Board

Anna Glasier BSc MD MRCOG
Director, Family Planning and Well Woman Services,
Edinburgh Healthcare NHS Trust; Senior Lecturer,
Department of Obstetrics and Gynaecology, University of Edinburgh

Ailsa Gebbie MB ChB DCH MRCOG MFFP
Senior Registrar in Community Gynaecology,
Edinburgh Healthcare NHS Trust

Foreword by
Sir Malcolm Macnaughton MD, LLD, FRCP, FROCG, FRSE
Past President of the Royal College of Obstetricians and Gynaecologists

THIRD EDITION

CHURCHILL LIVINGSTONE
EDINBURGH LONDON MADRID MELBOURNE NEW YORK AND TOKYO 1995

CHURCHILL LIVINGSTONE
Medical Division of Pearson Professional Limited

Distributed in the United States of America by
Churchill Livingstone Inc., 650 Avenue of the Americas,
New York, N.Y. 10011, and by associated companies,
branches and representatives throughout the world.

First published 1985
Second edition 1991
Third edition 1995

ISBN 0 443 05157 7

British Library Cataloguing in Publication Data
A catalogue record for this book is available from
the British Library.

Library of Congress Cataloging in Publication Data
A catalog record for this book is available from
the Library of Congress.

Printed in Singapore

Foreword

Easy access to all types of family planning is essential to enable women and men to control their reproductive lives. The major change over the years is that individuals now wish to know about the various methods available so they can select one that is appropriate for their needs. Today, family planning is an integral part of the National Health Service in the UK, and is internationally recognized as part of any programme of health care.

Population growth is one of the world's continuing environmental concerns; it was the major topic at the International Conference on Population and Development in Cairo in 1994. Women's reproductive health and population control are linked to the issue of poverty throughout the world. Moreover, the status of women in society pervades all aspects of reproductive health. No society treats women as well as it does men and often the health and well-being of women are compromised by a combination of neglect and abuse.

The teaching of family planning is now an established part of the curriculum in UK medical schools and general practitioners are expected to be able to advise individuals appropriately. Yet, in spite of the great growth in family planning there are still too many unplanned and unwanted pregnancies. In particular, the number of teenage pregnancies is far too high. During adolescence, people adopt a pattern of behaviour that affects health in later life. Unprotected sex can lead to unwanted pregnancy, unsafe abortion and sexually transmissible disease including HIV infection. It is vitally important that in the reorganization of the National Health Service there should be no cutback in family planning services. If family planning resources are reduced, the result will be an increase in demands for therapeutic abortion and the birth of unwanted babies.

In this, the third edition of her book, Dr Nancy Loudon, the doyenne of family planning in Edinburgh and beyond, her successor Dr Anna Glasier and her colleague Dr Ailsa Gebbie provide an up-to-date compendium of family planning methods and services.

The chapter on therapeutic abortion by Professor David Baird expands on 'medical abortion' which now gives women a choice regarding the method of abortion. Postcoital contraception is well established but is not used widely enough and in her chapter on this subject Dr Anna Glasier provides information to help those who advise women who have been exposed to unprotected intercourse. An interesting addition is the use of breastfeeding as a method of family spacing by Mrs Margaret Foxwell and Professor Peter Howie. This will be of particular interest to those in developing countries. The chapters on gynaecological problems and the menopause will be of great value since women attending a family planning consultation frequently ask questions about these related subjects.

Women have been using contraception since time immemorial but the real breakthrough came with the introduction of the contraceptive pill in the 1950s by Gregory Pincus and M. C. Chang. This has led to a great variety of hormonal methods, the most recent of which is Norplant. Future methods of contraception discussed by Dr Paul Van Look include preparations that will prevent implantation and a vaccine that will prevent conception. These methods will no doubt be elaborated on in later editions of this book.

Dr Nancy Loudon has been a major force in the development of efficient family planning services in the UK, and the foundation of the Faculty of Family Planning and Reproductive Health Care of the Royal College of Obstetricians and Gynaecologists is the fine result of her efforts and those of her colleagues over some 30 years. This volume is essential for the shelves of any health care professional involved in family planning.

1995   Sir Malcom Macnaughton

Preface

Ten years ago, the first edition of this handbook was written primarily for doctors and nurses working in family planning clinics, which at that time were offering a more comprehensive service than the family doctor. Nowadays, the general practice team is the main provider of family planning services and patients of both sexes, married and unmarried, are happy to get their contraceptive advice there.

However, a well organized clinic service remains essential and must be maintained and developed. Not only does it offer patients a choice, it also serves as a valuable support and complement to the family doctor service. Young people in particular still feel unsure about the response they will receive to a request for contraceptive help from their GP, and a clinic service designed to meet their special needs is essential. Clinics, now increasingly staffed by community gynaecologists, also act as referral centres for patients with contraceptive problems as well as providing contraceptive techniques and counselling not always available in general practice.

The establishment of the Faculty of Family Planning and Reproductive Health Care recognizes the changing role of clinics. Often led by a consultant in community gynaecology, more and more clinics offer open access help to women with menopausal and minor gynaecological problems and provide many other facilities such as colposcopy, ultrasound scanning, vasectomy and research into new methods of fertility control.

We have recognized these changes in the third edition of this handbook. It was obvious that there was no place for a special chapter on family planning in general practice and we have amalgamated other subjects to allow room for new chapters on the menopause and common gynaecological problems encountered in the course of a family planning consultation. The chapter on contraceptives of the future has been expanded to include many exciting prospects for world-wide fertility regulation.

We would like to thank Dr John Loudon for all the help he gave us at every stage in preparation of the book, from the early planning to the meticulous checking of manuscripts so necessary to produce a book in consistent synoptic style; and for coping with the disruption of his tranquil life in retirement by endless meetings in his home! Our thanks go also to our families for their support and forbearance over the past 18 months.

We are greatly indebted to Mr John Griffiths of Simpson & Marwick WS who advised us on legal matters, particularly about the differences between English and Scottish law, and for translating legal dogma into understandable English; Dr David Farquharson, consultant obstetrician and gynaecologist, for his advice; Mrs Margaret Harper for her secretarial assistance; Mrs Margaret Forest, the library services manager at the Health Education Board for Scotland, who so willingly checked addresses and references; and Mr Tom McFetters and Mr Ted Pinner of the Centre for Reproductive Biology in Edinburgh for drawing the additional diagrams.

We greatly appreciated all the help we received from Ms Lucy Gardner and the staff of Churchill Livingstone at every stage in the preparation of the book.

We hope that this handbook will serve as a clear, concise and accurate guide to current clinical practice in the field of family planning and reproductive health care, as a source of answers to contraceptive problems, and as a consensus of informed opinion in areas of doubt and uncertainty. If it contributes to a better service for patients, whether they seek contraceptive help at clinics, in general practice or in hospital, we shall be satisfied.

Edinburgh 1995   Nancy Loudon
                                                              Anna Glasier
                                                              Ailsa Gebbie

Contributors

Mary M. Anderson MB ChB, FRCOG
Consultant Obstetrician and Gynaecologist,
Lewisham Hospital; Chairman, Medico-Legal Committee,
Royal College of Obstetricians and Gynaecologists

David T. Baird DSc, FRCOG
MRC Professor of Reproductive Endocrinology,
University of Edinburgh

John Bancroft MA, MD, FRCP, FRCPsych
Clinical Scientist MRC Unit, Centre for Reproductive Biology,
Edinburgh; Honorary Senior Lecturer, Department of Psychiatry,
University of Edinburgh

James O. Drife BSc, MD, FRCS(Ed), FRCOG
Professor of Obstetrics and Gynaecology, University of Leeds

Margaret E. R. Foxwell RGN, FP Cert
Teacher, Scottish Association of Natural Family Planning;
formerly Nursing Officer, Family Planning and Well Woman
Services, Lothian Health Board

Ian S. Fraser MD, BSc, FRCOG, FRACOG
Professor of Reproductive Medicine, University of Sydney;
Director, Sydney Centre for Reproductive Health Research

Ailsa E. Gebbie MB ChB, DCH, MRCOG, MFFP
Senior Registrar in Community Gynaecology, Edinburgh
Healthcare NHS Trust

Anna Glasier BSc, MD, MRCOG
Director, Family Planning and Well Woman Services,
Edinburgh Healthcare NHS Trust; Senior Lecturer,
Department of Obstetrics and Gynaecology,
University of Edinburgh

John Guillebaud MA, FRCS(Ed), FRCOG, MFFP
Professor of Family Planning and Reproductive Health;
Medical Director, Margaret Pyke Centre for Study and Training
in Family Planning and Reproductive Heath Care

Mary Hepburn BSc, MD, MRCGP, MRCOG
Senior lecturer in Women's Reproductive Health,
University of Glasgow; Consultant Obstetrician and
Gynaecologist, Greater Glasgow Health Board

Peter Howie MD, FRCOG
Professor of Obstetrics and Gynaecology, University of Dundee

Patricia A. Last FRCS (G), FRCOG
Honorary Lecturer, Department of Obstetrics and Gynaecology,
St Bartholomew's Medical School, London; formerly Director of
Women's Screening for BUPA Medical Centres

Nancy B. Loudon OBE, MB ChB, FFFP
Vice Chairman Health Education Board for Scotland; formerly
Medical Coordinator Family Planning and Well Woman Services,
Lothian Health Board

Alexander McMillan BSc, MD, FRCPE
Consultant Physician, Department of Genitourinary Medicine,
Royal Infirmary NHS Trust; Part-time Senior Lecturer,
Department of Medicine, University of Edinburgh

Paul F. A. Van Look MD, PhD, MFFP
Associate Director, Special Programme of Research,
Development and Research Training in Human Reproduction,
World Health Organization

Penelope A. Watson BSc, MB ChB, DRCOG, MRCGP, MFFP
Principal in general practice; Clinical Medical Officer,
Family Planning and Well Woman Services,
Edinburgh Healthcare NHS Trust

Contents

1. Family planning in the United Kingdom:
    services and training   1
    Nancy Loudon, Penelope Watson

2. Factors influencing contraceptive choice   19
    Mary Hepburn

3. Combined hormonal contraception   37
    John Gillebaud

4. Progestogen-only contraception   91
    Ian Fraser

5. Intrauterine contraceptive devices   119
    James Drife

6. Barrier methods   147
    Ailsa Gebbie

7. Natural regulation of fertility   183
    Margaret Foxwell, Peter Howie

8. Sterilization   203
    Anna Glasier

9. Emergency postcoital contraception   229
    Anna Glasier

10. Theraputic abortion   241
    David Baird

11. Legal and ethical aspects of family planning   259
    Mary Anderson

12. Screening and reproductive health   279
    Patricia Last

13. Sexually transmissible diseases 301
Alexander McMillan

14. Sexuality and family planning 339
John Bancroft

15. Gynaecological problems in the family planning consulation 363
Anna Glasier

16. The menopause 383
Ailsa Gebbie

17. Contraceptives of the future 409
Paul Van Look

Abbreviations 435

Useful addresses and helplines 439

Index 447

1. Family planning in the United Kingdom: services and training

Nancy Loudon and Penelope Watson

Background
  Abortion Act 1967
  National Health Service (Family
    Planning) Act 1967
  National Health Service Reorganisation
    Act 1973
  Family Planning Association
  Brook Advisory Centres
  Joint Committee on Contraception
  National Association of Family Planning
    Doctors
  National Association of Family Planning
    Nurses
  Faculty of Family Planning and
    Reproductive Health Care

Current position

Family planning services
  General practice
    Routine consultation
    Practice FP clinic
    Home visits
    Emergency contraception
    Shared care
    The role of the nurse
    Remuneration
    Research
    Training

Family planning clinics
  Popularity of clinics
  Brook Advisory Centres
  Hospitals
  Private sector
  Pharmacists and other retail outlets

Professional family planning bodies
  Faculty of Family Planning and
    Reproductive Health Care of the
    Royal College of Obstetricians and
    Gynaecologists (FFPRHC)
  National Association of Family Planning
    Nurses (NAFPN)
  Royal College of Nursing (RCN)

Training
  Doctors
    Undergraduate
    Postgraduate
  Nurses
  Other professionals
  Natural family planning
  Psychosexual medicine
  SPOD

The future of family planning in the UK

BACKGROUND

The first 'Birth Control' clinic in the United Kingdom (UK) was opened in 1921. It took 53 years of publications, debates and law suits to establish a comprehensive, free family planning service.

The National Health Service Act 1946 empowered local health authorities and regional boards to open contraceptive clinics where advice could be provided for nursing mothers seeking help with family planning (FP) on medical grounds, or to contribute to organizations which undertook to give such advice. Few health authorities took any action and voluntary organizations, particularly the Family Planning Association (FPA), were left to develop contraceptive services by opening clinics throughout the country. These

1

clinics were used almost exclusively by married women, the majority of whom had to pay for the service and for contraceptive supplies, although payment for both was often waived for those in need.

Limitation of family size was achieved by abstinence, the rhythm method, coitus interruptus, chemical contraceptives, occlusive diaphragms, condoms, or by illegal abortion. Therapeutic termination of pregnancy was rare. Sterilization was unusual, the majority of operations being performed by tubal ligation in the puerperium or at caesarean section.

In the 1960s, with the introduction of oral contraception and modern intrauterine devices, and with the perfection of laparoscopy and vasectomy techniques permitting sterilization on a large scale, the scene gradually changed. Contraception was discussed openly and these 'respectable' methods found much more favour with doctors. Changing attitudes to premarital chastity led to demands by the unmarried for effective contraception.

Abortion Act 1967

This Act, implemented in April 1968, legalized termination of pregnancy (TOP) in England, Scotland and Wales, but does not apply to Northern Ireland (Ch. 11). It acted as a real spur to the acceptance of family planning, for it was recognized that unless good contraception was freely available the demand for termination of unwanted pregnancies would escalate (Ch. 10).

National Health Service (Family Planning) Act 1967

This enabled local authorities in England and Wales to give contraceptive advice, supplies and appliances to persons seeking contraception, from whom charges could be recovered. A similar service was introduced in Scotland in 1968 by the Public Health and Health Services Act.

These Acts were interpreted liberally by local authorities and, as a result of agency arrangements with the FPA, free contraception was provided for many women.

National Health Service Reorganisation Act 1973

A completely free family planning service at clinics and hospitals came with the reorganization of the National Health Service (NHS) in 1974, and was extended to primary care in 1975.

Thus, over a decade family planning services were revolutionized, so that in the UK there exists the first completely free, universally available contraceptive service in Western Europe.

Family Planning Association

In 1930 the National Birth Control Council was formed to coordinate the work of various birth control societies. In 1939 this became the Family Planning Association. The FPA was thereafter the major source of provision of contraceptive advice in this country until reorganization of the NHS in 1974 (see above).

The FPA, having obtained its primary objective, decided that its future role would lie in the field of public information and education, as well as training and support for professionals working in health education and social services in the public, private and voluntary sectors.

The FPA now acts as a consumer advocate, both monitoring and pressing for improvements in services. Its remit has broadened to encompass the promotion of sexual health as well as family planning in order to enable people to ensure sexual well-being and be free from the risks of unwanted pregnancy and infection.

Brook Advisory Centres

The first Brook Advisory Clinic was opened in London in 1964 with the aim of 'the prevention and mitigation of the suffering caused by unwanted pregnancy, by educating young persons in matters of sex and contraception and developing among them a sense of responsibility in regard to sexual behaviour'. Since then, centres have been set up in Bristol, Belfast, Birmingham, Coventry, Edinburgh and Liverpool.

Joint Committee on Contraception (JCC)

In 1972, when family planning was provided increasingly by local authorities, the Royal College of Obstetricians and Gynaecologists (RCOG) took the initiative of setting up a committee with the Royal College of General Practitioners (RCGP), the FPA, the Faculty of Community Medicine and, later, the National Association of Family Planning Doctors, in order to supervise standards of training in family planning and certification of doctors. It ceased to exist when its functions were taken over by the Faculty of Family Planning and Reproductive Health Care (see below).

National Association of Family Planning Doctors (NAFPD)

The objects of NAFPD, which was founded in 1974, were to advance the education of doctors in all matters pertaining to family planning and sexual medicine and to promote high standards of practice and research. It also published the *British Journal of Family Planning*. In 1994 it was disbanded, its role being encompassed in the new Faculty of Family Planning and Reproductive Health Care (see below).

National Association of Family Planning Nurses (NAFPN)

NAFPN and the Scottish Society of Family Planning Nurses perform, for nurses, functions similar to NAFPD (see above).

Faculty of Family Planning and Reproductive Health Care (FFPRHC)

In 1993 the Royal College of Obstetricians and Gynaecologists established the Faculty, which took over the functions of both NAFPD and the JCC (FFPRHC 1993).

CURRENT POSITION

It is government policy that family planning services should be available through general practitioners (GPs) and clinics in the community and in hospitals, with the aim of maximizing uptake by this dual provision and offering choice (Executive letter, Department of Health 1990).

In 1992 guidelines were issued to regional health authorities in England to assist in a review of FP services and giving advice on targeting and accessibility of services, information about services offered, sex education and the needs of the young.

In *The Health of the Nation* (Department of Health 1992) targets were set to reduce conceptions among the under 16-year-olds from 9.5 per 1000 girls aged 13 to 15 in 1989, to no more than 4.8 per 1000 by the year 2000. Similar strategies have been adopted by Northern Ireland, Scotland and Wales.

The reorganization of the NHS with the development of the internal market, the purchaser/provider split, the mushrooming of Trusts and the Management Executive's drive to increase and expand fund-holding within general practice almost certainly means that the provision of family planning and reproductive health care services will be subjected to increasing regional variability.

FAMILY PLANNING SERVICES

1. Free contraceptive services are available from GPs, in family planning clinics (FPCs), in hospitals and from some voluntary organizations such as the Brook Advisory Centres, which receive grants from central government or Health Authorities.
2. Patients have freedom of choice as to where they go for contraceptive advice and are entitled to attend a clinic and their GP at the same time. Attendance at a clinic does not preclude the GP from giving contraceptive advice or treatment and for claiming payment.
3. Male and female sterilization is currently free in NHS hospitals. Vasectomies are also carried out in some of the larger family planning clinics, and by a small number of general practitioners in the surgery. Reversal of sterilization under the NHS is available in some areas but not in an increasing number of others.
4. No charge is made for termination of pregnancy under the NHS, although facilities vary widely in different parts of the country. In some, patients have to resort to seeking abortions from gynaecologists in private practice or from voluntary agencies, such as the British Pregnancy Advisory Service (BPAS), which also undertakes abortions on an agency basis for some health authorities. The introduction of contracting and cross-charging is making it increasingly difficult for women to be referred for abortion by anyone other than their GP.
5. Contraceptive supplies are exempt from prescription charges. All are available free of charge from family planning clinics. All except condoms (other than in special circumstances, see p. 169) may be prescribed by GPs and are not currently subjected to cost-limited GP prescribing budgets.

   The proposal of a 'limited list' of contraceptives that may be prescribed by GPs free of charge under the NHS has not yet been implemented.

Services, however provided, should be comprehensive, easily accessible and 'user friendly'. Complicated appointment procedures, long waits to be seen, offhand staff and uncongenial surroundings do not encourage attendance. Advice should always be objective, patient-centred, sensitive and unhurried. Both men and women often prefer to see a doctor of their own sex, but it is really the attitude of staff which is more important than their gender.

All staff, whatever the setting, have a strong moral and legal responsibility to preserve confidentiality and privacy (Ch. 11). This is of particular importance for young people (BMA et al 1993).

Special provision for young people is essential. Although the current contraceptive prevalence rate is about 72%, the uptake of services among teenagers is particularly poor. Other groups among whom uptake is low should have their needs assessed at a national as well as local level (Ch. 2). Adequate statistics are required to provide a needs assessment.

General practice

'The provision of family planning is part of the core content of general practice' (RCGP 1991). As can be seen from Table 1.1, in 1991/1992 almost three times as many patients attended their GP for family planning services as went to family planning clinics.

Women attend the surgery on average four to five times each year in addition to those occasions when they bring their children. In general, parous women spacing their families get contraceptive advice for themselves – and their husbands – from their family doctor, while young, mobile, childless women tend to favour the clinics.

Reasons for an increased uptake of GP services may include:

1. Increased numbers of women GPs and practice nurses.
2. Increased emphasis on health promotion.
3. The required routine interview and medical examination of newly registered patients offer the opportunity to discuss contraception.
4. A reduction in the number of family planning clinics.

GPs work closely with all members of the primary care team, all of whom have a contribution to make towards an efficient FP service. Managers, secretaries, receptionists and telephonists should

Table 1.1 Number of patients seen for family planning services in clinics and by general practitioners, and number of general practitioners offering contraceptive services (FPA 1994). Total figures for England and Wales, and Scotland (figures for Northern Ireland not available).

Year	1975	1980	1985	1991/1992
Patients attending FPCs	1626793	1714436	1695814	1246585
GPs giving FP advice	22717	25199	28123	30920
Patients attending GPs for FP advice	1396048	2344153	2836279	3415392

all be able to advise patients of the facilities the practice provides and how to gain access to them.

Health visitors, community midwives, treatment room, practice-attached and district nurses should all be aware of the particular needs of diverse groups of patients, give basic advice and refer them as appropriate.

Ideally, all members of the team should be in general agreement with the practice policy, have the same attitude to patients' requests and give roughly the same advice. The standard and type of care a woman receives should not depend on which partner she happens to consult.

Publicity should be used to increase awareness of what is available, where, when and from whom. Posters in waiting rooms, baby clinics etc. can all advertise the services available.

GPs on the contraceptive list are identified by a 'C' after their name in the local register of family doctors, which is available to the public in post offices, public libraries etc.

GPs are required to make available information about services and facilities provided by the practice and to declare their gender and year of qualification. This provides a useful way of indicating their interest in FP and reproductive health care (RHC) and helps the patient to select the type of GP she or he prefers, although Newman showed in 1991 that there was no access to a woman doctor in almost half the practices in England.

A woman is free to register with another GP purely for contraceptive advice although few members of the public are aware of this fact. A woman who chooses to do this usually does so because her own doctor is one of the very few who decline to provide the service; or, for example, it may be more convenient to consult a doctor close to her place of work.

Almost all GPs prescribe the pill but not all provide a comprehensive service. A recent study found that 84% of women attending their GP were given the pill compared to 55% of clinic attenders. A disproportionately small number of GPs fit IUDs. This may be due to difficulty in arranging training and the need for assistance by a trained nurse, but also because they recognize that the occasional use of any skill increases the risk of complications. In larger practices one or two partners are often responsible for fitting IUDs and occlusive pessaries. A small number of GPs are trained to perform vasectomy.

Within the general practice setting, family planning can be provided in a variety of ways as discussed below.

Routine consultation

Most patients ask for contraceptive advice at an ordinary appointment – neither reception staff nor other patients then know the
reason for the visit. It does however require the GP to be both
mentally flexible and prepared with information leaflets, demon-
stration caps, coils and sheaths etc. It may be necessary to ask a
patient to return for a longer discussion on difficult topics such as
abortion counselling or to have an IUD fitted or a cervical smear
taken.

Notes can be marked to prompt the clinician to enquire about
family planning in women known to have poor uptake of contraceptive services, and GPs should be alert to a hidden need for
contraception.

Practice FP clinic

In some practices the number of patients seeking contraceptive
advice is sufficiently large to justify running a separate clinic. A
well-trained doctor and nurse team should be able to offer a
comprehensive service, with appointments allowing enough time
for discussion, counselling or fitting of devices.

Attendance at a special clinic does, however, mean that the reason
for the patient's visit is obvious and that appointment times are
inflexible.

Home visits

Home visiting is an integral part of primary care and FP advice is
often given in the home setting, particularly in the puerperium. But
it may also be appropriate for particular groups such as for the
patient with learning disabilities who cannot tolerate surgery visits
and for persistent defaulters, particularly those requiring 3-monthly
injections of Depo-Provera.

Emergency contraception

It is important that the whole practice team know the time limits
within which both hormonal treatment and IUD insertion may be
effective, and appreciate the need for an urgent appointment. A
sensitive, confidential way of enabling women to get an early
consultation should be established.

Shared care

Some patients will switch from their GP to the clinic and vice versa as the mood takes them. They may be happy to get the pill from the family doctor but prefer to have a cervical smear at a clinic, particularly if their GP is male. Because of the need for chaperoning, male GPs often encourage them to do this, although a trained practice nurse could easily take the smear.

GPs often have a good working arrangement with the local FP clinic and refer patients there for services they themselves do not provide or when contraceptive problems arise. Good communication between clinicians is essential but if a patient does not wish her GP to be told of her visit this should be respected. GPs can learn a lot from FP specialists and are often welcome to attend their clinical meetings.

The role of the nurse

The nurse is frequently the first professional to be asked for contraceptive advice. All primary care nurses should have a basic knowledge of FP and know what services are available locally. Nurses carrying out breast examinations and cervical smears are particularly likely to be asked questions about contraception.

Practice nurses   These professionals have a vital role to play. In 1994, in England and Wales, there were almost six times as many of them as in 1984. Most, if not all, should attend a FP course and be regularly updated. They can extend the range of service within the practice and accept a high level of clinical responsibility, undertaking much of the practice's routine FP workload such as fitting occlusive pessaries and seeing patients at their follow-up visit, and checking that all is well with patients on the pill at routine return visits before the doctor signs the prescription. Some are experienced enough to undertake routine checks in patients using the IUD, and to take vaginal swabs, and a few are trained to take blood.

With appropriate training, practice nurses could share with a doctor the counselling of patients considering sterilization, of those with problems in their personal or sexual relationships and of women seeking help with unwanted pregnancies. Many patients prefer to discuss such intimate matters with a nurse and feel more comfortable in doing so. The employing GP or community trust is responsible for ensuring that the nurse is adequately trained.

Table 1.2   Claim forms for remuneration for family planning services within general practice

FP 1001 (GP 102 in Scotland)	Pills, condom, cap and coil check, advice only, sterilization counselling and postcoital contraception.
FP 1002 (GP 103 in Scotland)	Coil insertion.
FP 1003 (GP 104 in Scotland)	Temporary residents receiving contraceptive advice only.

Remuneration

Contraceptive payments are made on an item of service basis. They are regarded as an integral part of a GP's income by government and pay review bodies and if a GP does not undertake FP work and claim for it, his NHS income is likely to be below average.

Claim forms signed by the patient not only allow remuneration of the GP but also form the basis for statistics on reproductive health care (Table 1.2) within primary care. They have to be submitted annually and are paid quarterly. There are cut off dates both for submission for payment and for how long before and after the actual date of renewal the claim can be signed to be continuous.

No claim can be made for advising a man alone.

A claim may be made for merely advising a woman to contact a clinic, for example, for IUD insertion.

Insertion of Norplant does not currently attract a fee additional to that for ordinary contraceptive advice.

No fee is payable for vasectomy as it is not considered a minor surgical procedure normally performed in general practice.

In 1990 target payments were introduced for cervical cytology, which include an allowance for patients having smears elsewhere.

Research

The RCGP has coordinated studies on the efficacy, side-effects and risks of oral contraception and on termination of pregnancy. There is great scope for further research in the GP setting.

Training

A small number of general practices are recognized for training in family planning, but this facility will have to expand to cope with increasing demand (p. 15).

Family planning clinics

FPCs vary from the small clinic open for only a few hours each month to a highly organized clinic network system with a comprehensive service provided by well-trained staff. Run by health authorities, boards and Trusts they are an important alternative source of advice and offer a wide range of services.

Doctors are usually employed on a sessional basis as clinic medical officers or senior clinic medical officers, depending on their training and the amount of administrative responsibility they accept. Increasingly, the larger area services are becoming consultant-led either by a dedicated gynaecologist, a community gynaecologist or a general obstetrician/gynaecologist working at a local hospital who takes responsibility for FP services. As with all medical staff who are not in a training-grade post, Trusts may devise their own contracts and conditions of service.

Nurses are also employed on a largely sessional basis and will have had post-basic training in family planning. They often have the first contact with patients, take the routine history and undertake an increasing amount of clinical responsibility. Many are trained to undertake counselling in relation to termination of pregnancy and sterilization. In some clinics, fitting of occlusive pessaries is almost exclusively done by nurses and they may undertake routine return visits in oral contraceptive users prior to the doctor issuing supplies.

Popularity of clinics

Clinics are popular for a variety of reasons including:

1. Self-referral.
2. Largely staffed by women.
3. Easier to talk about intimate matters without embarrassment to a stranger than to the GP.
4. Flexible opening times especially in the evenings and at weekends.
5. Perception that staff are more highly trained and that confidentiality will be assured.

Most clinics provide a comprehensive service, although small ones refer patients for special procedures to larger centres.

In addition to contraception, many FPCs now provide other help and advice in the field of reproductive health care:

1. Counselling for those with sexual, marital and personal problems, including disclosure of sexual abuse as a child.

2. Health screening: health promotion and education (Ch. 12).
3. Clinics specially designed to meet the needs of young people (Ch. 2).
4. Pregnancy testing.
5. Advice, counselling, referral and ongoing support for women before and after therapeutic abortion (Ch. 10).
6. Ready access to emergency contraception (Ch. 9).
7. A domiciliary service for the small number of patients who either lack the motivation or are unable to attend a clinic or GP surgery.
8. Special provision for those with disability.
9. Referral centre for those with contraceptive problems.
10. Pre-pregnancy counselling (Ch. 15).
11. Training facilities for medical and nursing staff and members of other disciplines.
12. Programmes of clinical and epidemiological research.
13. With the extension of clinic services to wider aspects of reproductive health care some clinics provide advice on menstrual problems and the menopause as well as colposcopy and ultrasound scanning (Ch. 15).

Brook Advisory Centres

At these clinics young people, particularly teenagers including young men, find sympathetic advice to help them with their contraceptive problems and their sexual and emotional relationships. They are designed to be more informal and less 'clinical'. They are staffed by fully-trained doctors, nurses and social workers, who may have additional training in the needs of the young and special counselling skills. Brook clinics tend to provide the same range of contraceptive services as other large city FPCs and see large numbers of girls with unwanted pregnancies.

Outreach work is done in community settings and peer group teaching used – interested youngsters are accurately informed on basic contraception, safer sex and sexual relationships and paid a small sum to undertake teaching among their contemporaries.

Hospitals

Routine advice should be offered to obstetric and gynaecological patients and provided at the appropriate time. Some hospitals run FP clinics staffed either by obstetric and gynaecological personnel or by community doctors and nurses. Although they are used primarily by women who have just had babies or abortions, all hospital patients should have access to them.

Female sterilization and therapeutic abortion are undertaken by gynaecologists; vasectomy by general surgeons or urologists.

An item of service fee is paid for IUD insertion and both the surgeon and anaesthetist may be paid for sterilization.

Emergency contraception should be available in accident and emergency departments; staff must know where to send patients for follow-up and further help.

Private sector

FP and health screening are both available from private practitioners.

Therapeutic abortion, both first and second trimester, is performed in licensed private hospitals and clinics. Where NHS provision for this is poor, more than 50% of abortions are dealt with in the private sector.

Pharmacists and other retail outlets

Condoms, spermicides, contraceptive sponges, female condoms and caps can all be bought over the counter (Ch. 6). Free or relatively cheap information on contraception, sexuality and safer sex is available in pamphlets (FPA 1992) or on video from the same sources.

PROFESSIONAL FAMILY PLANNING BODIES

Faculty of Family Planning and Reproductive Health Care of the Royal College of Obstetricians and Gynaecologists (FFPRHC)

The FFPRHC was established in 1993 incorporating the JCC and NAFPD. Primarily an educational body and one concerned with setting and maintaining standards, its aims are:

1. To give academic status to the discipline of family planning and reproductive health care and recognize the expertise within it.
2. To maintain and develop standards of care and training and ensure that a high quality of practice is maintained by all providers of FP and RHC.

3. To promote the effective interaction of reproductive health care with related disciplines.
4. To gather, collate and provide information in support of basic and continuing education in the discipline.
5. To advance medical knowledge in the discipline and encourage audit and research.
6. To support and represent those working in the discipline at regional, national and international levels.

The RCGP was originally involved in setting up the Faculty but has now no official involvement or representation.

The *British Journal of Family Planning* will continue to be produced by the Faculty and sent quarterly to all Fellows, Members and Diplomates.

The Faculty has affiliated groups of FP doctors throughout the UK, representatives of whom meet once a year in different parts of the country.

National Association of Family Planning Nurses (NAFPN)

Members of this association are nurses qualified in family planning.

Royal College of Nursing (RCN)

The RCN also has a family planning group.

TRAINING

This is in a state of flux throughout the UK. In 1994 the arrangements are as discussed below.

Doctors

Undergraduate

At present there is no national undergraduate curriculum and medical student teaching in family planning depends on the interest of individual university departments.

Postgraduate

Many postgraduates intending to pursue a career in general practice sit the Diploma of the Royal College of Obstetricians and Gynaecologists (DRCOG) which includes family planning as a part of the theoretical syllabus which may be examined but which, since 1990, has no requirement for practical training. Membership of the RCOG (MRCOG) currently requires attendance at eight family planning clinic sessions.

The FFPRHC awards two qualifications, Membership (MFFP) and Diploma (DFFP), and recognizes and issues certificates of equivalent training in the speciality. Qualification for the Diploma involves theoretical and practical training at approved premises and by faculty-approved instructing doctors. Entry to the Membership will be by examination.

Additional certification is required for competence in IUD insertion and may in the future be established for other 'special skills' such as Norplant insertion and abortion counselling.

Re-certification has now been formalized for most of the above qualifications.

There are no set requirements for FP training within general practice, but all GPs on the contraceptive list are required by their terms and conditions of service to be cognizant with current medical practice. There is therefore an implicit need to keep up to date. Examination for Membership of the Royal College of General Practitioners (MRCGP) does not include family planning as a core component. Although the Joint Committee on Training in General Practice (JCTGP) previously recommended the possession of the JCC certificate as necessary proof of competence to practise contraceptive work in general practice, it does not regard the FFP Diploma in the same light.

The RCGP is actively devising its own 'in-house' assessment and training in FP.

Nurses

FP training arrangements differ in different parts of the UK and detailed inquiry should be made to the relevant nursing board (see useful addresses). The UK Central Council advises on Post Registration Education and Professional Practice (PREPP). The common foundation courses for registered general nurses (RGNs), and the newer 'Project 2000' courses for adult, child, mental handicap or mental ill-health nursing training all contain a theoretical component on reproductive health care, as does the midwifery foundation course.

Post-basic FP training consists of both practical and theoretical components. The aim is to educate and train a first level nurse, midwife or health visitor to give advice, care and counselling to people of all ages in infertility, fertility control, sexuality and appropriate screening. More advanced training aims to enable experienced FP nurses to develop appropriate advanced skills and knowledge. Some experienced FP nurses have extra informal training to enable them to perform IUD checks, see pill return patients (but they are not legally able to prescribe), counsel couples on vasectomy, and those with an unplanned pregnancy. This has been termed the 'extended role' and obviously depends on a close relationship of trust with the medical clinical staff involved.

Midwives have only theoretical FP instruction in their course, as do other nurses in their basic training courses. The practice nurse course is a theoretical course on the basics of FP and screening including cervical screening.

Other professionals

Teachers, social workers, and police are all examples of other professional groups whose work will on occasions require a working knowledge of contraception and human sexuality. They will be required to be at ease when talking about such topics with their clients, to be accurately informed on basic facts and also when and where to refer people for specialist help. The FPA runs multi-disciplinary seminars for such professionals, and there is 'in house' training for individual groups on a somewhat variable and locally arranged basis, e.g. guidance teachers in secondary schools.

Natural family planning

Instruction is available from the Natural FP Centre in Birmingham, the National Association of Ovulation Method Instructors (NAOMI), and the Catholic Marriage Advisory Council (see useful addresses).

Psychosexual medicine

The Institute of Psychosexual Medicine promotes education and research in this field; it offers courses of training and issues a certificate of competence to medical practitioners.

The Association of Sexual and Marital Therapists publishes a journal of the same name and aims to establish high ethical standards in human values and professional skills. It also promotes interprofessional cooperation, training and research, and runs multidisciplinary seminars.

SPOD – Association to Aid the Sexual and Personal Relationships of People with a Disability

This body provides an advisory and counselling service for disabled people with sexual difficulty. It also arranges study days, courses and workshops on sexuality and disability.

THE FUTURE OF FAMILY PLANNING IN THE UK

The government has issued recent statements confirming their intention to continue to provide a dual source of supply of FP provision in the UK, and some groups such as pregnant teenagers are specifically targeted. The establishment of the FFPRHC and the appointment in a number of Trusts of consultants in community gynaecology or family planning demonstrates the profession's desire to improve the speciality. It therefore seems hopeful that services will be maintained, free at point of use.

'Routine' family planning is increasingly being provided by GPs, but FPCs still perform a vital role in specialist and alternative sources of service. The technology undoubtedly exists to prevent the vast majority of unplanned pregnancies and cervical cancers, but there are pockets of low uptake which deserve further examination.

The demand for financial savings within the reorganized NHS in which the emphasis is increasingly on GP provision of services threatens the survival of some family planning clinics. It will be necessary for the government and professional and voluntary bodies to press for adequate services that suit local needs and for the traditional clinics to diversify and expand into new areas of reproductive health care. The UK currently provides a free family planning service that few countries can emulate and which should be carefully protected.

REFERENCES

BMA, GMSC, HEA, Brook Advisory Centres, FPA and RCGP 1993
    Confidentiality and People under 16. Guidance issued jointly
Department of Health 1992 The Health of the Nation. A strategy for health in
    England. HMSO, London
Faculty of Family Planning and Reproductive Health Care of the RCOG, 1993
    'Introducing the Faculty'. RCOG, London

FPA 1992 Pharmacy Healthcare. Your choices – contraception. FPA, London
FPA 1994 Fact sheet 1B Use of Family Planning Services in the UK.
   FPA, London
Royal College of General Practitioners 1991 Family Planning and Sexual Health.
   A policy statement on clinical services provision. RCGP, London
Newman L 1992 Second among equals. British Journal of General Practice
   42.71/4

2. Factors influencing contraceptive choice

Mary Hepburn

Current trends and patterns of contraceptive use
  Oral contraception
  Sterilization
  Condoms
  Other methods

Social trends which influence choice
  Birth rates
  Age of mothers
  Family structure
  Social class
  Availability of abortion

Sexual behaviour which influences choice
  Age at first intercourse
    Gender
    Social class
    Educational level
    Changes in the role of women

  Ethnic background
  Religious background
  Use of contraception at first intercourse

Individual factors which influence choice
  Age
    Young women
    Young people
    Older women
  Disability
  Religion and culture
  Lifestyle
  Childbirth
  Provider's influence

Cost
  Methods
  Services

Conclusion

The method of contraception chosen by an individual woman and her partner will largely be determined by several personal considerations including:

1. Which methods of contraception are usable and medically safe
2. Which are acceptable to both partners
3. How anxious they are to avoid pregnancy at that time
4. Their plans or hopes regarding possible future pregnancies.

Such individual requirements will in turn be influenced by wider social trends. Behaviour may be influenced by health education campaigns; scientific reports; the opinions of friends; anecdotal information, or even misconceptions about the mode of action, side-effects, or risks of a contraceptive; and past experience of the individual, couple or their acquaintances. It is important to be aware of these influences when talking to women about contraception.

19

CURRENT TRENDS AND PATTERNS OF CONTRACEPTIVE USE

About one-third of pregnancies are unplanned, yet more than 85% of couples who are sexually active say that they are using a method of contraception. This is in contrast to an estimated 10% of women using contraception at the turn of the century (Wellings et al 1994).

There are wide variations in both contraceptive prevalence and the method used in different sections of society and by different age groups (Fig. 2.1). Three methods, the oral contraceptive pill, surgical sterilization (male or female) and the male condom, together accounted for almost two-thirds of reported contraceptive use in Britain in 1991 (Office of Population Censuses and Surveys (OPCS) 1993) and more than 75% in 1993 (Wellings et al 1994) although this latter figure probably includes couples using condoms for protection from infection.

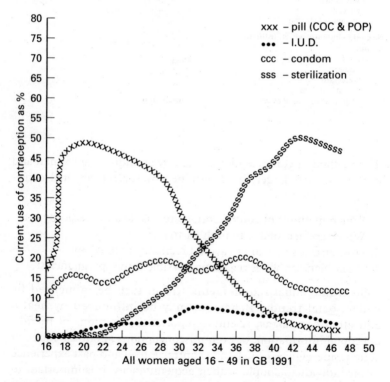

Fig. 2.1 Current use of contraception as % of all women aged 16 to 49 in Great Britain in 1991 (with acknowledgement to Dr Penelope Watson).

Oral contraception

Use of the pill increased almost steadily from its introduction in the 1960s until the late 1970s but thereafter fluctuated with the publication of reports of possible adverse effects. Levels of use since the mid 1980s have remained fairly constant overall but the pattern of use has altered with a steady rise in use by women under 30 years of age and a steady fall among those over 30 (Thorogood & Vessey 1990). Married women tend to use the pill less often than women who are single or cohabiting (Wellings et al 1994).

Sterilization

Sterilization is more common among married and older women and is the commonest method among women over 35 years of age (OPCS 1993). In 1991 almost 50% of women aged 40 to 49 years and using contraception were sterilized. Between 1986 and 1991 rates of female sterilization remained constant at 11–12%, and rates of male sterilization rose from 11% to 13%. Among couples under 45, male sterilization exceeds female sterilization but among those aged 45 to 49, female sterilization is commoner.

Condoms

The condom has reportedly overtaken sterilization as the method showing the greatest increase in popularity (Wellings et al 1994). The increased use of the condom since the mid 1980s reflects health promotion campaigns aimed at reducing the transmission of sexually transmissible diseases including human immunodeficiency virus (HIV). Some of the reported increase in condom use may therefore include use solely for protection from infection rather than for contraception. Nevertheless, an overall increase in condom use is observed. In the General Household Survey of 1991 (OPCS 1993) 8% of women using contraception had changed to the condom from another method during the preceding two years while only half as many had switched in the opposite direction. Single women were more likely to change to the condom (16%) than married/cohabiting women (6%). In 1993 a quarter of women and more than a third of men reported using condoms during the preceding year (Wellings et al 1994). The reported rate of condom use by women aged 16 to 24 was twice that of women aged 35 to 44 and more than three times that of women aged 45 to 59 years. Patterns of use among men were similar although higher than those reported by women in all age groups.

Other methods

All other methods of contraception are relatively less common with each method reportedly used by less than 10% of women (OPCS 1993).

The intrauterine device (IUD) is used by around 7% of women and is more popular among those who are married or cohabiting than single women; peak levels of use are seen among women aged 30 to 34, 9% of whom report using this method.

Some 4% of women use the diaphragm and similar percentages rely on injectable progestogens and natural family planning methods. The progestogen implant Norplant became available in the United Kingdom in late 1993 and has proved to be extremely popular. As yet no reliable data about Norplant use are available.

SOCIAL TRENDS WHICH INFLUENCE CHOICE

Birth rates

Birth rates in Britain have consistently exceeded death rates resulting in an increase of 51% in the population of the UK from the start of the century to mid 1991. However, from the mid 1990s onwards, a steady decline in birth rate is predicted with reversal of this ratio by the year 2028 (if migration trends remain constant). The total period fertility rate (TPFR) estimates the average number of children a woman would have if she experienced the age-specific fertility rate of the year in question throughout her reproductive life. By taking account of the number of women of childbearing age the TPFR provides an accurate measure of fertility. The TPFR in 1992 was 1.8 and is predicted to stabilize by the year 2000 at about 1.9, a figure which is below the population replacement level of 2.1. The current rate of 1.8 is nevertheless the second highest in the European Union (EU) after the Irish Republic.

Age of mothers

The mean age of mothers at childbirth is increasing. In England and Wales from 1981 to 1991 there was a drop in fecundity of women aged 20 to 29 years and although there was a rise among teenagers, there was an even greater rise in fecundity of women aged 30 to 39 and especially 35 to 39. Consequently, the mean age of mothers giving birth in England and Wales rose over this decade by almost one year to 27.9 years in 1992. Changing trends in maternal age will have implications for contraceptive choice.

Family structure

In Britain over the 20 years from 1971 to 1991, the number of marriages has declined by almost 16% while divorces have more than doubled. In the UK in 1991, for every two marriages there was one divorce. Divorces also occur sooner, with almost 10% of divorces occurring in the first two years of marriage.

Cohabitation has become much more common with 21% of non-married women aged 18 to 44 cohabiting in 1992 compared with only 11% in 1979 (OPCS 1994).

Births outside marriage increased to almost 1 in 3 by 1992, although 75% of these were registered by both parents. Nevertheless, over the same 20-year period, one parent families with dependent children as a proportion of all families more than doubled to almost 1 in 5. The vast majority of these were headed by single mothers who in 1991 accounted for one in six of all mothers. Single mothers head 17% of families with dependent children while single fathers account for just over 1%.

The rate of remarriage is also increasing but is much more common among men. Women have a limited reproductive lifespan, are more likely to have custody of their children after divorce and are less likely to remarry. These various trends will inevitably have implications for contraceptive choice especially of irreversible methods and particularly male sterilization.

Social class

Although the effect of social class on both contraceptive prevalence and choice of method has decreased, nevertheless a weak association remains. Women from social class I (Wellings et al 1994) are less likely to use the pill than women from lower social classes but more frequently report the use of the diaphragm and natural methods. Sterilization is common in all social classes but male sterilization predominates except in social classes IV and V where female sterilization is the commoner choice.

Availability of abortion

It is argued that the availability of abortion influences contraceptive choice. The anti-abortion lobby would have us believe that abortion on demand encourages promiscuity and removes the need for effective contraception.

In Great Britain the number of abortions performed increased by just over one-third (37%) between 1971 and 1992 (Central Statistical Office 1994). This rise was due to an increase in the number of abortions among single women which in 1992 was almost twice the number in 1971. In 1992 almost 7 out of 10 abortions were carried out on women aged 20 to 34 with very similar proportions among married and single women (Central Statistical Office 1994).

SEXUAL BEHAVIOUR WHICH INFLUENCES CHOICE

Age at first intercourse

Data from various studies all confirm that there has been a progressive reduction in age at first intercourse. The number of young people having sexual intercourse before the age of 16, the age of legal consent, has also increased. Age at first intercourse (coitarche) is influenced by a variety of factors.

Gender

Average age at first intercourse has always been lower among men than women but this difference is steadily diminishing (Wellings et al 1994). Although the pill is often regarded as the cause of the sexual revolution of the 1960s, Wellings et al (1994) found, as had others before them, that the greatest reduction in age at first intercourse actually took place in the 1950s.

Social class

Differences between social classes in age at first intercourse appear to have diminished in America and elsewhere in Europe while remaining quite marked in Britain. Wellings et al (1994) reported that average age at first intercourse was 19 for men and 20 for women from social class I compared with 16 and 18 respectively in social class V.

Educational level

This also has a separate effect with higher levels of education associated with greater age at first intercourse and less likelihood of intercourse before the age of 16 years.

Changes in the role of women

With changes in social attitudes and behaviour have come changes in the role of women. Increasing numbers of women go on to further education and have improved employment opportunities.

Ethnic background

In Britain age at coitarche (including first intercourse before the age of 16 years) is highest among those of Asian origin (particularly women) and lowest among those who are black (particularly men). Gender differences, although diminishing overall, are more marked among ethnic minority groups.

Religious background

Age at first intercourse is also influenced by religion. It is higher among those with some, as opposed to no, religious affiliation and highest among members of non-Christian religions (Wellings et al 1994).

Use of contraception at first intercourse

First intercourse is occurring more often outside marriage as a planned event within an established relationship and more often with use of contraception especially condoms (Wellings et al 1994). Contraception is less likely to be used if intercourse occurs on the first meeting. In such circumstances more than two-thirds of women reported using no contraception compared to less than one-third of women for whom first intercourse occurred within a regular relationship. This is of particular concern since an unplanned pregnancy is likely to be more of a problem among those who appear to be at greater risk.

INDIVIDUAL FACTORS WHICH INFLUENCE CHOICE

Age

Young women

No method is absolutely contraindicated for adolescents but young girls may have difficulty with, or lack of self-confidence in, intercourse-related methods which they often find embarrassing. Conversely, lifestyle or absence of a regular relationship may cause problems with methods requiring memory and/or discipline of use such as oral contraception. Protection from pregnancy and protection from sexually transmissible infections are both of vital importance and, particularly in this age group, must be clearly distinguished.

The combined oral contraceptive (COC)   This pill is often the method of choice provided the woman's lifestyle is sufficiently stable and provided she is able to remember to take the pill regularly. If her parents are unaware that she is using the pill, there is a risk of discovery. If taken properly, it provides the high level of protection young women require but with even a few memory lapses it will become unreliable. Poor compliance is a common cause of unplanned pregnancy among younger women using the pill. Young women often have relationships of relatively short duration. Stopping the pill when one relationship ends and failing to restart when another begins often results in unplanned pregnancy.

The progestogen-only pill (POP)   Generally less suitable for young women than the combined pill because of the higher failure rate and the even greater discipline required in taking it.

Injectable progestogen   A popular choice among young girls whose lifestyle makes the pill less suitable. Some consider the possible side-effect of weight gain a major disadvantage. The frequently associated amenorrhoea may cause anxiety but is not seen as a problem if adequately explained and discussed beforehand. Regular contact is required for follow-up.

Norplant   This will no doubt be increasingly used in Britain among young women. Side-effects, particularly irregular bleeding, may make it less attractive while its 5-year duration of action may limit its usefulness for some. It is important to ensure that its use by young women is not advocated for social reasons and that it is prescribed only after good counselling and with complete freedom of choice.

The intrauterine device (IUD)   Can be difficult to fit because the uterine cavity is often small. Moreover, there may be an increased risk of pelvic inflammatory disease among young women with short-lived relationships and, consequently, multiple partners. There is nevertheless a place for the IUD particularly for young women who have already had a pregnancy.

The diaphragm   Is unlikely to be acceptable or used properly.

Condoms   These should be encouraged at all times for protection from infection in addition to a more reliable method of contraception. The female condom is unlikely to prove popular in this age group.

Spermicides   Alone or impregnated into sponges they provide poor protection against pregnancy and only some protection against infection. While an inadequate method of contraception in this age group, they are better than nothing and have the advantage of being under the girl's own control. They are certainly worth using in conjunction with more reliable contraception as protection against infection for those unable to negotiate condom use by the partner.

Sterilization   Rarely appropriate for young people but it should not be absolutely ruled out on grounds of age alone. The newer, long acting, reversible methods will usually be more appropriate.

Emergency contraception   This will sometimes be necessary and young people should be informed about it before the need arises. For those using the combined pill it can be useful to keep a packet or part of a packet for 'spares' if they are away from home overnight.

Young people

Targets have been identified for reductions in teenage pregnancies and abortions as well as reductions in sexually transmissible diseases (Department of Health 1992). Achieving these targets will require effective sex education and imaginative development of services specifically targeted towards young people. Sex education does not encourage sexual activity and the value of a more open approach to education and service provision is demonstrated by the low rate of teenage pregnancies in other countries, notably the Netherlands. While many women who attend their general practitioners for family planning advice do so because of familiarity, it is for precisely this reason that many young girls choose not to do so. Familiarity may cause not only embarrassment but also concern about confidentiality and possible disclosure to parents. However, while attendance at community family planning services may provide anonymity it may feel like a public declaration of sexual activity. Moreover, many young girls find services, if not hostile, certainly inaccessible and unwelcoming.

Services for young people should have a wider remit. They should cater for both sexes and provide education, information, counselling and health care in a non-judgmental way. They should be concerned not just with contraception but with all issues relating to sexuality and its expression, to promotion of sexual health in general and to other health issues of relevance to young people. The value of peer group education should be recognized (p. 12). Services should be offered in a wide range of places and accessibility could be increased by providing them in sites or within services already used by young people. Uptake of services could be increased by including help with non-medical or social issues such as employment and benefits. Instant access without appointment must be available with, among other options, provision of emergency contraception.

The services should be widely publicized so that young people are aware not only of where and how to obtain information and help but also of their rights. Young people are entitled to sensitive, sympathetic and confidential treatment which meets *their* needs, not those of service providers.

Older women

Older women, particularly those in the perimenopause who are having troublesome irregular bleeding and women who for a variety of reasons can no longer use the combined pill, not infrequently have problems finding an acceptable method of contraception. Some women may also have problems deciding when they may stop using contraception. Provision of contraception for women around the menopause is covered in Chapter 16. Women in this age group who present for contraception often appreciate access to other types of reproductive health care including well woman screening and menopause clinics.

Disability

It is important to remember that men and women with a physical disability are often sexually active. People with learning disabilities, while especially vulnerable to exploitation, may also have close, fulfilling relationships. Those with a disability, whether physical or mental, may want and be capable of caring for children, but whether or not this is the case they need appropriate advice in controlling their fertility.

People with disabilities may have difficulties resulting from a poor body image, low self-esteem or depression. In addition, they may have special contraceptive needs. While an exhaustive list of disabilities and their implications for contraceptive choice is not possible, it is important to identify the precise problems posed by the disability and, therefore, which individual methods may or may not be appropriate.

The combined pill   Taken under supervision this may be a practical and effective method of contraception, but in the presence of moderate learning disability any method under the woman's control may be ineffective. The various medical conditions in which the pill is contraindicated are fully discussed elsewhere (Ch. 3). Many conditions may have secondary effects which make the pill unsuitable even if it is not contraindicated. For example, there have been theoretical concerns about the use of the COC by women with multiple sclerosis in case it might provoke relapse or progression, but this is no longer considered a significant contraindication. However, for those with paralysis who are immobilized, the COC may be unsuitable because of the greater risk of thromboembolism, signs of which might not be noted in the absence of sensation. The POP does not carry such risk.

Long-acting progestogens   These can overcome many of the problems of COC discussed above. They are not intercourse-related and do not require manual dexterity. Their long action is an advantage when compliance might be a problem. Amenorrhoea associated with the use of Depo-Provera can be a real benefit for women who have difficulties with personal hygiene.

The IUD   This is sometimes difficult to fit in the presence of deformity or limited mobility. Checking the threads of the coil, important in the absence of sensation when expulsion might not be felt by the woman, requires manual dexterity but can be done by the partner or health care worker. The risk of pelvic inflammatory disease can also be a problem if symptoms are masked by a lack of sensation, and is considered a contraindication to IUD use in the immuno-compromised and particularly the HIV positive woman. However, this contraindication should not be regarded as absolute in that, if an alternative method is less effective, the risks and consequences, physical and emotional, of an unplanned pregnancy must be taken into consideration.

Barrier methods   Manual dexterity is required to put on a male condom or insert a female condom or diaphragm into the vagina. The male condom can be damaged by an indwelling female catheter while, with lack of sensation, displacement of the diaphragm might not be detected.

Sterilization   This can be a good method for those who do not intend to have a further pregnancy and also for those who, for whatever reason, do not plan to have any children. If such a decision is related to disability or disease, and if circumstances and consequently choice are unlikely to change, sterilization can be appropriate at a younger age than might otherwise be considered. While controversial and with legal implications for those with learning disabilities (Ch. 11), sterilization can be appropriate in certain circumstances, particularly where the woman can give informed consent.

Religion and culture

Religion may influence but not necessarily dictate contraceptive choice. Different religions may have well defined rules on whether contraception of any kind, individual methods or abortion are acceptable. However, not only do different branches of the same religion hold differing beliefs (as, for example, in different branches of the Christian faith) but the same religion may be practised differently in different countries or modified by different cultures. In addition, teachings on contraception may be accepted wholly, partially or not at all by different individuals all professing allegiance to the same religion. Equally, others who profess no religious affiliation may hold strong views on contraception or abortion.

While it is useful to be aware of some of the major issues, and particularly those of local relevance, rather than identifying the individual's religion and assuming it to be an accurate predictor of behaviour, it is preferable, as always, to determine the methods acceptable to that individual. These views may not coincide with the view of the health professional and may even be deemed medically or socially inappropriate. However, it is important to avoid expressing an opinion in a way which makes the individual feel guilty or irresponsible. Factual information should be given in a non-judgmental way to allow an informed decision acceptable to the individual. Religious and cultural influences may be difficult to separate. Both may influence local availability and consequently choice among those who do not adhere to a particular religion or culture.

In general, Chinese, Sikhs and Hindus accept any form of contraception while Buddhists accept none believing family size to be a matter of destiny. Among Christians, Protestants are usually in favour of all methods, while Roman Catholics are directed by the papal encyclical *'Humanae Vitae'* to use only natural family planning or abstinence. Orthodox Muslims approve of contraception (but not permanent methods) to space families.

West Indians disapprove of abortion, while the Chinese use it as a method of contraception and Buddhists condemn it. In the

Christian faith, Protestants generally are in favour and Roman Catholics totally opposed to abortion.

Other cultural factors may be indirectly relevant. Hindus may not cook and Orthodox Muslims cannot attend the mosque if menstruating, while West Indians are unhappy with scanty periods. Hindus consider it important to have a son; to West Indians proof of fertility is important.

A woman doctor may be preferred on religious or cultural grounds. However, many individuals share this preference for other reasons such as a history of sexual abuse or simply embarrassment. Such women, whose need is arguably greater, are often less able to express their wishes and consequently may not avail themselves of the services available.

Lifestyle

Lifestyle may affect ability to use a particular method and consequently compromise compliance. While this is often attributed to poor motivation, inappropriate advice and choice of method are more often to blame.

Irregular lifestyle may be a problem for young people; those of any age not in a regular relationship; those whose partners are frequently absent; those who work irregular hours or those who travel a lot. All may have difficulty with a method such as the pill which requires a regular routine. Women whose lifestyles are chaotic because of social problems may also have difficulties with compliance regardless of motivation and yet they have particular need of reliable contraception. This is especially true for those who also have behavioural problems such as drug or alcohol abuse. Methods involving less rigid compliance will often be more appropriate for such women.

The combined pill   This requires disciplined compliance. While often a good method for the young, those with irregular or frankly chaotic lifestyles have difficulty taking it correctly. Drug-users may have malabsorption, vomiting or liver damage due to hepatitis. They frequently also smoke heavily.

The progestogen-only pill   This requires even greater regularity of use so is even less suitable.

Long-acting progestogens   By injection or implant, these overcome many of the compliance problems of the pill and can be used for women with contraindications to oestrogen although severe liver disease is still a contraindication. Regular follow-up is necessary with injectable methods and may be difficult to organize. Norplant has the advantage of being effective for 5 years although the irregular vaginal bleeding may not be very acceptable to this group. Among women with HIV infection, more frequent bleeding and, consequently, shedding of the virus, could increase the risk of sexual transmission during unprotected intercourse (Ch. 13).

The IUD   This offers some advantages. IUD users who fail to attend for follow-up are less likely to have an unplanned pregnancy than those on Depo-Provera who default. Most IUDs are at least partially effective for longer than the manufacturers say and the risks of expulsion and pelvic inflammatory disease are highest at the time when the device is changed. However, the risk of infection, including HIV, makes the coil relatively contraindicated for women having unprotected intercourse with numerous partners, such as women financing a drug habit by prostitution – a group who would particularly benefit from its reliability and minimal need for compliance. While many would consider HIV infection an absolute contraindication, among women with many medical and social problems for whom reliable contraception is vital, HIV infection can be no more than another factor in a very complicated equation, any solution to which involves compromise.

Barrier methods   Being intercourse related, these have advantages and disadvantages. Contact with services can be more opportunistic and a regular routine is not necessary for use. However, with male condoms, partner cooperation can be a problem while intoxication with drugs or alcohol may dull memory and awareness of a partner's behaviour. Consequently, drug-using prostitutes often use sponges, spermicidal pessaries or foam. Barrier methods do not provide reliable contraception while methods other than the condom do not provide reliable protection from infection. Although the two issues must be kept separate, any method which provides any degree of protection from either pregnancy or infection is better than nothing and should be encouraged.

Sterilization   This provides excellent contraception for the woman who does not want a family or whose family is complete. If her lifestyle is chaotic, sterilization of the woman will be more effective than sterilization of her partner and may be justified at a younger age than usual. Counselling about irreversibility is particularly important since she may change partners and circumstances may alter, but a woman should not be refused sterilization because health professionals fear she may change her mind. Equally, she should not be pressurized to accept sterilization if she is unsure and certainly never as a condition of termination of pregnancy even when she has had one or more pregnancies terminated before. Where repeated terminations are necessary, inappropriate postoperative contraceptive counselling may be as much to blame as patient irresponsibility.

Childbirth

The question of future contraception should be raised at an appropriate time preferably during the pregnancy so that a couple can decide which method they wish to use and when they should start it (Ch. 7). Some methods are contraindicated in the postpartum period.

The combined pill (COC)   Not recommended during the early months of lactation (Ch. 3) and, because of the risks of oestrogen soon after delivery, it is not usually given to those who bottle-feed until 3 to 4 weeks postpartum.

Injectable progestogens   Given early in the puerperium, these can be associated with troublesome bleeding (Ch. 4).

The IUD   This is not inserted until 6 to 8 weeks after delivery because of the increased risk of perforation or expulsion (Ch. 5).

The male condom   Effective for postpartum women who have minimal risk of pregnancy (ovulation has not been reported before 33 days postpartum) and often little desire for sexual activity.

Sterilization   Immediately postpartum, unless done at the time of caesarean section, this may be associated with increased risk of thromboembolism and regret (Ch. 8). However, a pragmatic approach is necessary and for those who may prove difficult to follow up it is often not practical to delay starting an effective method and it may be safer on balance to accept the increased risk of complications and side-effects and begin contraception immediately.

Provider's influence

Patterns of contraceptive use differ between women attending GPs and those who go to community family planning clinics (FPCs); 84% of women who attend their GP are prescribed the pill compared with 55% of those attending FPCs (FPA 1992a). GPs are much less likely to advise women to use the diaphragm and they cannot prescribe condoms for contraception. Women attending their GP tend to be older than clinic attenders, they often already have a child and are spacing their families. While different patient characteristics may account for differences in contraceptive prescribing, availability of a particular method and the views of the prescriber may also contribute.

Women sometimes choose a method of contraception they think will be approved of by health professionals or they may even be pressurized to accept such a method.

COST

At present all contraceptive methods except male condoms are free. Although the user does not therefore take into account the cost of a method, the provider may increasingly do so.

Methods

Comparison of the cost of different methods of contraception is difficult. Calculations must be made over a period of time at least as long as the duration of the longest-acting reversible method (Table 2.1). Such comparisons assume long-acting methods are not

Table 2.1 Comparative 5-year costs of methods of contraception

Method		5-year cost (£)
[1] Combined O.C. pill	(Marvelon)	91.40
	(Mercilon)	166.20
[1] Progestogen-only pill	(Femulen)	58.80
[1] Injectable Progestogen (Depo-Provera 150 mg/3 months)		91.00
[1] Norplant		179.00
[1] IUCD (Nova-T)		9.90
[1] Diaphragm (Durex Flat Spring × 1/6 months) + [1] spermicide (Duragel 1 tube/2 months)	[54.90] [78.00]	132.90
[2] Condoms (Durex Nuform Extrasafe 3/week) + [1] spermicide (Double Check Pessaries 3/week)	[34.06] [84.24]	118.30
[3] Female sterilization (laparoscopic, daycase)		399.00

Notes: [1] = NHS Price, MIMS, February 1994
[2] = Chemist and Druggist Price May 1994
[3] = Glasgow Royal Infirmary University and NHS Trust May 1994.

discontinued before their effectiveness ends. Comparative costs for intercourse-related barrier methods will depend on the frequency of intercourse. The cost of sterilization is related to the number of years after surgery until the woman reaches the menopause. The actual cost of sterilization procedures will depend on a number of variables, e.g. whether it is carried out as a day case. For all methods, costs will be influenced by local pricing agreements.

Costs will also vary according to who provides the service (see below). Table 2.1, therefore, provides theoretical comparisons, but the real cost in any individual situation may be quite different.

Services

Various studies in Britain and abroad have supported the view that provision of good family planning services is cost effective. Family planning has been available free under the NHS from clinics since 1974 and from general practitioners since 1975 (Ch. 1).

Some studies have suggested that services provided by family planning clinics are more cost effective than those provided by GPs but, since each offers a slightly different range of services to a different clientele, they are not strictly comparable. The two types of service should, therefore, be regarded as complementary rather than competitive and freedom of choice over where to obtain care should be maintained. The exact level of benefit from the provision of family planning is difficult to measure. In America, one study (Forrest & Singh 1990) estimated that for every government dollar spent on family planning services there is an average saving of $4.40. In an updated review in 1982, Laing suggested a benefit to cost ratio of at least 1.3:1 and possibly as high as 5.3:1. The lower ratio is based on estimated cost savings of avoiding a 'typical unwanted conception'. Unplanned pregnancies among single women or those who already have several children are assumed to lead to major demands on health and social services, hence the higher ratios. However, these calculations are to some extent conjectural. The FPA has reviewed some of the relevant studies (FPA 1992b) and research is ongoing. In any case, a high savings to cost ratio should not be the sole criterion for justification of family planning services; emotional costs are less easily measured but equally important.

CONCLUSION

The couple who, for whatever reason, are not entirely happy with their chosen method of contraception, are more likely to have problems using it and compliance will suffer. The method must be acceptable on social, cultural, and religious grounds with reliability appropriate to current need. Medical as well as contraceptive safety should be considered, and finally lifestyle, memory, and inter-personal skills must be such that the method can be used effectively. The ultimate choice may be a compromise accepting some risks if the alternatives are riskier. An unreliable method may be more effective than a reliable method unreliably used.

REFERENCES

Central Statistical Office 1994 Social Trends 24. HMSO, London
Department of Health 1992 The Health of the Nation. A Strategy for Health in
    England 1992. HMSO, London
Forrest J D, Singh S 1990 Public-Sector Savings Resulting from Expenditures for
    Contraceptive Services. Family Planning Perspectives 22 (1) : 6-15
FPA 1992a Use of Family Planning Services in the United Kingdom.
    Fact-sheet 1B August. Family Planning Association, London
FPA 1992b The Costs and Benefits of Family Planning services.
    Fact-sheet 3D June. Family Planning Association, London
Office of Population Censuses and Surveys: Social Survey Division 1993
    General Household Survey 1991: Series GHS no. 22. HMSO, London
Office of Population Censuses and Surveys 1994: General Household Survey 1992.
    HMSO, London
Thorogood M, Vessey M P 1990 Trends in Use of Oral Contraceptives in Britain.
    The British Journal of Family Planning 16 : 41-53.
Wellings K, Field J, Johnson A M, Wadsworth J 1994 Sexual Behaviour in Britain,
    The National Survey of Sexual Attitudes and Lifestyles. Penguin, London

3. Combined hormonal contraception

John Guillebaud

Preparations
Oestrogens
Progestogens
Monophasic pills
Biphasic pills
Triphasic pills

Endocrinology of the normal menstrual cycle

Mode of action

Practical prescribing

Effectiveness

Indications
Contraception
Gynaecological conditions

Contraindications
Absolute
Relative
Intercurrent disease
Sickle cell disorders
Diabetes mellitus

Advantages

Disadvantages
Metabolic effects
The liver
Cardiovascular system
Venous disease
Arterial disease
Relative risk of cardiovascular disease
Effects on other systems

Clinical management
History
Examination
Choice of pill
First choice of pill
Instructions to patients
Starting the pill
Postpartum
Changing preparations
Management of missed pills:
importance of the pill-free interval (PFI)
Vomiting, diarrhoea and short-term drug
interactions
Drug interaction
Long-term use of enzyme-inducing drugs

Discontinuing enzyme-inducing drugs
Effects of COCs on other drugs
Manipulation of the menstrual cycle
To postpone a period
The tricycle regimen
Follow-up
Indications for stopping COC

Complications and their management
Cardiovascular system
Hypertension
Central nervous system
Depression
Loss of libido
Headaches (including migraine)
Epilepsy
Chorea and benign intracranial pressure
Eyes
Gastrointestinal system
Nausea and vomiting
Weight gain
Jaundice
Gall stones
Liver tumours
Crohn's disease
Urinary system
Genital system
Breakthrough bleeding: spotting
Absence of withdrawal bleeding
Vaginal discharge
Fibroids
Carcinoma of the ovary and the
endometrium
Carcinoma of the cervix
Choriocarcinoma
Breasts
Enlargement and discomfort
Carcinoma of the breast
Clinical implications
Musculoskeletal system
Carpal-tunnel syndrome
Leg pains and cramps
Cutaneous system
Chloasma/melasma
Photosensitivity
Acne, greasy skin, hirsutism
Malignant melanoma
Other skin conditions
Infections and inflammations

37

Reversibility	Breaks in pill taking
Outcome of pregnancy	Risks/benefits
Exposure during pregnancy	

In 1921 Haberlandt was the first scientist to advocate that extracts from the ovaries and placenta of pregnant animals might be used for fertility control. In 1937 Kurzrok noted that ovulation was inhibited during treatment for dysmenorrhoea with ovarian oestrone, and suggested that this hormone might be of value in contraception. It was only in the 1950s, when potent orally active progestogens (first norethynodrel and then norethisterone) became available, that an oral contraceptive pill became possible. The research chemists chiefly responsible were Russell Marker, who first produced progesterone from diosgenin extracted from the Dioscorea plant, George Rosenkranz, Carl Djerassi and Frank Colton (Djerassi 1979).

Encouraged by Mrs Margaret Sanger and Mrs Page McCormick, Gregory Pincus started a screening programme of contraceptive steroids in animals. With Michael Chang and John Rock, Pincus developed the first oral contraceptive pill and reported the first trials in humans in Puerto Rico with Drs Rice-Wray and Garcia in January 1957 (Diczfalusy 1982).

The first pills were thought to contain only progestogen and gave good cycle control. When purified preparations were tried however, cycle control deteriorated. The impurity had been mestranol, and when this oestrogen was restored to the tablets the combined pill Enovid (norethynodrel plus mestranol) was created.

The combined oral contraceptive (COC) was approved for use in America in 1959, and in Britain 2 years later. For years its use appeared to be associated with only minor side-effects which were acceptable to most women in return for its high effectiveness. Cardiovascular problems, related to the dose of oestrogen, and attributed primarily to venous or arterial thrombosis, first came to light in 1969. Later, some of the synthetic progestogens were linked to the risk of arterial wall disease, primarily in smokers. The non-contraceptive benefits took longer to be established and have always received far less public attention.

At least 200 million women throughout the world have taken the pill since it first became available, and about 65 million are current users. In developed countries, 15–40% of women of reproductive age use it as a contraceptive, rising to 75% of those aged 20 to 30 years. In the United Kingdom (UK), it remains one of the most popular methods of fertility control, being used by about 3 million women.

PREPARATIONS

The combined oral contraceptive pill contains two steroid hormones, oestrogen and a progestogen (a synthetic progesterone). Over the years the composition of the pill has changed markedly. The total dose of steroid has been reduced, the oestrogen in some pills by a factor of seven, the progestogen by up to a factor of twenty. Mestranol has largely been replaced by the more potent ethinyl-oestradiol. Natural oestrogens, though probably associated with less thrombotic risk, have so far proved incapable of adequate cycle control or inhibition of ovulation. Some progestogens are no longer used as new preparations have been introduced.

Oestrogens

Most modern combined pills contain ethinyloestradiol; only two formulations in the UK still contain mestranol. Both oestrogens affect coagulation factors in such a way as to promote both arterial and venous thrombosis. These changes are dose-dependent. Thus oral contraceptive pills in Britain do not contain more than $50\,\mu g$ of oestrogen and the usual dose is in the $20\text{--}35\,\mu g$ range.

Progestogens

Those in current use are all derivatives of 19-nortestosterone and may be divided into two groups:

1. Second generation progestogens: norethisterone; norethisterone acetate; ethynodiol diacetate and levonorgestrel (known in the USA as d-norgestrel).
2. Third generation progestogens: desogestrel; gestodene and norgestimate. This group differs from the second generation progestogens in that they:
   a. Have a higher affinity for (bind more strongly to) the progesterone receptor thus increasing their effectiveness at inhibiting ovulation.
   b. Have a lower affinity for (bind less strongly to) androgen receptors thus having fewer androgenic effects.

Pills containing third generation progestogens produce fewer adverse effects on carbohydrate and lipid metabolism than earlier formulations. High density lipoprotein (particularly $HDL_2\text{-C}$) concentrations are increased while low density lipoproteins (particularly LDL-C) and insulin concentrations are decreased compared with pills containing second generation progestogens.

Table 3.1 Currently available preparations of combined and progestogen-only oral contraceptives (UK)

Pill type	Preparation	Oestrogen (μg)	Progestogen (mg)	
Combined				
Ethinyloestradiol/ norethisterone type	Loestrin 20	20	1	norethisterone acetate *
	Loestrin 30	30	1.5	norethisterone acetate *
	Conova 30	30	2	ethynodiol diacetate *
	Brevinor	35	0.5	norethisterone
	Ovysmen	35	0.5	norethisterone
	Neocon 1/35	35	1	norethisterone
	Norimin	35	1	norethisterone
Ethinyloestradiol/ levonorgestrel	Microgynon 30	30	0.15	
	Ovranette	30	0.15	
	Eugynon 30	30	0.25	
	Ovran 30	30	0.25	
	Ovran	50	0.25	
Ethinyloestradiol/ desogestrel	Mercilon	20	0.15	
	Marvelon	30	0.15	
Ethinyloestradiol/ gestodene	Femodene (also ED)	30	0.075	
	Minulet	30	0.075	
Ethinyloestradiol/ norgestimate	Cilest	35	0.25	
Mestranol/ norethisterone	Norinyl-1	50	1	
	Ortho-Novin 1/50	50	1	
Biphasic and Triphasic				
Ethinyloestradiol / norethisterone	BiNovum	35	0.5	(7 tabs)
		35	1	(14 tabs)
	Synphase	35	0.5	(7 tabs)
		35	1	(9 tabs)
		35	0.5	(5 tabs)

Table 3.1 *(cont'd)*

Pill type	Preparation	Oestrogen (µg)	Progestogen (mg)	
	TriNovum (also ED)	35	0.5	(7 tabs)
		35	0.75	(7 tabs)
		35	1	(7 tabs)
Ethinyloestradiol / levonorgestrel	Logynon (also ED)	30	0.05	(6 tabs)
		40	0.075	(5 tabs)
		30	0.125	(10 tabs)
	Trinordiol	30	0.05	(6 tabs)
		40	0.075	(5 tabs)
		30	0.125	(10 tabs)
Ethinyloestradiol / gestodene	Tri-Minulet	30	0.05	(6 tabs)
		40	0.07	(5 tabs)
		30	0.1	(10 tabs)
	Triadene	30	0.05	(6 tabs)
		40	0.07	(5 tabs)
		30	0.1	(10 tabs)
Progestogen only				
Norethisterone type	Micronor	–	0.35	norethisterone
	Noriday	–	0.35	norethisterone
	Femulen	–	0.5	ethynodiol diacetate *
Levonorgestrel	Microval	–	0.03	
	Norgeston	–	0.03	
	Neogest	–	0.075	norgestrel

* Converted (>90%) to norethisterone as the active metabolite.
Reproduced with the kind permission of MIMS.

Although these metabolic differences ought in theory to be associated with a reduction in the risk of arterial disease and hypertension, as yet there is no evidence that third generation progestogens confer a clinical advantage over the older, cheaper preparations. As the incidence of cardiovascular disease attributable to the pill is so small, millions of women will have to use the newer pills for many years before evidence of a clinical rather than just a biochemical benefit is demonstrated.

In the past the potency of steroids was considered to be important when choosing the brand of pill. With the advent of the more powerful third generation progestogens this is no longer of clinical relevance.

There are 26 different combined oral contraceptive (COC) preparations available and they are listed in Table 3.1. They can be divided into three groups, monophasic, biphasic and triphasic.

Monophasic pills

Preparations containing 20–35 μg of ethinyloestradiol (EE) are the most widely used. Only three preparations now contain 50 μg of oestrogen. Of the pills containing 20 μg of oestrogen, Loestrin 20 gives poor cycle control and has a higher failure rate. A 20 μg preparation containing gestodene is likely to become available soon.

Biphasic pills

These are not widely prescribed and there are only two preparations in current use. Gracial is a new 22-day product designed to produce oestrogen-dominance during the first 7 days and will be marketed sometime during 1995 for women with troublesome breakthrough bleeding (BTB).

Triphasic pills

The triphasic regimen was designed to reduce the total dose of steroids over 21 days, while at the same time mimicking the characteristic fluctuations in oestrogen and progesterone which occur during the menstrual cycle. Although a more normal-looking endometrium is demonstrated histologically, there is no good evidence of better cycle control over long-term use. Moreover, while the old triphasics do expose the user to a lower total dose of steroids, the newer ones (Tri-Minulet and Triadene) do not.

Phasic preparations are more complicated to use with respect to giving advice about missed pills or postponing withdrawal bleeds.

They are also expensive for the Health Service when prescribed by general practitioners (GPs) as each phase attracts a separate dispensing fee.

ENDOCRINOLOGY OF THE NORMAL MENSTRUAL CYCLE

At the start of the ovarian cycle (day 1 of the menstrual cycle) around 20 follicles begin to develop, stimulated by the intercycle rise in follicle stimulating hormone (FSH) from the pituitary gland. The growing follicles produce oestrogen, the concentrations of which rise over the next few days. As a result of the negative feedback effects of oestrogen, FSH concentrations fall, allowing only one follicle to continue developing to the point of ovulation. Oestrogen from the dominant follicle reaches a threshold which stimulates (by positive feedback) the mid-cycle surge of luteinizing hormone (LH). Once ovulation has taken place around day 14, the follicle becomes the corpus luteum and starts to secrete progesterone. Oestrogen concentrations gradually fall over the second half (luteal phase) of the cycle. Progesterone reaches a peak about 7 days after ovulation and then falls until day 28 of the cycle when menstruation starts (Fig 7.1 p. 185). If conception occurs, human chorionic gonadotrophin (hCG) produced by the embryo stimulates the continued secretion of progesterone from the corpus luteum until the placenta takes over.

In the first half of the cycle (follicular phase) when oestrogen is the predominant steroid, the endometrium 'proliferates' with a growth of glands, stroma and blood vessels. Progesterone matures the endometrium during the 'secretory phase', stimulating histological and biochemical changes essential for implantation. When progesterone concentrations fall at the end of the luteal phase, the endometrium can no longer be supported and is shed – thus, the onset of menses. In the presence of a pregnancy with persistence of the corpus luteum, the endometrium becomes decidualized and no bleeding occurs.

MODE OF ACTION

Hormonal contraceptives act both centrally and peripherally by:

1. Inhibition of ovulation – the oestrogen component inhibits pituitary FSH secretion thereby suppressing follicle growth while the progestogen inhibits the LH surge preventing ovulation.

2. Alteration in cervical mucus – it becomes scanty, viscous and cellular with low spinnbarkeit (stretchiness), thus impairing sperm transport and penetration. This type of cervical mucus is produced by COCs at all doses and provides an additional contraceptive action if breakthrough ovulation does occur.
3. Alteration of the endometrium – the usual development does not occur. An atrophic endometrium unreceptive to implantation is produced with microtubular glands and a fibroblastic condensation of the stroma. With prolonged COC use the endometrium becomes progressively thin and atrophic. Development of the vasculature is reduced and less of the uterotonic and vasoactive prostaglandins are produced which explains the scanty, less painful withdrawal bleeding in pill users.
4. Possible direct effects on the fallopian tubes impairing sperm migration and ovum transport are of doubtful importance.

PRACTICAL PRESCRIBING

Although the combined pill is easy to use, can provide maximum protection from pregnancy, and has many beneficial effects, it is neither suitable for, nor acceptable to, all couples. In the UK almost 95% of sexually active women under 30 have used it for at least a few months.

Anxiety about adverse effects and possible long-term consequences makes it necessary for all those who prescribe the pill to:

1. Form their own opinions based on scrutiny of published work.
2. Keep regularly updated.
3. Prescribe carefully after discussing anxieties, risks and benefits.
4. Reassure patients when appropriate, but leave the final decisions to them.
5. Supervise follow-up conscientiously.

EFFECTIVENESS

Provided the pill is taken correctly and consistently, is absorbed normally, and its metabolism is not affected by interaction with other medication, its reliability is nearly 100%. In practice the failure rate is 0.2–3 per 100 woman years (HWY), or higher, depending mainly on the population studied.

Many more errors in tablet-taking occur than are reported. Detailed questioning – including whether any pills might have been missed or not absorbed just before or just after, the pill-free interval – nearly always reveals the reason for any unexpected pregnancy.

Careful teaching of the woman (and sometimes her partner) accompanied by written information, is essential for effective use.

INDICATIONS

Contraception

The pill is indicated where maximum protection from pregnancy is required, or where the woman wishes to use a method independent of intercourse.

It is particularly valuable, and associated with lowest circulatory risk and fewest adverse side-effects, in healthy young women who do not smoke and who are sufficiently motivated to use it reliably.

Gynaecological conditions

The combined pill is commonly used in the treatment of the following conditions (Ch. 15):

1. Dysmenorrhoea.
2. Menorrhagia.
3. Premenstrual Syndrome.
4. Endometriosis – often as a continuous regimen.
5. To control functional ovarian cysts.

CONTRAINDICATIONS

Absolute

1. Past or present circulatory disease.
    a. Any proven past arterial or venous thrombosis.
    b. Ischaemic heart disease, including angina, and cardiomyopathies.
    c. Severe or combined risk factors for arterial disease (Table 3.2).
    d. Atherogenic lipid disorders: cholesterol above 7.5 mmol/l. Specialist advice should be taken if concentrations of other lipid fractions are abnormal.
    e. Known prothrombotic abnormality of coagulation or fibrinolysis including:
        i.   the congenital thrombophilias with abnormal levels of individual factors

Table 3.2 Risk factors for cardiovascular system (CVS) and arterial disease

Risk factor	Absolute contraindication	Relative contraindication	Remarks
Family history (FH) of CVS disease (arterial or venous) in a first-degree relative ≤ 45	Known atherogenic lipid profile or pro-thrombotic haemostatic profile; or test results not available	Normal blood profiles or first attack in relative > 45	If FH of arterial disease, test both for lipids and haemostatis
Diabetes mellitus (DM)	Poorly controlled, or diabetic complications present, e.g. retinopathy, renal damage	Well controlled, and no complications, young patient with short duration of DM	POP better choice See text
Hypertension	BP > 160/95 mmHg on repeated testing	Systolic BP 135–160 mmHg Diastolic BP 85–95 mmHg	See text
Cigarette smoking	> 40 cigarettes/day	5–40 cigarettes/day	
Increasing age	> 35 in all smokers. Age alone is not an absolute contraindication	40–50 years non-smokers	
Excess weight	> 50% above ideal for height (BMI > 35)	20–50% above ideal (BMI 30–35)	
Migraine	Focal, crescendo or requiring treatment with ergotamine	Uncomplicated/acceptable to the woman	1. Relates to stroke risk 2. Consider tricycling if uncomplicated headaches mainly in pill-free interval 3. Sumatriptan treatment is now considered a relative contraindication

Notes:
1. Some of the numbers selected are necessarily a little arbitrary and relate to use solely for contraception.
2. Use of COCs for medical indications entails a different risk–benefit analysis (see text).
3. Blood Group O is associated in some studies with a reduced risk of venous thromboembolism and myocardial infarction. Hence a woman with this group might be allowed to continue using the pill despite other less favourable factors.

       ii. development of the lupus anticoagulant/
antiphospholipid antibody

      iii. following splenectomy for any indication if the
subsequent platelet count is above 500×10^9/litre
(Machin S 1987, personal communication).

  f. Other conditions predisposing to thrombosis including:

       i. blood dyscrasias

      ii. autoimmune disorders with this risk such as polyarteritis
nodosa, scleroderma and severe systemic lupus
erythematosis (SLE)

      iii. Klippel Trenaunay syndrome

      iv. severe primary or secondary polycythaemia

      v. elective major or leg surgery

      vi. during leg immobilization

      vii. varicose vein treatments

      viii. residence above 4000 metres, which is associated with
raised blood viscosity due to haemoconcentration in the
short term and polycythaemia later (Ward 1986,
personal communication)

      ix. severe inflammatory bowel disease (including
Crohn's)(p. 83).

  g. Focal and crescendo migraine (p. 72) and migraine
requiring ergotamine treatment.

  h. Transient ischaemic attacks even without headache.

  i. Past cerebral haemorrhage (exceptionally the COC may be
permitted after successful surgery following a subarachnoid
haemorrhage).

  j. Vascular malformations of the brain.

  k. Most types of valvular heart disease (discuss each case with
the cardiologist first) because of risk of systemic emboli in
the presence of arrhythmias.

  l. Pulmonary hypertension.

2. Diseases of the liver.

  a. Active liver disease (i.e. currently abnormal liver function
tests; infiltrations and cirrhosis); recurrent cholestatic
jaundice, or a history of this in pregnancy; Dubin–Johnson
or Rotor syndrome. COCs may, however, be prescribed after
viral hepatitis once liver function tests have returned to
normal for at least three months.

  b. Liver adenoma or carcinoma.

  c. Gall stones (although COCs can be used after
cholecystectomy).

    d. The porphyrias (progestogen-only methods are also
       contraindicated).
3. History of a serious condition known to be affected by
   sex-steroids or by previous COC use.
    a. Chorea.
    b. COC-induced hypertension.
    c. COC-associated acute pancreatitis.
    d. Pemphigoid gestationis (formerly termed herpes gestationis).
    e. Haemolytic uraemic syndrome or thrombotic
       thrombocytopaenic purpura.
    f. Otosclerosis. Many authorities permit closely supervised
       COC use
    g. Stevens–Johnson syndrome (erythema multiforme) if
       COC-associated.
    h. Trophoblastic disease until hCG levels are undetectable
       (p. 78).
    i. Most cases of SLE.
   This is not necessarily a complete list. Certain criteria can used
   to assess the risk associated with any disease about which there
   is uncertainty (p. 50).
4. Pregnancy.
5. Undiagnosed genital tract bleeding.
6. Oestrogen-dependent neoplasms, e.g. breast cancer. (Some
   oncologists, however, permit selected women in prolonged
   remission to take COCs.)
7. If a woman's anxiety about COC safety is not relieved by
   counselling.

Relative

1. Risk factors for arterial disease (Table 3.2) are all only relative
   contraindications, provided, normally, that only one is present,
   and that it is not serious enough to make it an absolute
   contraindication.
2. Long-term partial immobilization, e.g. in a wheelchair.
3. Sex-steroid dependent cancer. The specialist's advice should be
   sought. A history of breast cancer is almost invariably
   considered an absolute contraindication. Breast biopsy showing
   premalignant epithelial atypia is considered by some to be a
   strong relative contraindication, and by others an absolute
   contraindication. Most authorities no longer consider
   malignant melanoma, after successful treatment, to be a

contraindication to starting or continuing with either the COC or the POP (p. 83).

4. Amenorrhoea or oligomenorrhoea should be investigated but the pill may subsequently be prescribed (Ch. 15).
5. Hyperprolactinaemia is now considered only a relative contraindication for patients under specialist supervision.
6. Very severe depression – but unwanted pregnancies can be very depressing too!
7. Chronic systemic diseases – see below.
8. Disease requiring long-term treatment with drugs which might interact with the pill (pp. 63–67).
9. Conditions which impair absorption of COCs, such as some operations for obesity. The lipoprotein HDL-C is reduced in some chronic malabsorption states with a well-recognized increased risk of arterial disease.

Intercurrent disease

There are some conditions in which COCs are absolutely contra-indicated, but others which are benefited or at least unaffected. There are persistent myths about some of the latter, and it is unfortunate that women are often wrongly or unnecessarily deprived of the pill for reasons such as hypo-oestrogenic amenorrhoea, thrush, uncomplicated varicose veins or fibroids.

Most medical conditions can be grouped into broad categories:

1. Disorders in which COCs are *not known* to have any effect. We can reassure the patient that the rate of deterioration is not known to be accelerated in:

Asthma
Carcinoma of the colon
Gilbert's disease
Hodgkin's disease
Multiple sclerosis
Myasthenia gravis
Neuroblastoma
Raynaud's syndrome (primary, no suspicion that it is secondary)
Renal dialysis (but HDL-C is lowered in some chronic renal disorders)
Retinitis pigmentosa
Rheumatoid arthritis

Sarcoidosis
Spherocytosis
Thyrotoxicosis
Thalassaemia major.

Most cancers in current remission are not affected by the combined pill provided hormone-dependency is not suspected and the thrombotic risk is not increased as it may be in advanced malignancy. Pill use should be discussed with the specialist responsible for the patient's management.

2. Disorders of varying degrees of seriousness in which the COC *might have* the potential to interact in a harmful way.
It is impossible to list every known disease which might have a bearing on pill prescribing. For many, data are not available or are contradictory. There are some useful criteria which can be applied if the prescriber first makes all necessary enquiries about the condition itself, however rare it may be. *Because they may summate with other risk factors*, COCs are absolutely contraindicated if the disorder:
   a. Increases the risk of arterial or venous thrombosis.
   b. Predisposes to arterial wall disease.
   c. Adversely affects liver function.
   d. Shows a tendency to significant sex-steroid hormone dependency (e.g. deterioration with previous administration of COCs or during pregnancy).
In some cases, the added risk of pregnancy in women with the condition, or the likelihood of deterioration of the disease in pregnancy, may fully justify some increased risk due to the COC – primarily because it is so effective. A good example of this is sickle cell disease (see below).

3. Conditions treated with drugs which may interact with COCs (pp. 63–67).

For further discussion of contraception and disease, the reader is referred to the excellent chapter with that title in the book by Sapire (1990).

Sickle cell disorders

Sickle cell trait is not a contraindication to COC use.
The situation regarding the homozygous conditions (SS and SC genes) is more uncertain. Both sickle cell disease and COCs independently lead to an increased risk of thrombosis, which may be exacerbated during the arterial stasis of a sickling crisis. Hence,

many authorities and most manufacturers have for many years included the frank sickling diseases among absolute contra-indications to COCs. However, more recent studies in West Africa and the West Indies suggest that sickle cell disease should be considered only a relative contraindication – especially when the benefits of COCs as a very effective contraceptive are balanced against the serious risks of pregnancy. Until this has been confirmed the injectable DMPA is an even better choice (p. 115).

Diabetes mellitus

It is well established that the combined pill may decrease glucose tolerance and cause a rise in insulin levels in healthy non-diabetic women. Despite this, the pill does not increase the risk of developing clinical diabetes. Much less is known about the effects of the pill on existing diabetes. Based on early studies, there has traditionally been a negative attitude toward the use of the combined pill by diabetic women. More recent work (Skouby 1989) suggests that low dose pills may be used by women in whom diabetic control is good and who do not have any serious complications of the disease.

ADVANTAGES

1. Reliable, reversible, convenient method which is independent of intercourse.
2. Periods become more regular. Blood loss is reduced, decreasing the incidence of iron deficiency anaemia.
3. Menstrual and premenstrual symptoms such as dysmenorrhoea and premenstrual tension are often relieved.
4. Ovulation pain is abolished.
5. Unlike most other commonly used drugs, there is no acute toxicity as a result of overdose except withdrawal bleeding in prepubertal girls, and vomiting.
6. Decreased incidence while on treatment of:
   a. Benign breast disease.
   b. Functional ovarian cysts.
   c. Pelvic inflammatory disease (PID).
   d. Ectopic pregnancy since ovulation is inhibited and PID reduced.
   e. Seborrhoeic conditions including acne.
   f. Endometriosis.
7. Protection against carcinoma of the ovary and endometrium. In at least nine studies a reduction in the risk of ovarian cancer

and in seven a reduction in the risk of endometrial cancer has been shown (Vessey 1989). The effect is related to the duration of use and provides reduction by a factor of three in the risk of both conditions after 5 years. The protective effect persists for at least 15 years after the pill is stopped.

8. Other possible benefits have been identified in one or two studies but have yet to be fully confirmed. These include protection against rheumatoid arthritis, thyroid disease, duodenal ulcer, trichomonal vaginitis and toxic shock syndrome.

DISADVANTAGES

It is not surprising that a combination of steroids which proves so effective in controlling reproduction also affects other physiological systems. Epidemiological evidence of adverse effects relates mainly to pills containing 50 µg or more of oestrogen, since the latter tends to promote intravascular thrombosis. Well over 90% of women on the pill now use brands containing only 20–35 µg of oestrogen, and most of those with risk factors are now prescribed, as recommended (pp. 39, 58), products with third generation progestogens. Coupled with improved assessment and monitoring this should reduce still further the already low rate of serious adverse effects.

Clinical experience suggests that modern low-dose preparations are also less likely to cause the so-called 'minor' side-effects such as nausea and weight gain.

Metabolic effects

These are many and varied (Table 3.3 p. 54). Many are similar to those found in normal pregnancy. Although this may be reassuring, it should be remembered that pregnancy has its own hazards, often not unlike those of the pill.

In the event of laboratory investigations being undertaken in a woman who is taking the pill, COC use should be mentioned on the accompanying request form as the pill alters serum binding of some circulating hormones.

The liver

Contraceptive steroids are metabolized by the liver and affect its function. The resultant effects on the metabolism of carbohydrates, lipids, plasma proteins, amino acids, vitamins, enzymes and the factors concerned with coagulation and fibrinolysis explain the majority of the adverse effects. Non-oral routes of administration which avoid the first pass through the liver are likely to be preferred for the future.

Increase in appetite and weight gain, with or without fluid retention, which occur in a proportion of COC users are also based on metabolic changes which are as yet not fully understood.

Cardiovascular system

The incidence of the conditions discussed below is increased in users of the pill.

Venous disease

Deep venous thrombosis; pulmonary embolism; thrombosis in other veins, e.g. mesenteric, hepatic or retinal. The metabolic basis for these problems is an oestrogen-induced alteration of clotting factor levels, tending to promote coagulation. One of the more important changes is a reduction in concentrations of antithrombin III. Platelet function is also modified. The changes are less marked in pills containing less than 50 µg of oestrogen. There is evidence of compensatory increased fibrinolytic activity which may explain the rarity of overt disease in most pill users. Increased fibrinolysis is, however, less marked among smokers.

The risks of venous thromboembolism are enhanced by tissue damage and immobility. There are also some rare conditions, known as congenital thrombophilias, in which a predisposition to thrombosis makes an overt event more probable if COCs are used. Examples include deficiency of Protein C, Protein S, antithrombin III and the newly-described Factor V Leiden (Vanderbroucke 1994). A family history of a thrombotic event (usually venous but occasionally arterial) occurring in a first-degree relative under 45 provides an indication for investigating haemostasis. If the result for an important factor is outside the normal range this would normally absolutely contraindicate COCs (see Table 3.2 p. 46).

Arterial disease

This includes myocardial infarction, thrombotic stroke, haemorrhagic stroke including subarachnoid haemorrhage (although the data here are less convincing), and other arterial events such as

Table 3.3 Some metabolic effects of combined oral contraceptives

	Blood level	Remarks
Liver		
Liver function		These many changes cause no apparent long-term damage to the liver itself. The liver is involved, however, in the production of most of the changes in blood levels of substances shown elsewhere in this table, including the important changes in carbohydrate and lipid metabolism, and coagulation factors.
a. generally	Altered in all users	
b. specifically		
Albumen	→	
Transaminases	→	
Amino acids	Altered	
Homocysteine	←	These changes, barely detectable with the latest pills, may partly explain the increased risk of arterial disease with earlier preparations.
Blood glucose after carbohydrate ingestion	↑	
Blood lipids	←	Altered, mostly ↑
HDL-cholesterol	→	
Clotting factors		
a. generally	mostly ↑	Both the pill and smoking affect these inter-related systems. Fibrinolysis is enhanced in the blood, but reduced in the vessel walls.
b. specifically		
Antithrombin III (anti-clotting factor)	→	
Fibrinolysis	←	
Tendency for platelet aggregation	↑	
Hormones		
Insulin	←	These hormone changes are related to those affecting blood sugar and blood lipids (above).
Growth hormone	←	
Adrenal steroids	←	
Thyroid hormones	←	
Prolactin	↑	
Luteinising hormone (LH)	→	These effects are integral to contraceptive actions. However, the first three tend to rise in some women during the pill-free week. Hence any effective lengthening of the pill-free time may lead to an LH surge and ovulation.
Follicle-stimulating hormone (FSH)	→	
Endogenous oestrogen	→	
Endogenous progesterone	→	

Table 3.3 (cont'd)

	Blood Level	Remarks
Minerals and vitamins		
Iron	↑	This is a good effect for women prone to iron-deficiency.
Copper	↑	
Zinc	↓	Effects unknown, but not believed to cause any health risk for most pill users. Pyridoxine is discussed on page 71.
Vitamins A, K	↑	
Riboflavine, folic acid	↓	
Vitamin B₆ (pyridoxine)	↓	
Vitamin B₁₂ (cyanocobalamin)	↓	
Vitamin C (ascorbic acid)	↓	
Binding globulins	↑	These globulins carry hormones and minerals in the blood. Because their levels increase in parallel with the latter, the effective blood levels of the hormones or minerals are usually not much altered.
Blood viscosity	↑	
Body water	↑	This retention of fluid explains some of the weight gain blamed on the pill (p. 74).
Factors affecting blood pressure		
Renin substrate	Altered	
Renin activity	↑	Changes do not correlate as well as expected with the incidence of frank hypertension (p. 70).
Angiotensin II		
Cardiac output		
Immunity / allergy		
Number of leucocytes	↑	
Immunoglobulins	Altered	See page 83.
Function of lymphocytes	Altered	

Notes:
1. In the table ↑ means the level usually goes up, ↓ down.
2. 'Altered' means that the changes are known to be more complex, with both increases and decreases occurring within the system.
3. The changes are generally (a) within the normal range, (b) similar to those of normal pregnancy.

thrombosis of mesenteric or retinal arteries. It appears that the predisposition to arterial thrombosis results both from the metabolic changes (principally progestogen-related) which may promote atherosclerosis in long-term users, and the oestrogenic changes affecting blood coagulability leading to thrombosis superimposed on the damaged arterial wall. Both the oestrogen and progestogen content are therefore potentially involved, particularly in smokers (p. 46).

Relative risk of cardiovascular disease

Epidemiological estimates vary, but from the prospective study of the Royal College of General Practitioners (RCGP 1981) the risk ratio for all vascular disease mortality was 4.0. Risk ratios for the individual conditions varied between 1.5 and 6.0. In this study there were very few deaths or incidents of disease under the age of 35. More recent research suggests that the risk ratio for modern formulations containing less than 50 μg of oestrogen has fallen to between 1 and 2. Indeed, Croft & Hannaford (1989), like some other researchers, found that current use of the pill had no detectable effect on the risk of myocardial infarction unless the woman also smoked in which case the risk was very high, over 20 for heavy smokers.

The stroke risk in current users is doubled in both smokers and non-smokers (Hannaford et al 1994). Smoking not only increases the risk of arterial diseases, but also the fatality rate (RCGP 1983).

See Table 3.2 (p. 46) for a detailed consideration of risk factor management.

Relative risks among current users   With the possible exception of strokes (RCGP 1983), the relative risk of cardio-vascular disease (CVS) does not appear to increase with increasing duration of pill use, provided those who develop hypertension are identified and stop using the combined pill. The important factor is the age of the woman, not the number of years that she has been on the pill.

Relative risks among ex-users   The increased risk of venous thromboembolism disappears around one month after stopping the pill. There is some evidence that former users continue to have an elevated risk of stroke, but that effect appears to be restricted to smokers. Stampfer and colleagues (1988) were unable to show any persistent effect on the risk of heart disease among ex-users.

Effects on other systems

COC also has effects on the central nervous system (pp. 71–74); gastrointestinal system (pp. 74–75); urinary tract (p. 75); genital tract (pp. 76–78); breast (pp. 78–81); musculoskeletal system (pp. 81–82); and on the skin (pp. 82–83).

CLINICAL MANAGEMENT

Suitability for the pill is based on history and physical examination. Allow time to discuss the concerns of each individual, raising the issues relating to circulatory disease and cancer at the appropriate time even if she does not mention them herself.

History

Take a full history. Pay particular attention to those conditions which might contraindicate COC use, and the importance for this individual of avoiding pregnancy, including:

1. Social factors, particularly those relating to the risk of sexually transmissible disease, including HIV and hepatitis B.
2. Family history especially of CVS disease including hypertension, and of breast cancer.
3. Obstetric history.
4. Past or current illnesses and investigations paying particular attention to contraindications.
5. Current drug therapy.
6. Allergies including skin conditions.
7. Headache or migraine: frequency, site, timing, severity, relation to menstrual cycle, initiating factors, therapy, presence of focal symptoms in the past.
8. Use of contact lenses – date of last check, any symptoms.

Examination

1. Observation on general health.
2. Record baseline weight and blood pressure (BP).
3. Although it may be reassuring to establish that the pelvis is normal, many women dislike pelvic examination. It should not be insisted upon at the first visit provided the patient gives a normal menstrual history with a normal last menstrual period, indicating that she is not pregnant.

4. A cervical smear should be taken according to the policy for a woman in that risk category (Ch. 12). This is good preventive medicine, but again a recent smear is not an essential pre-requisite for use of the pill or indeed any other method of contraception and should never be insisted upon.
5. Breast examination – a baseline examination is recommended in older women (age >35 years). Instruction can be given on breast self-examination.
6. Other investigations may be suggested by the history. A family history of heart disease may for example indicate the need for measurement of serum cholesterol.

Choice of pill

Much has been written in the past about matching pills to particular hormonal profiles, but the systems have no practical value for the initial selection of the low-dose pills now in use. The pill of choice should be the one containing the lowest suitable dose of oestrogen and progestogen which:

1. Provides effective contraception.
2. Produces acceptable cycle control.
3. Is associated with fewest side-effects.
4. Has the least known effect on haemostasis, carbohydrate and lipid metabolism and other metabolic parameters.

Each doctor needs to be familiar with the composition of available preparations. Women may react unpredictably, and several preparations may need to be tried before a suitable one is found. Some women are never suited. This is hardly surprising: individual variation in blood levels, and end-organ response (especially the endometrium), is well recognized (Guillebaud 1989). Thus it is a false expectation that any single pill will suit all women.

First choice of pill

The initial dose of oestrogen should normally be in the range 20–35 μg combined with the lowest dose of progestogen within each group (Table 3.1). In the presence of a cardiovascular risk factor (Table 3.2) the third generation progestogens should always be used, but low-dose norethisterone and levonorgestrel formulations remain acceptable for healthy individuals without risk factors. Special circumstances in which a 50 μg pill may be required include:

1. Long-term use of an enzyme-inducing drug
   (Table 3.5 pp. 64–65).
2. Past 'true' pill failures, suggesting unusually rapid metabolism
   or malabsorption. Tricycling (p. 67) should also be considered.
3. If a lower dose preparation cannot control the cycle after at
   least three months trial provided no other cause for
   breakthrough bleeding is found (p. 76).

The above policy should be applied flexibly. Psychology in pill prescription may be as important as physiology. One needs a good reason not to comply with the woman's personal choice if, for example, a particular preparation suited a friend or relative.

Instructions to patients

Although pills are dispensed in bubble packs, careful teaching and explanation are still essential. Some manufacturers have greatly improved their packaging and leaflets, but in other cases the leaflet in each packet is in very small print and often not up to date. The latest instruction leaflet produced by the Family Planning Information Service (FPIS) is clear and accurate.

The need for regular pill taking at a time of day when it is easy to remember, such as when cleaning one's teeth in the morning or evening, must be stressed. Being late in taking the pill(s) can lead to BTB, which may then be prolonged over many days and itself cause compliance problems leading to pregnancy.

Starting the pill

See Table 3.4 for a summary of starting routines.
   Monophasic pills   These are started as follows:

1. The first pill is taken on the first day of the next menstrual
   period. Manufacturers' literature still often suggests that
   starting should be delayed until the fifth day for some brands
   but this does not preclude the first day start which obviates the
   need for a secondary method.
2. The pill labelled for the appropriate day of the week is selected.
3. One pill is taken daily for 21 or 22 days at approximately the
   same time.
4. After the packet is finished, no pills are taken for 7 days (6 days
   with Gracial), then a new packet is started. It is important that
   the start of the next packet must never be delayed (pp. 61–63).

Table 3.4 Starting routines

	Start when?	Extra precautions?
1. Menstruating	On or after fifth day of cycle First day	Yes (see text) No*

2. Post-partum
  a. no lactation
  b. lactation
	Day 21 postpartum
	Not normally recommended at all (POP preferred)
		No

3. Therapeutic abortion / miscarriage	Same day/day 2	No
4. Post-trophoblastic tumour	1 month after no human chorionic gonadotrophin detected	As 1
5. Post-higher-dose COC	Instant switch	No ⎫ ⎬ see text
6. Post-lower or same-dose COC	After usual 7-day break	No ⎭
7. Post-POP	First day of period	No
8. Post-POP with secondary amenorrhoea / during lactation when infant starts solid feeds.	After last packet of POP	No
9. Other secondary amenorrhoea (pregnancy excluded)	Any day	Yes (7 days)
10. First cycle after postcoital contraception	1st day or by day 2 when sure flow is normal.	No

* Except in the case of ED pills, since the start-up routine entails the taking of a variable number of placebos.

5. Everyday (ED) varieties contain 7 placebo tablets which are taken during the 7 days that would otherwise be 'tablet-free'. With this regimen the next packet of pills is started immediately after the last one is finished.

6. Contraceptive protection is immediate if the pill is started on the first day of a period. If starting is delayed beyond the third day there is a very small risk that a graafian follicle will continue to develop so additional contraceptive precautions are advised for the first 7 days of the first packet. Extra precautions are also recommended for the first 14 days with ED varieties.

Biphasic and triphasic pills   Each packet contains 21 (or 22) tablets of two or three different doses, identified by different colours. It is most important that pills are taken in the correct order.

Postpartum

The combined pill is contraindicated during breastfeeding (Ch. 7). Women who choose to bottle feed their babies are usually advised to start at 3 or 4 weeks postpartum. This timing allows for the occurrence of the natural fall in circulating oestrogens (extremely high during pregnancy), thus reducing the risk of thromboembolism while initiating a reliable method of contraception before ovulation resumes.

After therapeutic abortion or miscarriage   The pill should be started immediately (day 1 or 2), without extra precautions. This is similar to the advice in a normal cycle, since ovulation can occur within 3 weeks after a first trimester abortion (Ch. 10). COCs will not interfere with recovery, nor increase morbidity.

Other starting routines are shown in Table 3.4.

Changing preparations

When changing from one COC to another one of lower dose the following regimens may be used. The first pill of the new packet is taken:

1. On the day immediately after the old packet is completed without a pill-free interval. This way no extra precautions are necessary. This is the preferred advice (Table 3.4).
2. On the first day of withdrawal bleeding following completion of the last pack: no additional precautions are required. Warn the woman that if withdrawal bleeding does not occur she should not wait longer than 7 days before starting a new packet and should then follow the instructions in (3) below.
3. After the usual 7 tablet-free days. Additional precautions are then required for 7 days if the new pill has a lower dose of either oestrogen or progestogen, or if there is any doubt about its equivalence.

Management of missed pills: importance of the pill-free interval (PFI)

It is now well established that in many women on current low-dose COCs there is a variable degree of restoration of ovarian function during the PFI, shown not only by follicular activity on ultrasound but also by rising concentrations of both gonadotrophins and endogenous oestradiol.

It follows, therefore, that breakthrough ovulation is most likely to occur at the end of any PFI which is lengthened, the lengthening

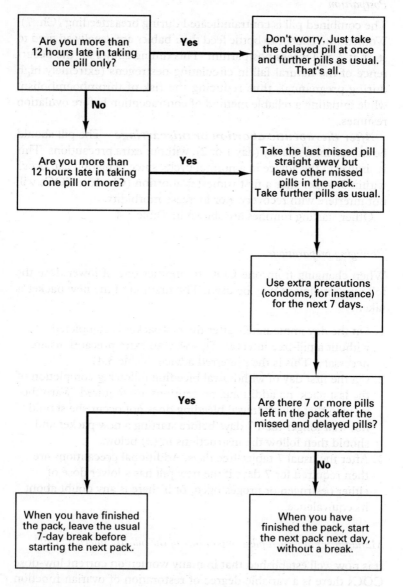

Fig. 3.1 Advice for missed pills (21-day packaging).

being caused by missed pills either just prior to the 7-day break or immediately following it; 7 pill-free days are acceptable, but in some women anything more will permit ovulation.

The routine advice for missed pills is shown in Figure 3.1.

Vomiting, diarrhoea and short-term drug interactions

Similar advice is appropriate when the bio-availability of contraceptive steroids is temporarily reduced by vomiting within three hours of ingestion of tablet(s), very severe diarrhoea or during short-term use of interacting drugs (Table 3.5 and discussion below). 'Stomach upsets' have been shown to be particularly important in this context, accounting for 1 in 3 breakthrough conceptions in apparently compliant women. *Extra contraceptive precautions should start from the onset of the illness and continue for seven days thereafter, with elimination of the PFI as indicated by the advice above.*

Drug interaction

The importance of the potential reduction in the effectiveness of COCs resulting from the simultaneous use of other medications has come to light since the introduction of low-oestrogen pills. Complex mechanisms are involved: induction of liver enzymes, competition for binding sites, and reduced enterohepatic recirculation of oestrogen if the relevant bowel flora are altered by broad spectrum antibiotics.

Enzyme-inducing drugs can affect both the oestrogen and the progestogen. Broad spectrum antibiotics have a lesser effect since they only influence the recycling of ethinyloestradiol. This also means that they can have no significant interaction with the POP.

Table 3.5 shows the more important interactions of this type and their clinical implications.

Women show enormous variability in their circulating concentrations of contraceptive steroids and demonstrate different degrees of interaction with other drugs. Many are unaffected, particularly by antibiotics. Nevertheless the individual response cannot be predicted clinically and it is wise to assume reduced protection in every case. Fortunately, with antibiotics the large bowel flora responsible for recycling oestrogens are reconstituted with resistant organisms in about two weeks (Orme 1992, personal communication). In practice therefore, if the COC is commenced in a woman who has been taking a tetracycline long-term (e.g. for acne), there

Table 3.5 The more important drug interactions with COCs

Class of drug	Approved names of important examples	Main action	Clinical implications for COC use
Drug which may reduce COC efficacy Anticonvulsants	Barbiturates (esp. phenobarbitone) Phenytoin Primidone Carbamazepine	Induction of liver enzymes increasing their ability to metabolise *both* COC steroids.	Preferably tricycling with shortened pill-free interval. 50µg oestrogen COCs can be used, increasing to 90µg if BTB occurs. Sodium valproate, clonazepam and all the newly-introduced anti-convulsants are not enzyme inducers.
Antibiotics a. Antitubercle	Rifampicin	Marked induction of liver enzymes.	Use of alternative contraception is preferred, e.g. DMPA with 8-week injection interval.
b. Antifungal	Griseofulvin	Induction of liver enzymes.	Short courses – additional contraception during treatment, and follow 7-day rule. Long courses – as for anticonvulsants.

Table 3.5 *(cont'd)*

Class of drug	Approved names of important examples	Main action	Clinical implications for COC use
c. Broad spectrum	Ampicillin and relatives Tetracyclines	Change in bowel flora, reducing enterohepatic recirculation of ethinyloestradiol (EE) only, after hydrolysis of its conjugates.	Short courses – wisest to use additional contraception during treatment up to 14 days (see text) plus follow 7-day rule. POP is unaffected.
Hypnotics / tranquillisers	Meprobamate Glutethimide Dichloral phenazone	Induction of liver enzymes.	Avoid these drugs in COC-users (alternatives available).
Drugs which may increase COC efficacy			
	Ascorbic acid	Theoretically, drug competes in bowel wall for conjugation to sulphate. Hence more EE available for absorption.	Recent research suggests that this effect is immeasurable and can be disregarded.
	Co-trimoxazole	Inhibits EE metabolism.	None, if short course given to low-dose COC user.

is no need to advise extra precautions. When a tetracycline is first started by a woman already taking the pill extra precautions need only be taken for about 2 weeks.

In conditions such as cystic fibrosis managed with recurrent long-term courses of potent antibiotics, there is a potential problem – managed as in the last paragraph – only at each change of antibiotic.

Long-term use of enzyme-inducing drugs

This applies chiefly to epileptics and women being treated for tuberculosis. For patients treated with rifampicin, since it is such a powerful enzyme inducer, an alternative method of contraception is preferable such as an IUD or the injectable DMPA with a reduced (8-week) injection interval. Otherwise, a 50 μg oestrogen preparation such as Ovran should be chosen along with elimination of most of the PFIs by advising the tricycle regimen. This is particularly appropriate for epileptics since the frequency of convulsions is often reduced by the maintenance of steady hormone levels.

If the preferred progestogen for a woman with a risk factor is not marketed as a 50 μg pill a logical, if expensive, alternative is a combination of tablets e.g. one Mercilon plus one Marvelon daily.

Discontinuing enzyme-inducing drugs

Enzyme-induction may take many days to reach its peak after a drug is introduced, and it may take up to 12 weeks before liver function reverts to normal when it is withdrawn (Guillebaud 1989). Hence, if the enzyme-inducer is used for a month or more, loss of contra-ceptive activity must be assumed to continue for several weeks. After long-term use of any drug which induces liver enzymes, or any use at all of rifampicin, Orme recommends a delay of about 4 weeks before the woman returns to a standard low-dose pill regimen. This might reasonably be increased to 8 weeks after very prolonged use of barbiturates. Logically there should then be no gap when changing from higher to low-dose preparations.

Effects of COCs on other drugs

COCs slightly lower the clearance of diazepam, prednisolone and probably other drugs. This may increase the risk of side-effects, but the effect is very unlikely to be clinically significant. COCs impair the metabolism of warfarin, and at the same time alter clotting factors. Since the interaction is completely unpredictable, this combination of drugs is best avoided.

Manipulation of the menstrual cycle

To postpone a period

The pill may be used to postpone menstrual bleeding for the social convenience of the woman. She takes two packets of monophasic pills consecutively with no break.

Phasic preparations cannot be used in this way because if the woman takes two packets of these pills one after the other she is liable to bleed, since the first pills from the second packet contain a lower dose of progestogen than those she has just finished. Women on phasic preparations may delay menstruation in one of two ways:

1. Continuing to take further tablets from the final phase of another packet of the same brand of the phasic preparation.
2. Transferring directly to a packet of the monophasic brand most similar to the relevant final phase e.g. Logynon to Microgynon, or Tri-Minulet to Minulet. The original phasic pill can be restarted after the usual 7-day break. Contraceptive efficacy will be maintained throughout.

The tricycle regimen

This has been mentioned above as an integral part of the modern management of the long-term use of enzyme-inducers among pill users. Three packets of a monophasic pill are taken consecutively followed by a 4–5-day break. This leads to a longer pill cycle and means that the woman only has 4 or 5 withdrawal bleeds per year. This regimen obviously involves a larger annual intake of contraceptive steroids and the majority of women are probably best advised to adhere to the normal pill cycle. The tricycle regimen should be reserved for the specific indications listed in Table 3.6.

Follow-up

Patients should be seen 3 months after starting the pill (earlier if there are any relative contraindications) and 6-monthly thereafter. At each visit it is important to assess the acceptability of the method and to check that it is being used correctly. Any newly apparent risk

Table 3.6   COCs – Indications for eliminating pill-free interval (PFI)

Short-term – holidays etc
Long-term – tricycle regimens

1. Severe headaches or non-focal migraines occurring after hormone withdrawal.
2. The occurrence of annoying or heavy withdrawal bleeding, especially in women given the COC to help menorrhagia.
3. Endometriosis – especially when using a progestogen-dominant pill for maintenance treatment.
4. Epilepsy (reduces hormone fluctuations triggering attacks, and increases efficacy if enzyme-inducing drug is in use, see 5).
5. Any cause for suspicion of reduced efficacy of the COC – e.g. past 'breakthrough' pregnancy, or during long-term use of an enzyme-inducing drug.
6. At the woman's choice.

---

factors must be noted. The most clinically significant side-effects are rise in BP (p. 70) and change in headache pattern (p. 72).

Where no problems arise, routine checks should be kept to a minimum and can be delegated to a family planning trained nurse.

1. Routine weighing and bimanual examinations are unnecessary. (The pill protects against almost all conditions that can be identified bimanually).
2. BP should be recorded regularly during the first year and usually 6-monthly thereafter. After the first year, the interval between visits can be increased to annually in selected women.
3. Screening tests should be carried out (Ch. 12).
4. In the presence of symptoms, the appropriate investigations should be performed.

Women with risk factors for cardiovascular disease, or suffering from any chronic medical condition on which the effect of COCs is not definitely known, need to be monitored more closely.

Indications for stopping COC

1. Onset of any of the sudden major symptoms listed on p. 70, if a serious cause is suspected.
2. A sustained BP above 160/95 mmHg or even 85-90 mmHg diastolic, if other risk factors associated with CVS disease risk are present.

3. Appearance of a new risk factor(s) constituting a risk of CVS disease that is unacceptable for that particular woman. The commonest of these is increasing age in women who smoke.
4. Onset of jaundice.
5. Before elective surgery – COCs should be stopped at least 2 and preferably 4 weeks before major or leg surgery or any other surgery known to be associated with an intrinsic increased risk of thrombosis. They should be re-started no less than 2 weeks after the woman is ambulant. COCs should also be stopped for 4 weeks before and 4 weeks after completion of treatment for varicose veins whether by surgery or sclerotherapy.
   Injectable progestogens are a good alternative while the woman is waiting for admission.
   Major emergency surgery may be carried out under subcutaneous heparin cover.
   The surgeon should always be told if the woman is taking the pill.
   It is not necessary to stop the POP before major surgery, or COC before minor surgery, including sterilization.
6. Long-term immobilization e.g. associated with orthopaedic injury or operation.
7. When pregnancy is desired.
8. When contraception is no longer needed.

COMPLICATIONS AND THEIR MANAGEMENT

In general terms, if a change of pill seems appropriate to cope with a specific side-effect, try empirically:

1. Changing to a pill with a lower dose of the same progestogen and/or oestrogen. If appropriate, oestrogen can be eliminated altogether by trying a progestogen-only pill POP (Ch. 4).
2. Changing to a different progestogen, again starting with the lowest available dose.

Using other drugs to treat pill-induced side-effects is almost always bad practice. For example, if a woman complains of headaches, try changing her pill or recommending the tricycle regimen rather than prescribing analgesics.

If every brand of combined pill one tries causes side-effects, the POP may prove satisfactory, but bear in mind that emotional and psychological factors may play a part in the inability to find an acceptable pill.

Whenever a patient presents with symptoms or signs suggestive of a major side-effect relating to pill use, the pill should be stopped immediately with appropriate investigation and treatment arranged. Pill users should be warned in advance about the action to take if these symptoms were to occur:

1. Painful swelling in the calf.
2. Pain in the chest or stomach.
3. Breathlessness or cough with blood-stained sputum.
4. A bad fainting attack or collapse, or focal epilepsy.
5. Unusual headache or disturbance of speech or visual field especially if this is asymmetrical.
6. Numbness or weakness of a limb.

Cardiovascular system

Hypertension

Hypertension is in itself an important risk factor for heart disease and for both types of stroke. In most women on the pill there is a slight but not significant increase in both systolic and diastolic blood pressure. Approximately 1–3% become clinically hypertensive; probably nearer 1% with modern formulations. The incidence increases with age and duration of use. Specific changes in the renin–angiotensin system have not been identified in women who develop hypertension on the combined pill.

Predisposing factors for pill-induced hypertension include a strong family history, obesity and any tendency to water retention.

Pregnancy-induced hypertension does not predispose to hypertension during COC use. However the RCGP study (Croft & Hannaford 1989) showed an increased risk of myocardial infarction among all women with a history of toxaemia of pregnancy, independent of that associated with continuing hypertension. This requires confirmation, but a past history of toxaemia of pregnancy in a woman who smokes clearly makes careful monitoring essential.

Management   All patients on the pill should have their BP recorded regularly, and this should be repeated if necessary to obtain a true record.

1. Repeated elevated BP readings are important as a marker of the risk of circulatory disease, even if not above the level (160/95 mmHg) at which the COC would be absolutely contraindicated. This is particularly so if superimposed on

other risk factors. For example, a 33-year-old smoker with a BP 140/85 mmHg would be best advised to stop the COC.
2. Repeated recordings of BP above 160 mmHg systolic or 95 mmHg diastolic are considered an indication for stopping the pill.
3. Patients with a gradual rise in BP should be changed to a lower-dose pill or a progestogen-only preparation. BP levels should be rechecked within 3 months in both cases.
4. Pill-induced hypertension should not be treated with antihypertensive drugs.
5. Young women with essential hypertension, which is well controlled by therapy, may sometimes be given a low-dose combined pill under the supervision of a consultant physician.

Central nervous system

Depression

This used to be a relatively common complaint among women on high-dose pills but is less frequently reported by those using modern low-dose preparations. Although depression appears to be more common among women who take the pill than among non-users, the causal factors may be related to the general lifestyle rather than to the pill itself. Paradoxically, some depressed women find the pill relieves them of one of their greatest fears – that of unwanted pregnancy – and they therefore find it a very acceptable form of contraception.

   Management   Depression may be alleviated by:

1. Lowering the dose of or changing the progestogen.
2. Pyridoxine (vitamin B_6) 50 mg daily. This may take up to 2 months to be effective.

Loss of libido

Loss of libido is occasionally reported (Ch. 14), particularly among those who are also depressed. This may sometimes be associated with psychological problems associated with pill-taking, such as anxiety about its dangers, fears about subsequent fertility or guilt about using contraception at all. For other women, libido may be increased because the method is reliable, requires no action related to sexual activity, and often reduces premenstrual tension.

Management   Marital and family circumstances and psycho-sexual aspects of the relationship should always be discussed fully (Ch. 14). If vaginal soreness and dryness are caused by thrush, the infection should be treated. Lubrication with a bland jelly (e.g. KY) may help.

Headaches (including migraine)

In the RCGP study, headache was the second most common reason (after depression) for women stopping COCs. Careful assessment is essential since it is believed that some headaches can give early warning of the risk of a thrombotic stroke and hence absolutely contraindicate starting or continuing with the combined pill. The following characteristics should be considered serious:

1. Crescendo or any very severe migraine which is unremitting for days.
2. In a migraine sufferer, asymmetry of symptoms or a change in the character of associated symptoms from diffuse to focal. These are symptoms suggesting transient cerebral ischaemia and may include:
   a. Unilateral loss of sensation or severe paraesthesiae on one side of the body, or affecting one limb, or one side of the tongue.
   b. Weakness on one side of the body, or of a limb.
   c. Nominal dysphasia.
   d. Focal epilepsy.
   e. Diplopia.
   f. Ataxia, drop attacks.
   g. Loss of a field of vision including teichopsia (a field defect surrounded by a bright flashing line) and tunnel vision.
   Asymmetry is the significant feature shared by these symptoms. Symmetrical blurring of vision, generalized flashing lights and photophobia are not causes for concern. Unilateral headache is, of course, a diagnostic feature for migraine and likewise does not have this significance.
3. Any similar symptoms suggestive of a transient ischaemic attack even in the absence of headache.
4. Any migraine severe enough to require ergotamine therapy.
5. The occurrence of what appears to be a woman's first ever migraine attack while taking COC. However, if no further problems develop and if there were no focal symptoms, it is

acceptable to try reintroducing COC. Explicit warnings must be given about stopping the method if any of the above symptoms should develop.

Oestrogen causes prothrombotic changes which might be sufficient to summate with the transient cerebral ischaemia of migraine and result in permanent ischaemia – a thrombotic stroke. Progestogen-only methods of contraception, which do not increase the risk of stroke, are not contraindicated even if headaches continue.

Management   Since migraine headaches are possibly associated with an increased risk of stroke, any woman reporting headaches on the pill must be taken seriously.

1. The headache pattern should be carefully assessed and compared with the pattern of headaches before starting the pill. It is often very helpful to keep a diary.
2. If a woman reports severe migraine for the first time, or if focal (asymmetrical) symptoms suggestive of transient ischaemia occur, the pill should be stopped immediately and replaced by another method of contraception.
3. If headaches appear to be pill-induced try the effect of:
   a. A different variety of pill.
   b. The tricycle regimen. This is particularly effective in reducing the frequency of headaches which occur during pill-free days.
   c. Changing to a POP.
   d. Changing to a non-hormonal method.

Epilepsy

This condition is not initiated by the combined pill. In someone who has epilepsy, the frequency of convulsions is often reduced, especially if hormone fluctuations are lessened by reducing the number of pill-free intervals. Rarely, the frequency of convulsions may be increased. Anti-epileptic therapy with an enzyme inducer is one of the few indications for a relatively high-dose pill (p. 66).

Chorea and benign intracranial pressure

The incidence of these rare conditions is increased in users of the pill, but both improve if COCs are discontinued. The method should be avoided thereafter.

Eyes

Minimal water retention can lead to slight corneal oedema, and result in discomfort or corneal damage in those who wear contact lenses. With modern soft lenses and low-dose pills this problem is now rare.

The catastrophes of retinal artery or vein thrombosis and bleeding are even rarer but may be related to COC use.

Management   If any acute visual disturbance occurs, the pill should be stopped pending further investigation.

If corneal irritation occurs in wearers of contact lenses, prescribe a pill containing the lowest possible dose of both steroids. If symptoms persist, the wearer has to decide whether to give up her contact lenses or the pill, otherwise corneal ulceration and scarring may result.

Gastrointestinal system

Nausea and vomiting

Nausea may occur in the first cycle and occasionally recurs with the first few pills of each packet. Vomiting is most unusual.

Both symptoms are related to the oestrogen component and are rare with low-dose preparations. Severe vomiting may interfere with COC absorption and lead to breakthrough bleeding or spotting (p. 76).

Management   Nausea and vomiting usually resolve with time; if not it may be helpful to alter the timing of pill taking. If nausea occurs in the morning try taking the pill at night and vice versa. If persistent nausea occurs, try changing to a pill with less oestrogen.

Vomiting starting for the first time after months or years of trouble-free pill taking should not be attributed to the pill. Consider the possibility of pregnancy.

Weight gain

Increase in weight is unusual with modern pills, although it is frequently and unjustifiably expected. It is sometimes associated with an increase in appetite on starting the pill.

Management   The patient should be advised about her diet, and if this does not produce the desired result, the pill should be changed to one containing a lower dose of the same progestogen, or to one with a different progestogen. The POP can be tried if the problem persists on different brands of COC.

Jaundice

If a user becomes jaundiced, the pill must be stopped at once. With a diagnosis of infective hepatitis, the pill should not be restarted until 3 months after liver function tests return to normal.

Cholestatic jaundice is commoner among COC users, as it is in pregnancy. A past history in either context is a contraindication to the pill. A diagnosis of cholestatic jaundice means that the pill is contraindicated and an alternative method of contraception should be chosen.

Gall stones

Latest reports imply that the increased risk of gallstones among COC users is significant only during the early years of pill use. This suggests that the risk applies only to predisposed women.

It is reasonable for a woman who has had a cholecystectomy to take a low-dose pill provided there have been no complications.

Liver tumours

The relative risk of benign adenoma or hamartoma is increased by COC use. However, the background incidence is so small (1–3 per 1 million women per year) that the COC-attributable risk is minimal. Most reported cases have been in long-term users of relatively high-dose pills.

Three case control studies support the view that primary hepatocellular carcinoma (unrelated to cirrhosis or hepatitis B infection) is less rare in COC users than it is in controls. The maximum attributable incidence would be about 4 per million users per year (Vessey 1989).

Crohn's disease

See 'Infections and inflammations' (p. 83).

Urinary system

Several studies show that urinary tract infections are more common in COC users than in controls. Although women on the pill may have more frequent intercourse, predisposing them to 'honeymoon' cystitis, evidence of an increased incidence of symptomless bacteriuria in COC users suggests an additional causal link.

Genital system

Breakthrough bleeding: spotting

Breakthrough bleeding (BTB) or spotting (Sp) may result from circulating concentrations of steroids which are insufficient to maintain the endometrium. It is not usually an indication of an increased risk of pregnancy. Most women who become pregnant on the pill have no previous BTB just as most patients with BTB do not become pregnant. Until the BTB problem is resolved, they should perhaps be warned to be unusually compliant.

BTB is common during the first two or three cycles of pill use. Women should be forewarned, and advised to continue regular pill taking and not to stop in the middle of a packet. If spotting or BTB do occur, a chart may be given on which to record further episodes of bleeding, and the situation reviewed after 3 months.

Management Persistent BTB should be investigated. The following check list is modified from Sapire (1990):

1. Disease – examine the cervix. Irregular bleeding from invasive cancer can be wrongly attributed to COC use. Also consider chlamydia.
2. Disorder of pregnancy causing bleeding. e.g. abortion, trophoblastic disease.
3. Default – poor compliance.
4. Drugs which interact, primarily enzyme inducers.
5. Diarrhoea (though this has to be extremely severe) and/or vomiting.
6. Disturbance of absorption, e.g. after major gut resection.
7. Diet – in vegetarians the gut flora involved in recycling of oestrogen may be reduced although this is rare.
8. Duration too short – minimal BTB which is tolerable may resolve after 2-3 months.
9. Dose – after the above causes have been excluded:
   a. If she is taking a monophasic pill try a triphasic or biphasic pill.
   b. Increase the dose of progestogen and/or oestrogen.
   c. Try a different progestogen.
   d. Consider using a 50 µg pill such as Ovran.
   e. After rechecking this check-list and following careful discussion, prescribe two lower-dose pills a day. Careful records should be kept.

Absence of withdrawal bleeding

This is not dangerous, does not signify overdosage, nor is it related to 'post-pill amenorrhoea'.

Management The best management is reassurance.

Check that the woman is not pregnant, particularly if pills have been missed or where drug interactions may have occurred.

If a patient misses a single withdrawal bleed it is normal for her to be advised to restart the next packet as planned unless the history suggests the risk of pregnancy. However, if two withdrawal bleeds have been missed the patient should not start her next packet of pills until pregnancy has been excluded.

The incidence of absent withdrawal bleeding is lower with triphasic pills.

Vaginal discharge

Low-dose pills usually do not affect vaginal discharge. While some women may complain of vaginal dryness others may notice a more profuse, clear mucoid discharge with or without cervical ectopy. There is no causal link between genital candidiasis and use of modern COCs.

Management Vaginal discharge (Ch. 13). Cervical erosion (ectropion) (Ch. 15).

The combined pill may provide some as yet unexplained protection against trichomonal vaginitis (p. 52) but not against other sexually transmissible diseases. COCs do, however, protect the upper genital tract from pelvic infection. This is believed to be mediated by the effect of progestogens on cervical mucus.

Fibroids

The combined pill may stimulate the growth of pre-existing fibroids. Low-dose preparations, however, appear to have the opposite effect, and reduce the frequency of all the associated symptoms and the need for hospital referral. Patients with fibroids may therefore be given the pill, with monitoring, ideally by the same observer.

Carcinoma of the ovary and the endometrium

A protective effect is well established (pp. 51, 52).

Carcinoma of the cervix

The literature is complex and often contradictory. Some studies show an association between pre-malignant cervical cancer and oral contraceptive therapy. Vessey showed an effect of duration of pill use in a prospective study involving about 10000 women. After 8 years the risk ratio in comparison with controls who were using the IUD was about 2.0, and all 13 cases of invasive cancer occurred in the COC group (Vessey 1989).

The majority of the more recent studies also suggest that the pill could be a co-factor in causing this disease. But there is no certainty that in any of them the confounding variables – especially young age at first intercourse and multiple sexual partners of the index case or of her partner – were not more frequent in COC users than in controls. These confounding factors have a far greater effect on the risk than the two- to threefold increase after 8 years demonstrated in Vessey's study. Cigarette-smoking is also a far stronger co-factor.

The main implication for prescribers is to ensure that pill users are screened following agreed guidelines, as in Chapter 12. It is acceptable practice to continue COC during the careful monitoring of any abnormality, or after definitive treatment of cervical intraepithelial neoplasia (CIN).

Choriocarcinoma

There are no data suggesting any increase in the risk of trophoblastic disease in women who have taken the pill. When trophoblastic disease has been diagnosed, however, in the UK it is strongly recommended that all sex hormones (including progestogen-only methods) should be avoided while hCG levels are raised.

Breast

Enlargement and discomfort

While some women find that the COC improves cyclical breast symptoms, others complain of breast tenderness and swelling associated with pill use. These symptoms can occur with any pill formulation, but seem to be particularly associated with the last phase of triphasic and biphasic brands.

Management   Sudden enlargement of the breasts may be the first sign of pregnancy.

1. Breasts which are tender to touch or pressure, whether they are enlarged or not, often respond to a change of formulation.
2. Breast symptoms may continue no matter which preparation is prescribed and sometimes oral contraceptives have to be abandoned.
3. Management of the patient in whom a discrete breast lump is found is dealt with in Chapter 12.

   Galactorrhoea among pill takers is rare and needs investigation.

Carcinoma of the breast

The literature is copious, complex and contradictory. In assessing a possible link between the pill and breast cancer many factors have to be taken into account including:

1. The long latent period between pill use or repeated pill use and the disease.
2. That different effects are possible according to the time of life when pill use occurred.
3. Early menarche and late first delivery are established risk factors for breast cancer and these may be compounded by pill use.
4. Other risk factors, especially a family history of breast cancer or personal history of benign breast disease.
5. Change in pill formulation – both the oestrogen and progestogen content of pills have changed over the years and different preparations have been used in different countries.
6. Confounding factors – the pill may act as a marker for some other unknown risk factor.

   The World Health Organization convened a scientific group in 1990 to advise on the risks of oral contraceptives and neoplasia. The resultant publication (WHO 1992) provides a comprehensive and extremely useful review of the subject. A meta-analysis of all the available published data on pill use and breast cancer reached the conclusions quoted below:

1. Numerous studies have found no overall association between oral contraceptive use and risk of breast cancer.
2. A number of recent studies have found a weak association between long-term use of oral contraceptives and breast cancer diagnosed before the age of 36, and perhaps up to the age of 45. Such cancers represent a very small proportion of all breast

cancers. It is unclear whether this observed association is attributable to bias, the development of new cases of cancer, or accelerated growth of existing cancers.

3. Evidence indicates no increased risk of breast cancer associated with prior use of oral contraceptives in women over 45 years of age.
4. Oral contraception does not appear to alter the risk of breast cancer to a greater or lesser extent in subgroups of women at high or low risk of this disease (such as those with a family history of breast cancer).
5. Varying hormonal composition of oral contraceptives does not appear to influence the risk of breast cancer.
6. Use of combined oral contraceptives appears to decrease the risk of biopsy-confirmed fibrocystic disease and fibroadenoma. The degree of protection is related to duration of use.

The risk, if any, of breast cancer among pill users would seem then to be of relevance only to young women who take it for a long time. It seems likely that the pill, rather than causing breast cancer, simply accelerates its development.

In 1989 the UK National Case Control Study (UK NCCS 1989) reported an excess of early pill use among women developing breast cancer under the age of 36. The increased risk was significantly duration-dependent, whether exposure was before the first term pregnancy or after it, and reached 74% at 8 years. Pills containing less than 50 μg oestrogen seemed to be associated with a lower risk, contrary to the WHO conclusion (5) above. Later work on the same database showed no difference in the increasing effect of duration of use (about 7% per year up to age 35) whether exposure was continuous or intermittent.

The risk could yet be found to persist into older ages among the cohort of women who were exposed when young (in their teens or early twenties), not enough of whom have yet reached the years of peak incidence of this cancer. To date however, all studies including mortality studies remain very reassuring about older age groups, despite the steadily increasing proportion of their populations who have used the combined pill at a young age.

The background rate for breast cancer in women under 35 is 2 per 1000. The UK NCCS data mean that an extra 1 in 1000 women would be under treatment for breast cancer by the age of 35 years as a result of having used the pill for more than 4 years.

UK cancer registration data, however, still show no clear increase in the age groups who have had access to the pill (including the under-40s). It is not yet clear whether or not this is because the register is seriously incomplete for young women. But much of the data allows us to remain confident that women exposed to the pill after the age of 25 or so have no cause for concern, regardless of duration of use.

The clinical implications are as follows:

1. If the COC does truly increase breast cancer risk in certain categories of women, it is possible that this will be minimized by the use of low-dose pills containing modern progestogens.
2. No study suggests that COC use by young women with benign breast disease or with a family history of a first-degree relative with breast cancer gives them a greater increment of risk than other young women.
3. Breast cancer risks should now be addressed as a routine part of normal pill counselling and dealt with in a proactive, sensitive and opportune way, in context with the protective effects of COCs against ovarian and endometrial cancer. This would rarely be at the first visit by a teenager who has no concerns about cancer. We should present the risks and benefits as fairly as we can to young women, but leave the decision whether or not to use the pill to them. Presented with the facts, many see the contraceptive and non-contraceptive benefits of COCs as being enough to compensate for almost any likely lifetime risk of breast cancer.
4. All women should be taught the concept of breast awareness. It is appropriate for older women (>age 35 years) to be examined to exclude any pre-existing breast tumour before the pill, or indeed hormone replacement therapy (HRT), is first prescribed. Unless an examination is requested it is unnecessary and can be intrusive in a teenager.

Musculoskeletal system

Oestrogen given in high doses to young female animals can lead to premature closure of the epiphyses. There is no evidence that a daily dose of 30 µg or even 50 µg of ethinyloestradiol has this effect in postpubertal girls. Their growth will not be stunted if they take the pill.

Carpal-tunnel syndrome

More frequent in pill takers.

Leg pains and cramps

Careful examination and assessment of patients presenting with these symptoms is important. If bilateral, note any altered physical activity, water retention, weight increase, varicose veins, chilblains or Raynaud's disease. If unilateral, venous thrombosis must be excluded. Superficial, as well as deep venous, thrombosis is of relevance to a thrombotic tendency and to the woman's contraceptive future.

If in any doubt about the diagnosis, the pill should be stopped and the patient referred for further investigation including venogram if possible. Her contraceptive future depends on an accurate diagnosis being made.

Cutaneous system

Chloasma/melasma

'Pregnancy mask' may develop in women on the pill, after excessive exposure to sunlight, irrespective of whether or not it occurred in a previous pregnancy. It appears that both oestrogen and progestogen can be contributory. The condition may be slow to fade after the pill is stopped.

Management   Mild degrees of chloasma can be masked by carefully applied cosmetics. If it is causing the woman distress, a different pill can be tried but often no benefit is gained by changing from one low-dose preparation to another. A POP benefits some women although many will have to stop using hormonal contraception. Even then the pigmentation may be slow to fade. Depigmenting creams and lotions should be avoided.

Photosensitivity

This may occur on its own or, rarely, be the first manifestation of one of the porphyrias and hence contraindicate continued use of steroidal contraception.

Acne, greasy skin, hirsutism

These androgenic effects are more commonly associated with pills containing second generation progestogens (norethisterone and levonorgestrel)

Management   Change to a different pill. Good results have been reported with Marvelon and may be expected from Gracial.

Dianette, which contains an anti-androgen (cyproterone acetate) in place of a progestogen together with 35 µg ethinyloestradiol, is marketed for the treatment of acne particularly in association with polycystic ovarian syndrome (PCOS). It is an effective contraceptive and can be used in selected, well-supervised women for the same duration as other combined pills. If the patient is given a prescription for Dianette, she will be charged for the pills unless it is stated on the form that it is being used for contraception (a female symbol will suffice).

Malignant melanoma

While there is some evidence of an increase in the number of skin naevi among women who have used the COC, there is no evidence for an association between pill use and malignant melanoma.

Other skin conditions

Telangiectasia, rosacea, eczema, neurodermatitis, erythema nodosum, erythema multiforme and herpes gestationis may all be causally associated with or exacerbated by oral contraceptives.

Infections and inflammations

Some studies suggest that COC users are more likely to suffer from infections such as chickenpox, 'gastric flu', respiratory and urinary tract infections, and also inflammations such as tenosynovitis and a form of allergic polyarthritis.

There is also evidence that Crohn's disease may be more frequent in pill takers. This is usually the non-granulomatous type and resolves if the pill is stopped. If Crohn's disease is severe, there is an added risk of thrombosis.

These and other effects, including the unconfirmed beneficial effect on rheumatoid arthritis and thyroid disease, are believed to indicate that the pill can modify immune mechanisms.

REVERSIBILITY

In general, when women stop COCs they regain, after a delay of about 1 to 3 months, the fertility that they would have had if they had never used the method. Vessey (1986) showed that about half of his population of ex-users stopping the method above the age of

30 took up to a year longer to conceive than a control group stopping barrier methods. The combined pill does not cause any permanent loss of fertility.

The first period after stopping the pill is often delayed. A very few women have amenorrhoea for 6 months or more, unrelated to the type of pill or duration of use.

Secondary amenorrhoea after stopping the pill is not uncommon, especially in women who have had a late menarche, previous episodes of amenorrhoea or very irregular cycles. Abnormalities which would normally lead to amenorrhoea are masked by regular withdrawal bleeds while on the pill. Women who fail to menstruate for over 6 months after stopping the pill should be investigated in the same way as any other case of secondary amenorrhoea (Ch. 15).

OUTCOME OF PREGNANCY

Some authorities advise that women should discontinue the pill and use a barrier method of contraception for two to three cycles before a planned conception to allow mineral and vitamin metabolism to return to normal. Although this would do no harm, there is no objective evidence that it is of any benefit. With universal obstetric diagnostic ultrasound, accurate identification of the last menstrual period (LMP) has become less important for calculating gestation. Certainly, any woman who does find herself pregnant less than 3 months after stopping the pill should be strongly reassured about risk to the baby.

After discontinuing the COC, there is no increased risk of miscarriage, ectopic pregnancy or stillbirth, and no alteration in the sex ratio or birth weight. WHO (1981) declared categorically that there was no evidence of any adverse effect on the fetus of pill use prior to conception. No subsequent publications have seriously challenged this view.

Exposure during pregnancy

No attributable risk of teratogenesis was shown in Bracken's 1990 meta-analysis (risk ratio 0.99). In the Oxford/FPA and RCGP studies the incidence of birth defects following COC exposure was no higher than expected among any group of women having a planned baby.

The rule that a pregnant woman should avoid all drugs, especially in the first trimester, remains the ideal.

Although common fetal abnormalities are not more frequent among women who take the pill during pregnancy, some uncertainty inevitably remains about rare abnormalities. No woman can ever be promised a normal baby, whether she has inadvertently taken the pill or not; after all, 2% of all babies do have a significant abnormality. The consensus of opinion is that this risk is small enough to be considered negligible and the concept of COC-related teratogenesis should not be used as grounds for recommending therapeutic abortion.

BREAKS IN PILL TAKING

Fertility is not enhanced by breaks in pill taking.

Most risks such as venous thromboembolism, and benefits such as relief from menstrual symptoms apply only while the pill is being used. There does appear to be a duration of use effect relating to certain cardiovascular diseases; nevertheless, there is no evidence that by taking breaks the risk is reduced unless these are long enough to have a real impact on total accumulated years on the pill. In other words, if a pill user takes a 6 month break every 2 years, she will accumulate 10 years of use in 12 years. This will not, so far as is known, reduce her CVS risk compared with a matched woman taking the pill continuously for 10 years, but it will certainly increase her risk of unplanned pregnancy.

The studies suggesting that COC use promotes breast cancer under 35 years also show a duration of use effect. Conversely, if the pill reduces a risk, as it does for carcinoma of the ovary and endometrium, the protective effect is clearly greater the longer the pill is used.

The benefits of long-term use tend to balance the risks. Of great potential relevance to this whole discussion is the fact that any woman who has been on the pill for 10 years has in fact taken 130 breaks, each lasting a week. They may well be beneficial to the method's reversibility, to metabolism and perhaps to overall health (Guillebaud 1987).

RISKS/BENEFITS

For many women the combined pill provides highly acceptable and reliable contraception as well as many benefits to general health. It is not possible to enjoy these advantages without some disadvantages and, although the risks associated with the pill are real and should not be denied, their incidence is small. It is important to put these risks into perspective comparing them with risks of other methods of contraception and with pregnancy should a less effective method fail. Table 3.7 compares annual morbidity in terms of hospital admissions among 100 000 users of COC and of the condom. The risks must also be put into perspective with the other risks that women run in their lives (Fig. 3.2).

Table 3.7   Morbidity (in terms of hospital admissions) experienced by women aged 25 to 39 years using either COCs or relying on the condom to try to prevent pregnancy for 1 year. Based partly on data from the Oxford/FPA study.

Reason for hospital admission	Number of hospital admissions in one year among 100 000 women relying on:	
	Combined oral contraceptives	Condom
Beneficial effects of COCs		
Menstrual problems	375	500
Anaemia	22	30
Benign breast disease	115	230
Pelvic inflammatory disease*	60	60
Functional ovarian cysts	15	60
Ovarian cancer	5	10
Endometrial cancer	2	4
Harmful effects of COCs		
Acute myocardial infarction	10	5
Thrombotic stroke	50	10
Haemorrhagic stroke	7	5
Venous thromboembolism	100	20
Hepatocellular adenoma	2	0
Hepatocellular carcinoma	0	0
Accidental pregnancy†		
Term birth	300	3040
Spontaneous abortion	63	640
Extra-uterine pregnancy	3	20
Induced abortion	134	1300

* These rates are equal because both COCs and a condom offer protection against pelvic inflammatory disease.
† The failure rate for COCs has been taken to be 5 per 1000 per year and for the condom to be 50 per 1000 per year.

Mortality not considered. Morbidity due to sexually-transmitted viruses omitted. For other assumptions see source.

Source: Vessey M P, Jephcott lecture of the Royal Society of Medicine, 1989. Published in Proceedings of meeting 'Oral contraceptives and breast cancer' 17–19 July, 1989. Parthenon Publishing.

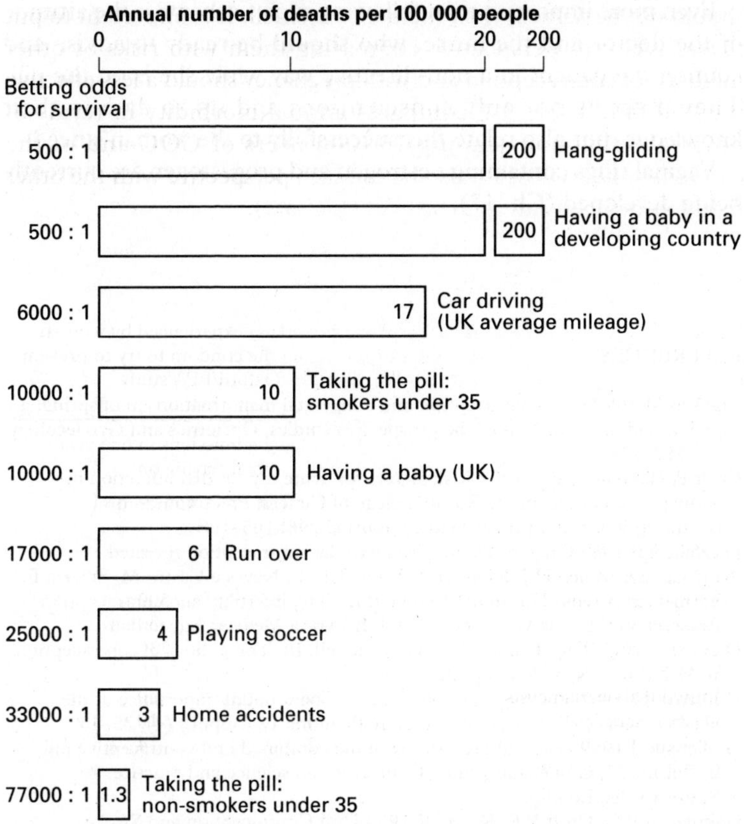

Fig. 3.2 Pill risks compared with other risks women run (reproduced with kind permission from Guillebaud J 1987 The Pill, 3rd edn. Oxford University Press, Oxford).

The safety of the pill can be further increased by:

1. Prescribing it primarily for healthy women.
2. Ensuring extra care and supervision for women with risk factors.
3. Using pills containing the lowest suitable dose of both oestrogen and progestogen.
4. Careful monitoring of:
   a. Any change in risk factors or new medical diagnoses.
   b. New circumstances of risk, e.g. elective surgery.
   c. Blood pressure.
   d. Headache pattern.
5. Appropriate well woman screening (Ch. 12).

Even more important than following such a scheme is the attitude of the doctor and the nurse, who should be ready to advise and counsel the patient in a non-directive way while she is on the pill. They must be not only conscientious and up to date in their knowledge, but also relate this successfully to the woman's needs.

Vaginal rings containing oestrogen and progestogen are currently being developed (Ch. 17).

REFERENCES

Bracken M 1990 Oral contraception and congenital malformations in offspring: a review and meta-analysis of the prospective studies. Obstetrics and Gynaecology 76: 552–557

Croft P, Hannaford P C 1989 Risk factors for acute myocardial infarction in women: evidence from the Royal College of General Practitioners' oral contraception study. British Medical Journal 298: 165–168

Diczfalusy E 1982 Gregory Pincus and steroidal contraception revisited.
In: Van der Molen H J, Klopper A, Lunenfeld B, Neves e Castro M, Sciarra F, Vermeulen A (eds) Hormonal factors in fertility, infertility and contraception. Research in Steroids Vol X. pp. 75–90. Excerpta Medica, Amsterdam

Djerassi C 1979 The chemical history of the pill. In: The politics of contraception. W W Norton, New York, pp. 227–255

Guillebaud J 1987 The forgotten pill – and the paramount importance of the pill-free week. British Journal of Family Planning 12 (Suppl.) (4): 35–43

Guillebaud J 1989 Practical prescribing of the combined oral contraceptive pill.
In: Filshie M, Guillebaud J (eds) Contraception science and practice. Butterworths, London

Hannaford P C, Croft P R, Kay C R 1994 Oral Contraception and Stroke.
Evidence from the Royal College of General Practitioners' oral contraception study. Stroke 25: 935–942

Royal College of General Practitioners 1981 Oral contraception study.
Further analyses of mortality in oral contraceptive users. Lancet i: 541–546

Royal College of General Practitioners 1983 Oral contraception study. Incidence of arterial disease among oral contraceptive users. Journal of Royal College of General Practitioners 33: 75–82

Sapire K E (adapted Belfield T, Guillebaud J) 1990 Combined oral contraceptives.
Contraception and sexuality in health and disease. McGraw-Hill, London

Skouby SO 1989 Oral contraceptives in Diabetic Women. In: Sutherland H W, Stowers J M, Pearson D W M (Eds) Carbohydrate Metabolism in Pregnancy and the Newborn IV pp. 319–325 Springer–Verlag, Berlin

Stampfer M J, Willett W C, Colditz G A, Speizer F E, Hennekens C H 1988
A prospective study of past use of oral contraceptive agents and risk of cardiovascular diseases. New England Journal of Medicine 319: 1313–1317

UK National Case Control Study (Chilvers C, McPherson K, Peto J et al) 1989
Oral contraceptive use and breast cancer risk in young women. Lancet i: 973–982

Vanderbroucke J P, Koster T, Reisma P H, Bertine R M, Rosendaal F R 1994
Increased risk of venous thrombosis in oral contraception users who are carriers of factor V Leiden mutation. Lancet 344: 1453–7

Vessey M P, Smith M A, Yeates D 1986 Return of fertility after discontinuation of oral contraceptives. British Journal of Family Planning 11: 120–124

Vessey M P 1989 Oral contraception and cancer. In: Filshie M, Guillebaud J (eds) Contraception – science and practice. Butterworths, London

World Health Organization 1981 The effect of female sex hormones on fetal development and infant health: report of a WHO scientific group. Technical report series 657, WHO, Geneva

World Health Organization 1992 Oral contraceptives and neoplasia. WHO Technical Report Series 871. WHO, Geneva

4. Progestogen-only contraception

Ian Fraser

Mode of action

Effectiveness
 Progestogen-only pills
 Long-acting injectables
 Norplant
 Levonorgestrel-releasing IUD
 Other methods

Indications

Contraindications
 Absolute
 Relative

Advantages

Disadvantages

Specific attributes of each method
 Progeston-only pills
 Injectables
 Subdermal implants
 Intrauterine devices
 Vaginal rings

Controversial aspects of Depo-Provera (DMPA)
 Animal toxicology
 Cancers
 In utero and neonatal exposure
 Bone loss
 Feminist and consumer concerns

Clinical management
 Assessment
  History
  Examination
 Choice of method
 Administration
  Progestogen-only pills
  Injectables

 Subdermal implants
 Hormonal IUDs
 Vaginal rings
 Follow-up

Side-effects, complications and their management
 Disturbances of the menstual cycle
  Prolonged or frequent spotting or bleeding
  Amenorrhoea
  Post-treatment menstual disturbance
 Ovarian persistent follicles or follicular cysts
 Other side-effects
  Weight gain
  Acne
 Delay in return to fertility

Special considerations
 Adolescents
 Older women and the perimenopause
 Women with pre-existing medical disorders
  Cardiovascular system
  Breasts
  Genital tract
  Liver
  Autoimmune system
  Nervous system
  Skin
  Diabetes mellitus
  Sickle cell disease
 Drug interactions
 Future fertility and pregnancy
 Interpretation of laboratory tests
 Indications for stopping progestogen-only contraception

Conclusion

Progestogen-only methods of contraception were introduced to avoid the side-effects of oestrogen and to reduce total exposure to steroids. With modern very low-dose oestrogen–progestogen regimens these reasons have become less of an issue, but the progestogen-only approach has encouraged the development of a range of useful devices allowing very prolonged duration of action and low-dose steroid exposure, while maintaining high contraceptive efficacy.

Progestogen-only contraception has had considerable promise for many years, but has only begun to achieve its full potential in the last decade. The use of injectable contraceptives (the most widespread of the long-acting progestogen-only methods) has until very recently only accounted for 1–2% of worldwide contraceptive use, although in a few countries it has been used more extensively. A number of social concerns have been expressed by consumer and feminist groups mainly regarding lack of informed consent and 'potential for abuse'. Social issues are still relevant to all methods, but have come sharply into focus with the introduction of very long-acting methods, e.g. implants and hormonal IUDs, which require a health professional to terminate their use.

Now a variety of modern delivery systems for low and high-dose progestogens provides women wishing to use hormonal contraception with a wide choice – pills, injections, subcutaneous implants, IUDs and vaginal rings. A large number of different progestogens are marketed in different countries for various indications, but only a limited number are used in progestogen-only contraceptive methods. These include levonorgestrel, norethisterone and its derivative ethynodiol diacetate, medroxyprogesterone acetate and 3-ketodesogestrel.

Methods of delivering progestogens which are now widely available or are likely to become so in the next few years are listed in Table 4.1. Of these the progestogen-only pill (POP, minipill), depot medroxyprogesterone acetate (DMPA, Depo-Provera), norethisterone enanthate (NET-EN), Norplant and the levonorgestrel-releasing IUD are the most important. These different methods offer a range of durations of action, routes of

Table 4.1 Progestogen-only delivery systems

High dose	Low dose	Very low dose		
Injectables	*Subcutaneous implants*	*Oral*	*Vaginal rings*	*IUDs*
Monthly	Norplant	POPs	Progestogen	Levonorgestrel
2-monthly	Implanon		-only	Progesterone
3-monthly			Combined	

Table 4.2 Progestogen-only pills

Name	Progestogen	Dose	No. of pills per packet	Manufacturer
Femulen	Ethynodiol diacetate	500 μg	28	Gold Cross
Noriday	Norethisterone	350 μg	28	Syntex
Micronor	Norethisterone	350 μg	28	Cilag
Neogest	Levonorgestrel	37.5 μg*	35	Schering
Microval	Levonorgestrel	30 μg	35	Wyeth
Norgeston	Levonorgestrel	30 μg	35	Schering

* Plus 37.5 μg of inactive isomer.

administration, efficacy, menstrual effects and ease of reversibility which will have varying appeal to different individuals and couples at different times in their reproductive lives.

POPs in current use in the UK (1995) are listed in Table 4.2.

MODE OF ACTION

Progestogens have a multiplicity of actions within the human reproductive system. The importance of each action probably depends on dosage and type of progestogen. The more important actions are thought to be:

1. Local ovarian effects:
   a. Suppression of follicular growth.
   b. Inhibition of ovulation.
   c. Suppression of luteal activity.
2. Cervical mucus modification inhibiting sperm penetration.
3. Endometrial modification sufficient to prevent implantation.
4. Hypothalamic and pituitary effects to inhibit cyclical release of FSH and LH, and hence contribute to suppression of follicular development and ovulation.
5. Effects on fallopian tubal function and fertilization are probably relatively unimportant.

Very low-dose progestogen-only methods probably act mainly by interfering with cervical mucus structure and endometrial function, with less predictable effects on luteal and follicular function, while high-dose methods usually reliably suppress follicular development and ovulation (Brache et al 1990). Direct effects also occur on the ovary; the most sensitive appears to be an effect on luteal function resulting in defective progesterone secretion.

EFFECTIVENESS

Contraceptive efficacy varies greatly depending on the delivery system.

Progestogen-only pills

Maximum effectiveness depends on meticulous tablet taking and individual motivation of the woman. Efficacy is clearly related to age with failure rates (FRs) being of the order of 3 per 100 woman years (HWY) in a motivated population aged 25 to 29, but only 0.3 per HWY in women aged 40 years or over (Vessey et al 1985). Higher FRs occur when tablet taking is poor, and in some studies have been as high as 10 per HWY.

Preliminary evidence that failure is more common in women who are overweight has not been confirmed.

Efficacy is very high in lactating women.

Some studies have suggested that the rate of ectopic pregnancy might be increased compared with the normal population. This has not been confirmed. It seems likely that POPs do not decrease the risk of ectopics as much as they do intrauterine pregnancies.

Long-acting injectables

Failure rates below 0.5 per HWY for DMPA have been reported in almost all large-scale studies in a wide variety of communities (Fraser & Weisberg 1981). FRs with NET-EN are slightly higher, but are still usually less than 1 per HWY. The incidence of ectopic pregnancy is very low. Once-a-month injectables also have a very low FR of less than 0.5 per HWY.

Norplant

Excellent long-term efficacy data demonstrate that this is one of the two most effective reversible contraceptives currently marketed. Most studies have demonstrated pregnancy rates of less than 0.5 per HWY even after 5 years of use (Sivin 1988). Early data indicating somewhat lower efficacy in women over 70 kg after 3 years of use (due to reduced blood levels) appear to have been corrected by modifications to the device.

Ectopic pregnancies are rare.

Levonorgestrel-releasing IUD

Increasing large-scale evidence confirms that this device is as effective as Norplant. FRs as low as 0.1 per HWY after 5 years of use have been reported (Luukkainen 1994).

Ectopic pregnancy rates are very low.

Other methods

Data on newer methods still at clinical trial stage, but due for marketing in the near future, are more limited. New implants and injectables will probably provide high efficacy (less than 0.5 pregnancies per HWY).

Combined oestrogen–progestogen vaginal rings are likely to be highly effective, but low-dose progestogen-only rings may have somewhat lesser efficacy depending on progestogen dosage.

INDICATIONS

1. As first choice contraceptives, where the attributes of the method appeal to the woman and no contraindications exist; local regulations may need to be considered e.g. in some countries DMPA is still licensed for contraception only for those women for whom other contraceptives have proved unsuitable. In the UK, DMPA (Depo-Provera) was licensed for generalized usage in 1995.
   NET-EN is licensed in the UK for short-term use (up to 2 injections):
   a. In conjunction with rubella immunization.
   b. For the partners of men undergoing vasectomy and for postpartum women awaiting interval sterilization.
2. Where the woman expresses a wish to use hormonal contraception, but:
   a. Oestrogens are contraindicated.
   b. Oestrogens are not well tolerated.
   c. The profile of oestrogenic side-effects or complications is disliked.
3. For older women and smokers. It is well established that smokers over the age of 35 run an increased risk of cardiovascular incidents, and this is exacerbated by simultaneous use of combined oral contraceptives (Ch. 3). This risk does not appear to be enhanced by progestogen-only methods, although long-term data are not so extensive as for

combined pills. These methods can be used up to menopause, and may even ameliorate the onset of perimenopausal symptoms.

4. During lactation. Progestogen-only methods are preferable to those containing oestrogen (p. 200).
5. For women with:
   a. Diabetes mellitus (p. 115).
   b. Mild hypertension or where blood pressure is well controlled (p. 113).
   c. Homozygous sickle cell disease (p. 115).
   d. Migraine, including focal types (pp. 72–73).
6. As an alternative to COCs prior to elective major surgery (p. 69).
7. For unreliable or unwilling pill takers. The long-acting delivery systems provide excellent reassurance for this group.
8. Where there is a need for highly effective, but reversible contraception. The long-acting progestogen-only systems are the most effective yet easily reversible methods currently available.

CONTRAINDICATIONS

In many countries, regulatory authorities still insist on a lengthy list of contraindications to progestogen-only methods which more accurately reflect the risks with combined preparations. Many are precautionary, and have little epidemiological evidence to support them. However, these warnings need to be carefully considered, and if necessary, discussed with the woman.

Absolute

1. Known or suspected pregnancy, even though there is no convincing evidence of risk to the fetus or mother. Androgenic progestogens in moderate dosage, e.g. NET-EN, may carry a very small risk of masculinization of a female fetus if inadvertently given during the first 4–5 months of pregnancy.
2. Menstrual disturbance of uncertain cause, at least until this has been investigated. Most progestogen-only methods will confuse the clinical picture.
3. Any serious side-effect which is not clearly oestrogen-related, e.g. hepatic adenoma, and certain other acute or chronic liver conditions such as porphyria.

4. Current history of serious cardiovascular disease, until this has been thoroughly assessed.
5. Injectable methods should not be used in women with coagulation disorders, including long-term anticoagulation, because of the risk of haematomas at the injection site.
6. DMPA should not be used in women wishing to conceive soon after the presumed end of the 3-month contraceptive effect.

Relative

1. Those who find irregular bleeding or amenorrhoea unacceptable, especially for cultural or other social reasons.
2. Severe obesity may reduce the efficacy of systemic low-dose methods, and may sometimes be exacerbated by injectables.
3. Malignant disease of the breast. Some doctors include this as an absolute contraindication, but recent evidence suggests that those women who have had their disease adequately treated are at little or no increased risk of a recurrence with use of progestogens (p. 113). Specialist consultation is always advisable.
4. After hydatidiform mole until the urine is free of chorionic gonadotrophin (p. 114).
5. Drugs which may interact (pp. 98–99).
6. A history of recurrent functional ovarian cysts. Very low-dose methods may exacerbate these, although data are anecdotal (p. 111).
7. POPs should generally be avoided in teenagers (p. 112).
8. The immediate postpartum period. A tiny amount of progestogen is transferred into breast milk, and some clinicians advise delaying the start of this contraceptive until 6 weeks postpartum to avoid possible theoretical effects on the neonatal hypothalamus and liver. Although progestogens usually have no effect on lactation, and may even enhance it, *the occasional woman* gives a history of interference by progestogens with the milk supply during the early weeks of breast-feeding.
9. Severe hypertension should be well controlled before use of low-dose progestogens, and then carefully monitored.
10. Chronic liver conditions, such as obstetric cholestasis or cirrhosis, which may occasionally be exacerbated (p. 114).

ADVANTAGES

Non-contraceptive health benefits Apart from their high contraceptive efficacy, COCs have been shown to confer a number of substantial non-contraceptive benefits on long-term users. The evidence for similar benefits in progestogen-only users is limited, and such benefits will probably vary with dosage and route of administration.

There is *strong* evidence for a major degree of protection against endometrial cancer, especially with DMPA.

DMPA also appears to protect against the development of acute pelvic inflammatory disease and vaginal candidiasis.

All progestogen methods probably exert some benefit on dysmenorrhoea, premenstrual syndrome, Mittelschmerz (ovulation pain) and mastalgia.

Diseases for which a degree of protection is likely, but unproven, include endometriosis, uterine myomas, benign breast disease and ovarian cancer.

There are some medical conditions which are occasionally caused or exacerbated by COCs, but which progestogen-only methods do not usually influence. One of the most important of these is thromboembolic disease. Others include chloasma, hypertension, systemic lupus erythematosis and other autoimmune diseases, and migraine. Conditions for which we have limited data on long-term interactions during or after progestogen use, but where some progestogens may have an advantage include most cardiovascular diseases, obesity, cigarette smoking, contact lens use, epilepsy, non-granulomatous Crohn's disease, obstetric cholestasis, gallstones and possible immunological interactions.

Final answers on these points will require careful case-control studies once there is extensive usage of these methods in specific populations.

Breastfeeding One of the most useful advantages of progestogen-only methods over COCs is the lack of adverse effect on lactation, with no evidence of reduction in milk volume and quality and no effect on infant growth and development (p. 200).

Drug interactions A substantial number of drug interactions have been described with COC. Much less information is available for progestogens alone. For example, we have little good information about possible interactions between cigarette smoking and progestogens, but expect them to be less.

Hepatic enzyme-inducing drugs, such as rifampicin and several anti-epileptic drugs, may sometimes reduce the efficacy of low-dose progestogens such as minipills, Norplant and vaginal rings, although this appears to be less of a problem than with combined pills.

Interactions do not appear to occur with antibiotics or with sodium valproate or clonazepam. Other minor drug interactions are possible.

Tolerance   Progestogen-only methods are generally well tolerated and continuation rates are good. Subjective side-effects generally present few problems apart from menstrual disturbances, although higher dose methods such as DMPA and NET-EN can be associated with other effects.

Metabolic effects   In general, progestogens induce fewer metabolic changes than COCs. Effects on lipids (such as total serum cholesterol, HDL and LDL-cholesterol, triglycerides, free fatty acids or phospholipids) are minimal, even with DMPA and NET-EN. Minor changes in the insulin response to a glucose load may occur with higher-dose methods, but precipitation of a diabetic state must be rare. There is little or no effect on liver, thyroid, pituitary or adrenal function.

Low-dose methods do not appear to influence body weight, although high-dose methods may.

Hypertension   Development of hypertension while using progestogens is uncommon, and is usually not related to use (p. 116).

Coagulation factors   Adverse effects on all parts of the coagulation and fibrinolytic cascades appear to be minimal, and there does not appear to be any induction of a hypercoagulable state even with higher-dose methods. Thromboembolic events are not increased (Thorogood &Vessey 1990).

Compliance   This is particularly easy with the long-acting methods, but may be a problem with POPs. The requirement for daily pill-taking is frequently associated with errors in compliance, and these errors are thought to account for the majority of unplanned pregnancies in pill users.

Major surgery   Progestogens do not affect blood coagulation and the risk of thrombosis, and therefore do not need to be stopped before major surgery.

Overdosage   No harmful effects appear to result from overdosage of any method, even when POPs are taken by a child.

DISADVANTAGES

Menstrual changes   All progestogen-only contraceptive systems alter the normal menstrual pattern, but relatively little is known about the mechanism of menstrual disturbance. The changes are unpredictable, vary to some extent with method, and vary greatly between individual women. In most users, there is an increased incidence of erratic and scanty spotting or breakthrough bleeding, sometimes with prolonged episodes, and sometimes with oligo-menorrhoea or even amenorrhoea (Belsey 1988). The pattern may change with time. Heavy bleeding with progestogens is unusual, although it may sometimes occur when progestogen contraception is started in the early postpartum period (within 3 weeks of delivery).

Ovarian follicular cysts and persistent follicles   Women using low-dose progestogen methods sometimes experience temporary breast tenderness and lower abdominal discomfort associated with persisting oestradiol-secreting follicles. Symptoms may fluctuate over a period of a few weeks, but specific therapy is rarely necessary. Torsion or rupture of these cysts is uncommon. A vaginal ultrasound scan will usually demonstrate a unilocular cyst of 5–7 cm diameter. The scan can be repeated 1 to 2 months later to confirm spontaneous disappearance.

Other side-effects   High-dose methods such as DMPA may sometimes be associated with weight gain, mood symptoms and reduction in libido. These are less likely to be reported with lower-dose methods.

Acne is sometimes reported, especially with the mildly androgenic progestogens, such as levonorgestrel and norethisterone.

SPECIFIC ATTRIBUTES OF EACH METHOD

Progestogen-only pills

These have the advantage of familiarity in a pill-taking society, as well as the flexibility to allow the woman to stop and start whenever she wishes. This very flexibility is also the major disadvantage, since the low dosage of minipills means that there may be little margin for delay in taking each tablet. In some women, the effect on cervical mucus is already wearing off by 24 hours.

Injectables

The major advantage is simplicity of administration combined with prolonged action. A 3-monthly injection schedule seems to suit many women well, with shorter intervals being less convenient. The oestrogen-containing once-a-month methods may have the benefit of more regular menstrual bleeding patterns, but the inconvenience of relatively frequent injections.

Amenorrhoea becomes prominent with prolonged use of DMPA – this is seen as a major advantage by some and unacceptable by others. The effect of DMPA may take many months to wear off after the last injection, resulting in an unpredictable delay in return of fertility. The effects of NET-EN are less pronounced than DMPA. DMPA may have a small effect on the rate of loss of bone mineral over many years. This issue remains to be resolved.

All these agents may have a number of non-contraceptive health benefits.

Subdermal implants

These systems have very prolonged duration of action (2–5 years) and very high contraceptive efficacy. They require a small operation under local anaesthesia for insertion and removal. They provide very constant and low blood levels of contraceptive steroid which decline very slowly over the lifespan of the device. They can be removed when required with very rapid return of fertility.

Menstrual bleeding patterns tend to be erratic in the first few months following insertion, but become more regular with time.

Intrauterine devices

The IUD appears to be a superb route for administration of low-dose long-acting contraceptive progestogen, with delivery of a sufficiently high local dose to be a very effective contraceptive as well as greatly reducing the volume of the menstrual periods (Ch. 5).

Vaginal rings

This approach carries great promise as a convenient, constant-rate delivery system over which the woman herself has complete control. It is anticipated that over the next few years several rings will be marketed, containing either progestogens alone or combined with an oestrogen, enabling the contraceptive steroids to be delivered at high or low dose (Ch. 17).

CONTROVERSIAL ASPECTS OF DEPO-PROVERA (DMPA)

DMPA (marketed by Upjohn as Depo-Provera) has been the major focus of a number of concerns arising from different groups in society over the past three decades. Much of the controversy has arisen in the USA where DMPA was first manufactured, but where marketing approval for contraception was only given in 1992 after a lengthy saga in which political, media, and feminist agendas played a more prominent role than science or clinical medicine. These same influences have resulted in the contraceptive availability of DMPA being restricted in the UK, Australia and some other countries.

Animal toxicology

There have been a number of real concerns about the possible effects of DMPA on the body, most of which have now been dismissed or put in sensible context. These began with the difficulties of extrapolating from excessive-dose animal toxicology, where female beagles on long-term, high-dose DMPA developed increased rates of breast cancer, and rhesus monkeys on lifetime treatment were found to have developed the occasional endometrial cancer. Although these animal cancers have now been demonstrated to have no predictive value for human risk and such toxicology is no longer required by drug regulatory agencies, the stigma caused by repeated negative media publicity has persisted against DMPA.

Cancers

There are now extensive WHO epidemiological data on women who have used a variety of hormonal contraceptives. All demonstrate a very similar situation in relation to reproductive cancers (Meirik 1994).

1. DMPA provides a major degree of protection against the development of endometrial adenocarcinoma, and possibly against ovarian cancer (not yet confirmed).
2. There is no *overall increase* in the risk of breast cancer in DMPA or POP users, but a possible very small risk in long-term users.
3. Carcinoma of the cervix risks are very difficult to sort out because of multiple confounding factors, but hormonal contraception, including DMPA, may play a very small promoting role. Data from other long-acting methods will take many years to accumulate.
4. There is no evidence of an increase in risk of liver, pituitary or other tumours.

In utero and neonatal exposure

Concern was expressed at one stage that inadvertent exposure to progestogens of the fetus in utero or of the breast-fed neonate could cause adverse effects on growth and development. This has been extremely difficult to disprove, but adequate long-term data now exist to be reasonably reassuring on both these concerns.

The only uncertain issue is the possible risk of masculinization of a female fetus exposed continuously over the first 4–5 months of pregnancy to a weakly androgenic progestogen, such as NET-EN.

Bone loss

The possibility that long-term DMPA use may increase the rate of bone mineral loss (Cundy et al 1991), resulting in a slightly increased risk of osteoporosis in later life, has still to be resolved. This study has been criticized on the grounds of inadequately matched controls and its cross-sectional nature. It was suggested that the low levels of circulating oestradiol in some DMPA users may allow this bone loss, but in other situations progestogens, including MPA, usually have some bone-conserving effect. This issue will require a good longitudinal study before it can be resolved, but in the meantime it may be appropriate to check bone mineral density in the occasional long-term DMPA user who has other risk factors for osteoporosis.

Feminist and consumer concerns

As the first of the successful long-acting methods, DMPA has drawn the attention of a number of feminist and consumer groups spanning a wide spectrum of philosophies. All of the above issues have attracted public attack from some group at some time in the past. These groups still express real worries about the potential for misuse or even abuse of some methods, and they point to the difference between 'informed consent' and 'informed choice' of method.

There is a need for women to feel that they have control over their decisions, particularly in relation to technology which they do not understand. This requires the provision of simple but full information about the advantages and disadvantages of new methods, and this may include brief discussion of controversies. A willingness for dialogue on the part of feminist, consumer and media groups may be important for successful introduction of new technologies where consumer choice is involved.

CLINICAL MANAGEMENT

Assessment

Suitability for progestogen methods will be determined on history, examination and patient preference.

History

This should always include details of age, obstetric history, previous contraceptive history, current contraceptive requirements and motivation, and details of those medical conditions which might influence choice of different methods.

Examination

This should generally include the components of a regular health check, although many experts do not consider them mandatory for every progestogen-only method especially at the first visit.

1. Record weight and BP.
2. Examine breasts to exclude pathology (according to local practice).
3. Perform pelvic examination to check perineum, vagina, uterus and adnexa.
4. Take a cervical smear according to local screening policy.

Choice of method

This will usually be determined by the woman's preference for the attributes of a particular method. Motivation for a specific method is more likely to lead to correct long-term use.

There is little to choose between different POPs, and first choice is usually a matter of physician or patient preference based on familiarity rather than actual differences between pills. Change to another pill will usually be a matter of trial and error. There is no evidence that one pill is more effective than another, or that one has a different side-effect profile. Nevertheless, some women will often feel better on one particular pill or progestogen.

Choice of one of the very long-acting methods such as Norplant or the levonorgestrel-releasing IUD presupposes that the woman does not plan to become pregnant within the next 4–5 years. Removal of the device prior to this time may not be cost-effective, although a multitude of unexpected reasons may make premature removal appropriate.

Administration

This is a crucial part of the woman's first visit, and requires time and careful explanation.

Progestogen-only pills

The pill-taking regimen must be carefully explained. Patient information leaflets are not always clear, and do not replace careful one-to-one instruction. Meticulous attention to timing of daily pill-taking must be emphasized.

Pills are dispensed in bubble packs with the day of the week and direction arrows clearly marked. The number of pills per packet may vary.

Starting When the first pill is taken depends on the circumstances.

1. The first pill should be taken:
   a. When starting for the first time: on the first day of the next period.
   b. When changing from a combined pill: on the day following the last active pill in the COC packet.
   c. After pregnancy: generally 3–4 weeks after delivery. Lactation should preferably be well established, since some women notice changes in milk volume in the early weeks. POP may occasionally cause postpartum bleeding disturbances if given before 3 weeks. It is not necessary to await the return of menstruation.
   d. After termination of pregnancy: within 24 hours.
2. Further pills are taken every day thereafter without a break.

Pills should ideally be taken at the same time every day
The best time is between 4 and 10 hours before intercourse is likely to take place, when the effect on cervical mucus is maximal. However, timings between 2 and 20 hours should be reasonably safe. For most women the optimum time would be a set hour in the late afternoon or early evening, but each woman will need to work out the preferable time for herself. For the 40% of women who continue to ovulate apparently normally while taking POPs, these considerations of timing may be very important.

Extra contraceptive precautions These are recommended for 7 days in the following circumstances:

1. If the pill is taken more than 3 hours late.

2. If a pill is forgotten. The missed pill should be taken as soon as
   the mistake is recognized, and the regular pill for the next day
   at the usual time.
3. If vomiting occurs within 3 hours of pill taking, another tablet
   should be taken. If this pill is also vomited additional
   contraceptive precautions should be used during the upset and
   for 7 days after symptoms have subsided.
4. If an attack of severe diarrhoea occurs, the pill may not be
   completely absorbed. Extra contraceptive precautions and
   normal pill taking should be continued through the upset and
   for 7 days afterwards.
5. Extra precautions may be needed to cover short-term drug
   interactions (pp. 98–99).

Postcoital contraception   This should be considered if two or
more POPs have been missed and intercourse has already taken
place. POP use should be resumed 1 day after postcoital contraceptive use, and follow-up planned to exclude pregnancy.

When transferring from POP to COC   The first new active
pill should be taken on the day after stopping POP, and should
usually begin during menstruation (unless the woman has lactational
or other amenorrhoea).

Injectables

Only DMPA and NET-EN will be considered here, because other
injectables have very limited availability in most parts of the world.

Deep intramuscular injections are given into the gluteal region
(or occasionally into the deltoid, especially in the very obese). The
injection site should not be massaged, since this sometimes dissi-
pates the depot resulting in higher initial blood levels and shortened
duration of action.

The recommended dosage of DMPA is 150 mg and of NET-EN
is 200 mg.

1. The DMPA vial should be shaken well before loading the
   syringe; new administration procedures include preloaded
   syringes in some countries.
2. The NET-EN vial should be warmed close to body
   temperature.
3. The first injection must be given within the first 5 days of the
   menstrual cycle.
4. Subsequent injections should be given according to a schedule
   marked on a calendar for the patient; DMPA is usually given

every 90±7 days, while the optimal NET-EN schedule is more complicated. For the first 6 months NET-EN should be given once every 60±5 days, and then at 84±7 day intervals to maximize efficacy and minimize side-effects.

5. DMPA has a much greater safety margin for delay in the next injection than NET-EN, and can be left with reasonable confidence up to 16 weeks. Longer intervals may still be quite safe, but patients need to be advised about a possible small increased risk of contraceptive failure. For medico-legal reasons it is wiser to do a pregnancy test if the interval is prolonged beyond 12 weeks.

Subdermal implants

Norplant is a six-capsule system, but newer systems will only consist of one or two rods or capsules. Health professionals need to be carefully trained in the techniques of insertion and removal (WHO 1990), and users need to be given thorough counselling and written information prior to insertion.

Authorities in most countries where Norplant has been marketed have developed formal training programmes with certification of competence to ensure that this high technology method is used optimally.

Insertion   This is carried out using standard sterile precautions and local anaesthesia (LA) through a 3–5 mm incision made with a fine point scalpel in the skin of the inner aspect of the upper arm (Fig. 4.1). The capsules are inserted one at a time through a purpose-designed trocar in a fan shape immediately under the

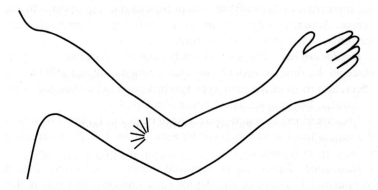

Fig 4.1   Norplant insertion.

dermis, so that they can be palpated easily but not seen. Insertion usually takes 10–15 minutes. Different insertion techniques are likely to be developed for newer systems.

Removal   This is also carried out with sterile precautions and LA through a 3–5 mm incision at the site of original insertion. Removal is usually very straightforward if the capsules have been inserted correctly in the first place. Each capsule is palpated and manipulated in turn so that the lower end protrudes at the incision. The tip is grasped with forceps, the thin overlying fibrous sheath is split with a second pair of forceps and the Norplant capsule withdrawn. Several variations on the removal technique have been developed. Occasionally removal may be very difficult, and this usually occurs because of an incorrect insertion technique.

Removal and insertion of a new set of implants should be planned for approximately 5 years after the original insertion. A reminder system should be clearly developed for the woman and for the clinic, and should be reinforced at annual visits. It seems probable that there will be a substantial safety margin for delay in next insertion.

Hormonal IUDs

Insertion and removal techniques for these devices do not differ from related copper-containing devices.

Vaginal rings

One of the major advantages of these devices is that the woman herself has control of insertion and removal. However, careful instruction in insertion and removal is essential for correct use.

Initial insertion   This should occur within the first 3 days of the menstrual cycle, with placement high in the vagina close to the cervix. Actual position of the device will depend on individual anatomy, shape and size of the ring.

Replacement   Progestogen-only rings are designed to stay in place all the time, in order to provide a long-acting minipill type of effect, and most of the prototype systems need to be changed every 3 months. 1-year systems are being developed.

Combination oestrogen–progestogen rings are designed to stay in the vagina for 3 weeks followed by removal for 1 week, to mimic a COC-type of regimen.

Removal   Rings can be removed before sexual intercourse if the partner is aware of the device (uncommon), but this is not recommended because the need for reinsertion within 2 hours may be overlooked. Removal of the ring for more than 2 hours may be followed by breakthrough bleeding and perhaps an increased risk of pregnancy.

Follow-up

In general, the woman should be seen for the first visit at a suitable time, which depends on the particular method. At that time, BP should be checked. Routine weighing is unnecessary. All women should be advised to return *at any time* if they perceive a possible problem related to their contraception.

POPs   The first visit should be planned for 3 months with annual follow-up thereafter.

DMPA   Regular visits should be planned at 12-week intervals for repeat injections, and reinforcement of counselling support about menstrual changes. Regular weighing may be useful to reinforce advice about diet and exercise.

NET-EN   Regular visits should be planned at 8-weekly intervals for the first 6 months and then 12-weekly for repeat injections and menstrual advice. Weighing is less likely to be needed than for DMPA users.

Norplant   The first visit should be scheduled for 3 months for general review and advice about menstrual patterns, and annually thereafter.

Levonorgestrel IUD   The first visit should be scheduled for 3 months for general review and advice about menstrual patterns, and annually thereafter.

SIDE EFFECTS, COMPLICATIONS AND THEIR MANAGEMENT

Disturbances of the menstrual cycle

Prolonged or frequent spotting or bleeding

These symptoms are common accompaniments of progestogen therapy particularly in the first few months of use, and are a major cause of premature discontinuation.

Pathological causes should be kept in mind, especially in older women. Pelvic infection (especially chlamydia) and surface lesions of the genital tract (including cervical ectopy, cervical or endometrial polyps, submucous fibroids and cervical or endometrial cancer) should be considered. The risk of endometrial cancer is reduced by most, if not all, progestogen methods.

If the risk of intrauterine pathology is felt to be significant, a careful transvaginal ultrasound scan will exclude thickened 'endometrium' due to polyps or cancer. A hysteroscopy and endometrial biopsy will give even more precise information about possible intrauterine and endocervical pathology. It must be borne in mind that these causes of abnormal bleeding in progestogen users are very uncommon compared with the breakthrough bleeding and spotting associated with the methods themselves.

Treatment Treating progestogen-associated breakthrough bleeding can be difficult. There is limited evidence to confirm that a 3-week course of oral oestrogen (ethinyloestradiol 50μg daily or, probably, a course of COC) will stop an episode of prolonged bleeding and perhaps improve the long-term menstrual pattern in Norplant users (Diaz et al 1990). The same effect will probably apply with other methods. Oestrogen should not be given to women using very low-dose methods such as POPs, because it may counteract the contraceptive effect of the progestogen on cervical mucus.

Amenorrhoea

This is common with DMPA and NET-EN, but can also occur with all other methods. Pregnancy may need to be excluded, although it is uncommon with the long-acting methods: if in doubt, a pregnancy test should be carried out. Prolonged amenorrhoea with progestogens is not known to be harmful, and many women find it highly acceptable. For those who feel that amenorrhoea is unnatural, a reasonable analogy can be drawn with lactational amenorrhoea.

Pre-treatment counselling about the range of possible menstrual changes, including amenorrhoea, is important with all progestogen-only methods.

Post-treatment menstrual disturbance

Once the effect of the progestogen itself has worn off, menstrual disturbance following any of these methods is uncommon. DMPA users may find that the depot preparation continues to work for many months after the last injection (p. 112), but once the progestogen has been cleared from the body the menstrual cycle usually returns to its previous pattern. Continuing menstrual disturbances should be investigated in the same way as in women who have never used these methods.

Ovarian persistent follicles or follicular cysts

Usually, no active treatment is required but rarely, if pain is persistent or severe, transvaginal drainage under ultrasound guidance can be considered. In older women, it is essential to ensure that more serious ovarian pathology is not present.

Other side-effects

Headaches, dizziness, nausea, mood changes, abdominal bloating, breast tenderness or a number of vague symptoms may be reported with any progestogen-only method. These usually subside within the first few months. If they do not, a different POP may be tried.

No simple guidelines exist for management of these symptoms with long-acting methods, but temporary symptomatic treatment and counselling may be remarkably effective in allowing continuation of a method which is otherwise highly suitable for the woman. If symptoms are persistent and troublesome the method may need to be terminated. With DMPA and NET-EN the woman will need to wait until the progestogen is completely out of the system, which may take many weeks, but it is surprising how infrequently this lack of flexibility causes real problems.

Weight gain

This is rarely caused by *low-dose* progestogens, but may be a problem for a minority of DMPA and NET-EN users. A small gain of 1–2 kg often stabilizes during continued use, but a very small number of women continue to gain moderate amounts of weight as long as they use the method. The main mechanism appears to be an increase in appetite with laying down of increased fat stores, but a small anabolic effect can occur.

Strict dieting and an exercise programme will help, but many women find this difficult to pursue in the long-term. The weight gain is not due to 'fluid retention' and diuretics do not help.

Acne

Acne can sometimes be caused or exacerbated by the slightly androgenic progestogens such as levonorgestrel or NET. Good skin care will usually carry the woman through a period of adjustment to the new method, although the rare user may need to discontinue.

Delay in return of fertility

This is only a problem for DMPA users, who may experience a prolonged period of waiting for normal ovulation to return. The delay is due to persistence of medroxyprogesterone acetate (MPA) in the circulation, because microcrystals in the injected depot may sometimes dissolve very slowly. The average delay in return of fertility is 7–8 months beyond the calculated 3–4 month effect of the last injection. This means that some women will take well over a year to conceive. There is no evidence that DMPA causes permanent sterility. NET-EN causes a very small delay, but the other methods are not known to have any lasting effect following the last dose or following removal.

SPECIAL CONSIDERATIONS

Adolescents

While the compliance necessary for POP use probably precludes this method for many teenagers, some may find long-acting methods such as Norplant and DMPA to be highly acceptable (Ch. 2).

Older women and the perimenopause

Progestogen-only methods of all types may be very suitable for older women (Ch. 16).

Women with pre-existing medical disorders

Progestogen-only methods may be the best choice for many such women, although patient information leaflets often still provide a counsel of excessive caution against their use. It is also essential to weigh up the risks of unplanned pregnancy in women with these conditions, while balancing the small uncertainties about long-term progestogen use.

Women with pre-existing medical conditions must be given reasonable information about the advantages and disadvantages of the relevant contraceptive choices in the light of their own particular condition, bearing in mind that there will always be a small degree of uncertainty about how a method will affect any individual.

Cardiovascular system

1. A history of superficial or deep thromboembolism does not appear to be a contraindication to the use of any progestogen-only method. Pregnancy may be a significant risk for these women.
2. Myocardial infarction or stroke are not thought to be contraindications to progestogen use, although extensive data do not exist. Low-dose methods are probably preferable, because they allow secretion of endogenous ovarian oestradiol which is important for normal vascular endothelial cell function and protection against further cardiovascular episodes. Norplant is a satisfactory choice in these circumstances because of its very high contraceptive efficacy.
3. Hypertension:
   a. Mild hypertension or where BP is well controlled. Progestogen-only methods are generally suitable, and the low-dose methods are preferable. BP control should be kept under regular review.
   b. Moderate or severe hypertension. Low-dose progestogens may be prescribed under careful supervision. It may be sensible to begin with a method which can easily be stopped if the woman experiences a significant rise in BP attributable to the method. This risk appears to be small.
   It is uncertain whether long-term progestogen use interacts adversely with severe hypertension on the risk of cardiovascular disease.

Breasts

1. Benign breast disease may improve with progestogens, although the response is variable.
2. Women with breast cancer should probably avoid use of progestogen-only methods, unless alternatives are unsuitable. It is possible that a small proportion of breast cancers in young women may be stimulated by progestogen exposure, although others may even be inhibited. Data on these effects are, as yet, limited.

Genital tract

1. Women with pre-existing endometriosis, adenomyosis or uterine myomas may benefit from progestogen-only contraception compared with COCs.

Endometriosis is most likely to benefit from high dose treatment.

Adenomyosis often continues to cause symptoms of erratic and painful bleeding, but in some patients will improve.

Myomas may continue to grow, but some will stabilize in size and symptoms may reduce.

2. Malignant diseases of the genital tract are not contraindications to progestogen use. It is usually recommended that hormonal contraceptives are avoided in women who have had a hydatidiform mole until β-hCG levels have returned to zero, and in women with choriocarcinoma until cure is confirmed. High-dose progestogens like DMPA and NET-EN may be contraceptives of choice in women with a history of endometrial hyperplasia or adenocarcinoma.

Liver

1. Women with a previous history of hepatic adenoma should not use steroid contraception of any kind, although the risk of recurrence with low-dose progestogens must be very small.
2. Severe active hepatitis could be exacerbated by progestogens, as may poor hepatic function in chronic cirrhosis. If progestogens are to be used in women with any degree of liver failure low-dose preparations should be chosen, and liver function monitored.
3. Previous hepatitis with normal liver function is not a contraindication.
4. Porphyria is usually felt to be a contraindication to the use of any hormonal contraceptive.
5. There is no evidence that gallstones are exacerbated or precipitated by progestogen-only methods, but data are limited.
6. Obstetric cholestasis is less likely to recur with low-dose progestogens than with COCs.

Autoimmune system

Exacerbations of autoimmune diseases, such as systemic lupus erythematosis, are not usually increased during progestogen-only contraceptive use, although progress of the condition should be monitored carefully during the first few months of use of any new medication.

Nervous system

1. Focal migraine (with unilateral neurological signs) is another phenomenon which is often exacerbated by oestrogen, but rarely by progestogen. Therefore, low-dose progestogens may be suitable contraceptives for these women.
2. Epilepsy is rarely exacerbated by progestogens, but higher-dose progestogens should generally be used because of occasional drug interactions which may reduce the contraceptive efficacy of the lower-dose preparations (see above).

Skin

Chloasma is an oestrogen-stimulated phenomenon and will usually fade steadily during progestogen use. These women should be advised to wear hats and use 'block-out' sunscreens when exposed to direct sunlight for any length of time.

Diabetes mellitus

Low-dose progestogen-only methods do not appear to make the management of diabetes more difficult or increase risk of complications. Injectables may alter the dosage requirements for diabetic control, but there is no evidence of increase in complications.

Sickle cell disease

There is good evidence that DMPA will improve the haematological picture and reduce the incidence of painful sickling crises, and this may be the contraceptive of choice for them (DeCeulaer et al 1982). Other progestogens may provide acceptable alternatives, while oestrogen should be avoided.

There are no data on other haemoglobinopathies, or other progestogens in sickle-cell disease.

Drug interactions

These are less of a problem for progestogen users than COC users, although women using low-dose methods such as POPs, implants or vaginal rings may run some risk with certain drugs (pp. 98–99). Higher-dose methods, such as DMPA or NET-EN, are preferable in women using rifampicin or most anti-epileptic drugs.

If doctors are suspicious that an interaction is occurring between progestogen contraceptives and any other drug, they should notify the Committee on Safety of Medicines on the appropriate yellow card.

Future fertility and pregnancy

There is no evidence to suggest that any progestogen method causes infertility following the end of expected contraceptive effect. It must be remembered that 10–15% of all couples will consult a doctor at some time about difficulty in conceiving, and several studies have indicated that this rate does not appear to be increased after hormonal contraception.

Before starting DMPA, potential users must be warned that there may be a temporary delay in return of fertility beyond the normal duration of effective action of the drug (p. 112).

There is no evidence that women who become pregnant immediately after stopping a progestogen method are at increased risk of fetal abnormality, and there is no justification for advising any delay before attempting to conceive.

Occasionally, a woman may inadvertently continue with use of her hormonal contraceptive after conceiving. There is no evidence of a significant increase in risk of birth defects in these women.

Interpretation of laboratory tests

Progestogen-only methods have little or no effect on common biochemical tests.

Indications for stopping progestogen-only contraception

There are few medical indications for stopping progestogen-only methods. These include:

1. Confirmed pregnancy when the woman does not wish to consider termination.
2. Acute liver disease.
3. Significant and maintained increase in BP which requires treatment.
4. Side-effects which are unacceptable to the patient.
5. When another pregnancy is desired.
6. When contraception is no longer required. With very long-acting methods, such as implants or IUD, the woman

may wish to leave her system in place in case of future requirement for contraception.
7. When menopause is reached (Ch. 16).

CONCLUSION

In many countries, progestogen-only methods have not yet gained the popularity that might have been expected, and this applies particularly to minipills. These pills have not been widely promoted by manufacturers, but deserve more widespread use, especially in older age groups. The resolution of several controversies, the introduction of new delivery systems and increasing community awareness will undoubtedly lead to a steady increase in usage. With this increased use will come many more questions about side-effects, and especially about the management of menstrual bleeding disturbances. The provision of clear and simple information at the time of starting, with reinforcement at follow-up has been shown to lead to high rates of satisfaction and excellent continuation rates of use with all these methods.

REFERENCES

Belsey E, Task Force on Long-Acting Systemic Agents for Fertility Regulation 1988 Vaginal bleeding patterns among women using one natural and eight hormonal methods of contraception. Contraception 38: 181–206

Brache V, Alvarez-Sanchez F, Faundes A, Tejada A S, Cochon L 1990 Ovarian endocrine function through five years of continuous treatment with Norplant subdermal implants. Contraception 41: 169–177

Cundy T, Evans M, Roberts H, Wattie D, Ames R, Reid I R. 1991 Bone density in women receiving depot medroxyprogesterone acetate for contraception. British Medical Journal 303: 13–16

DeCeulaer K, Gruber C, Hayes R, Serjeant G R 1982 Medroxyprogesterone acetate and homozygous sickle cell disease. Lancet 1: 229–231

Diaz S, Croxatto H B, Pavez M, Belhadj H, Stern J, Sivin I 1990 Clinical assessment of treatments for prolonged bleeding in users of Norplant implants. Contraception 42: 97–109

Fraser I S, Weisberg E 1981 A comprehensive review of injectable contraception with special emphasis on depot medroxyprogesterone acetate. The Medical Journal of Australia Jan. 24, 1 (Suppl 1): 1–19

Luukkainen T 1994 Progestin-releasing intrauterine contraceptive device. In: Bardin C W, Mishell D R (eds) Proceedings from the fourth International Conference on IUDs. Butterworth-Heinemann, Boston, pp. 32–41

Meirik O 1994 Updating DMPA safety. Preface to an issue on DMPA and Cancer. Contraception 49 pp. 185–188

Sivin I 1988 International experience with Norplant and Norplant-II contraceptives. Studies in Family Planning 19: 81–94

Thorogood M, Vessey M P 1990 An epidemiological survey of cardiovascular disease in women taking oral contraceptives. American Journal of Obstetrics and Gynaecology 163: 274–281

Vessey M P, Lawless M, Yeates D, McPherson K 1985 Progestogen-only oral contraception. Findings in a large prospective study with special reference to effectiveness. British Journal of Family Planning 10: 117–121

World Health Organization 1990 Norplant contraceptive subdermal implants: managerial and technical guidelines. WHO, Geneva

5. Intrauterine contraceptive devices

James Drife

Historical aspects

Types of IUD
Inert (non-medicated) devices
Copper-bearing devices
Flexible devices
Medicated devices

Mode of action

Effectiveness

Advantages

Disadvantages

Indications

Contraindications
Absolute
Relative
Debatable

Clinical Management
Assessment
History
Examination
Choice of IUD
Insertion
Timing of insertion

General advice about technique
Problems at insertion
Resuscitation measures in IUD clinics
Instructions to patients
Follow-up
Removal
Technique

Complications and their management
Abnormal bleeding
Pain
Vaginal discharge
Pelvic infection
Diagnosis
Management
Pregnancy
Intrauterine pregnancy
Extrauterine or ectopic pregnancy

Lost threads and lost devices
Lost threads
Expulsion of an IUD
Complete expulsion
Partial expulsion
The lost IUD
Displaced IUD within the uterine cavity

Future prospects

More than most methods of contraception, the intrauterine contraceptive device (IUD) is the subject of myth and prejudice. Recent studies have shown that the IUD does not cause pelvic inflammatory disease, ectopic pregnancy or infertility, that it acts by preventing fertilization and that some IUDs can be used to treat menorrhagia. Nevertheless, public perceptions lag well behind these research findings.

HISTORICAL ASPECTS

The first IUD, a ring of silkworm gut, was described in 1909. Graefenberg in 1931 and Ota in 1934 described metal devices, but large-scale studies were not published until 1959. In 1960 the plastic IUD was introduced and in 1962 came the Lippes Loop, the first to include a tail to facilitate removal. Flexible Silastic IUDs were introduced in the 1960s, followed in the 1970s by copper-bearing devices. In the 1980s hormone-releasing IUDs were developed. Worldwide, the IUD is now the second most common, reliable, reversible method of contraception: only the pill is more popular. IUDs are used by over 80 million women, mainly in China, where 29% of married women of reproductive age use them. Similarly high levels of use are found in Norway and Finland. In the UK they are used by about 7% of women and in the USA by an even lower proportion (Bromham 1993).

TYPES OF IUD

IUDs fall into three categories: inert, copper-bearing and medicated. All IUDs used in the UK have one or two threads attached. Thread colours have changed over the years and are therefore not helpful in identifying the device.

Inert (non-medicated) devices

Ring devices made of stainless steel are used mainly in China.

In the UK, inert IUDs had various 'open' designs and were made of Silastic, usually with barium sulphate to make them radio-opaque. The Lippes Loop was the most widely used. No inert IUDs are now marketed in the UK.

Copper-bearing devices

All IUDs currently available in the UK contain copper, which increases contraceptive efficacy and allows the devices to be smaller and easier to fit (Fig. 5.1). All have monofilament threads. The surface area of the copper determines the active life of the device.

The manufacturers recommend replacement at different intervals which may vary from country to country. Clinical trials have shown that for several devices the lifespan exceeds the recommendations and it is now generally accepted that all modern copper-bearing IUDs may be left in situ for 5 years (Bromham 1993). The Ortho-Gyne T 380 S device has been approved for up to 8 years continuous use. Even these lifespans are probably conservative.

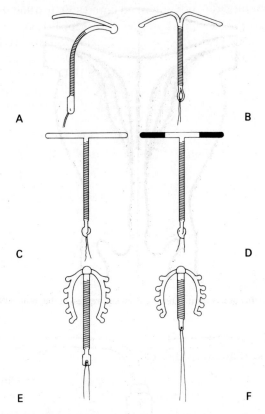

Fig. 5.1 Copper-bearing IUDs: **A**. Gravigard (Cu7) – no longer marketed in UK (1990); **B**. Novagard Nova-T; **C**. Ortho-Gyne T; **D**. Ortho-Gyne T 380 S; **E**. Multiload Cu 250; **F**. Multiload Cu 250 Short.

Flexible devices

The next logical step was to take away the Silastic frame, leaving only the copper. The Cu-Fix or Flexigard (GyneFix) has six copper sleeves threaded on a prolene filament (Fig. 5.2). A knot at one end of the filament is pushed into the myometrium with an introducer. The device can be left in place for 5 years and removal is apparently not a problem.

Pregnancy and expulsion rates are less than 1% per year (Wildemeersch et al 1994).

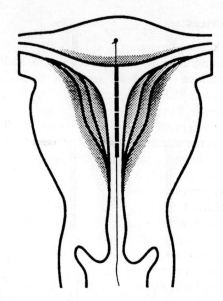

Fig. 5.2 GyneFix at insertion. The line drawings represent different cavity shapes.

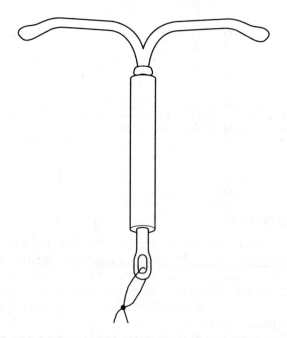

Fig. 5.3 The levonorgestrel IUD. 20 µg of levonorgestrel is released from the Silastic sleeve around the stem of a Nova-T plastic frame.

Medicated devices

Some IUDs contain a progestogen which is slowly released into the uterus, increasing contraceptive effectiveness and diminishing menstrual blood loss. (It has been suggested that such IUDs could be the ideal way to deliver progestogens to the endometrium in women who require 'opposed' hormone replacement therapy.)

A device releasing progesterone – the Progestasert – was marketed in the UK but its use was discontinued because of concern about an increased risk of ectopic pregnancy. It is still available in the USA, and indeed for a time was the only IUD marketed there.

The levonorgestrel IUD (Fig. 5.3) was developed in Finland and consists of a Nova-T frame carrying a silastic sheath impregnated with levonorgestrel, which is released at the rate of 20 µg/day. It can be left in place for up to 5 years. Pregnancy rates as low as 0.2% have been reported, with no increase in the rate of ectopic pregnancy. Fertility returns immediately after the device is removed.

This device markedly reduces menstrual flow and dysmenorrhoea and is an effective treatment for menorrhagia (Fig. 5.4). It has also

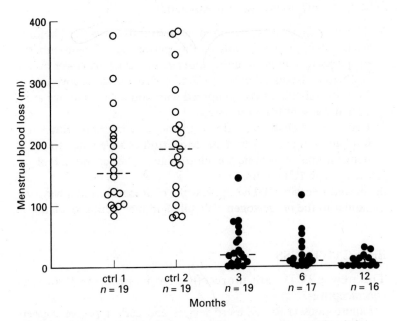

Fig. 5.4 Menstrual blood loss in menorrhagic women at two control periods (ctrl) before levonorgestrel IUD insertion and after 3, 6 and 12 months of use. All individual values are indicated, and median values are marked (from Anderson & Rybo 1990).

been reported to have a lower incidence of pelvic infection than the copper-bearing IUD, particularly in women under the age of 25. This may be due to the effect of progestogen on cervical mucus, menstrual loss or endometrial thickness. It can cause amenorrhoea or spotting and this worries some women. Removal rates for these problems are about 7% and users should be counselled about the change in bleeding pattern (Luukkainen 1993).

The levonorgestrel IUD is a potentially important advance in providing effective contraception along with another health benefit – reduction in menorrhagia. It was licensed in the UK in 1995 under the trade name Mirena.

MODE OF ACTION

All IUDs cause a foreign-body reaction in the endometrium, with increased numbers of leucocytes. This reaction is enhanced by copper, which affects endometrial enzymes, glycogen metabolism and oestrogen uptake and may inhibit sperm transport. Uterine and tubal fluids are altered and this impairs the viability of the gametes. IUDs probably do not affect tubal motility.

1. The main antifertility action of modern IUDs is exerted before fertilization, predominantly on the spermatozoa. The numbers of spermatozoa reaching the upper genital tract are fewer in IUD users. Reduced numbers of fertilized ova are recovered from the fallopian tube compared with non-users, and ova are virtually absent from the uterus.
2. Endometrial changes produced by the IUD interfere with implantation at an early stage. Most studies have failed to detect human chorionic gonadotrophin in the second half of the cycle in IUD users.
3. Steroid-releasing IUDs suppress the endometrium in a way similar to the progestogen-only pill, and may inhibit ovulation.

EFFECTIVENESS

The newer IUDs are more effective in practice than oral contraceptives.

Failure rates (FRs) of inert devices and early types of copper-containing IUDs were above 2 per 100 women at one year of use.

FRs of the Nova-T and Multiload 250 are between 1 and 2 per 100 users at one year.

The newer devices with larger surface areas of copper, such as the TCu-380, have FRs of less than 1 per 100 at 1 year.

The levonorgestrel IUD has a FR less than 1 per 100 women at 5 years of use.

Effect of duration of use

After the first year of use the annual FR of most modern devices is less than 1 per 100 woman years (HWY). For all devices, the rates of pregnancy and removal for bleeding tend to fall slowly with time after insertion; the expulsion rate falls dramatically with time. Data from the Oxford/FPA study show a noticeable decline in failure rates with increasing age and duration of use.

ADVANTAGES

1. IUDs are becoming increasingly effective and have very low failure rates (see above).
2. With the IUD, repeated action by the user, either daily or at the time of coitus, is not required.
3. The rapid return of fertility after IUD removal contrasts with the less predictable restoration of fertility after injectable contraception is discontinued. The modern IUD can be described as the most effective, rapidly reversible form of contraception.
4. Inert devices can be left in place until menstruation ceases; copper devices or the levonorgestrel IUD, for 5 years. During that time, visits for medical check-ups are infrequent.
5. The levonorgestrel IUD reduces menstrual loss, anaemia and the risk of pelvic infection. Nova-T mirena
6. More than 70% of users have few or no side-effects. There is no evidence of increased rates of cervical cancer or dysplasia or any other malignancy in IUD users. The risk of infection and other complications will be minimized by careful selection and counselling of patients. Expert fitting and understanding follow-up will contribute greatly to successful long-term use.

DISADVANTAGES

1. Unlike hormonal contraceptives, most IUDs (apart from the levonorgestrel IUD) confer no positive health benefits apart from preventing pregnancy.

2. The main disadvantage of the IUD is that for a woman with multiple partners, it increases the risk of pelvic infection.
3. Menstrual irregularities, menorrhagia, vaginal discharge and lower abdominal pain are often little more than a nuisance, although if they persist they may lead to a request for removal of the device (pp. 134–137).
4. Pelvic infection and pregnancy require careful assessment and management (pp. 137–140).

INDICATIONS

The IUD is a reasonable first choice of contraceptive for a mutually monogamous couple, even if the woman is nulliparous. It is particularly appropriate for women who are not good at remembering to take pills regularly and for those who see their partner sporadically.

The levonorgestrel IUD may be indicated for women with menorrhagia.

CONTRAINDICATIONS

Absolute

1. Known or suspected pregnancy.
2. Undiagnosed abnormal vaginal bleeding. Once malignancy or other uterine pathology is excluded and menstruation returns to normal, an IUD can be fitted.
3. Suspected malignancy of the genital tract. Appropriate gynaecological investigation should be instituted without delay. After local therapy for early lesions of the cervix (cervical intraepithelial neoplasia (CIN), carcinoma in situ) an IUD can be fitted.
4. Active pelvic inflammatory disease (PID). Fitting an IUD will increase the severity of the infection.
5. Copper allergy (rare) or Wilson's disease – for copper devices only.

Relative

1. Previous ectopic pregnancy. Although the new IUDs do not increase the risk of ectopic pregnancy, some authorities would regard an ectopic as an absolute contraindication if a woman has never had a successful pregnancy.

2. Cervical or vaginal infection. After successful treatment an IUD can be inserted. Ectropion (erosion) of the cervix is not a contraindication.
3. Uterine fibroids. Provided they are not large and periods are not excessively heavy, an IUD can be used. Yearly pelvic examination is necessary to assess any change in the size of the fibroids.
4. Abnormality of the uterine cavity. The shape of the uterine cavity may be distorted and necessitate modification of the IUD before fitting, e.g. shortening of the transverse arm. With a double uterus two IUDs need to be fitted.
5. A recent history of treated pelvic infection. A single episode of confirmed PID adequately treated is not a contraindication to IUD use provided it has not occurred within the previous 6 months. However, several attacks, confirmed or otherwise, must be viewed with suspicion and alternative methods of contraception advised. Some authorities regard an episode of sexually transmissible disease in the previous 12 months as an absolute contraindication to IUD insertion in nulliparous women.
6. Uterine scars from surgery other than caesarean section.
7. Menorrhagia. This is a relative contraindication to most devices but an indication for the levonorgestrel IUD.
8. Anaemia. The comments in the previous paragraph apply.
9. Valvular heart disease. There is a risk of sub-acute bacterial endocarditis. Appropriate antibiotic cover at the time of insertion should be given to patients with a prosthetic valve if the decision is made to use an IUD.
10. Multiple sexual partners. Although the IUD does not cause infection in a monogamous couple it can exacerbate PID caused by sexually transmissible disease. In a woman with multiple sexual partners the risks of PID and possible impairment of future fertility have to be weighed against her inability or unwillingness to use another method.
11. Youth and nulliparity. In general, younger women are at higher risk of pelvic infection than older women, due to higher levels of sexual activity and more sexual partners. The same comments apply as in the previous paragraph. Nulliparity in a woman with no other risk factors is not a contraindication to the IUD.
12. Systemic corticosteroid treatment, immunosuppressive therapy and HIV infection. These affect the immune system thereby increasing the risk of infection (Ch. 14).

Debatable

The suggestion that IUDs have a higher failure rate in women with insulin-dependent diabetes has not been confirmed, and the IUD is an acceptable method of contraception for this group (Mestman & Schmidt-Sarosi 1993).

There is some evidence that the risk of uterine perforation at insertion is greater in women who are breastfeeding, but a recent study of the Copper T-380A showed no uterine perforations, fewer insertion-related problems and lower removal rates among breast-feeding than non-lactating women. IUDs are particularly suitable for lactating women since they do not affect milk production, but *particular care is required with insertion* (Chi 1993).

CLINICAL MANAGEMENT

Assessment

Suitability for an IUD is based on history and examination.

History

Take a history, particularly in relation to the need to avoid preg-nancy, past use of contraceptives, the acceptability of the method to the patient, and those conditions – such as pelvic infection – which might contraindicate its use. Only after full discussion of the possible risks and benefits should an IUD be fitted.

Examination

1. Perform a pelvic examination to determine the size, shape and position of the uterus and to confirm that the appendages are normal.
2. Examine the vagina and cervix with a speculum to exclude abnormality and infection.
3. Take a cervical smear and examine the breasts, if indicated by clinic or practice screening policy for women in the age group
4. Record the blood pressure (BP) if the woman is over 40 and has not had a normal reading in the previous 3 years.

Choice of IUD

There are no firm rules for selecting the right IUD for an individual patient. Smaller devices, e.g. Novagard or Nova-T, are better suited to the nulliparous uterus. The woman's previous experience with IUDs may determine the choice; e.g. unexplained expulsion of a small device – try a larger one (and vice versa). Problems with a current IUD may dictate a change; e.g. menorrhagia or pain – change to a smaller device.

Insertion

Instruments needed for insertion:

Light source
Bivalve speculum
Bacteriological swabs (when appropriate)
Kidney dish (receptacle for insertion instruments)
10-inch sponge-holding forceps
Pair of scissors, Sims curved on flat, 8-inch blunt-ended
Malleable uterine sound graduated in centimetres
12-inch tissue forceps or single-toothed tenaculum with blunted tips.

Timing of insertion

Stage of the cycle   An IUD may be inserted at any time during the menstrual cycle, but this should not be done later than day 19 of a 28-day cycle unless the possibility of pregnancy can be confidently excluded.

Insertion during or shortly after a menstrual period has conventionally been recommended for the following reasons: pregnancy is unlikely; the cervix is softer and the os open, making insertion easier; post-insertion discomfort is less and bleeding is not noticed.

After unprotected intercourse   An IUD may be used as a postcoital contraceptive (Ch. 9).   up to 5days.

After delivery   IUD insertion immediately after delivery is associated with unacceptable expulsion rates, though rates of perforation, bleeding or infection are not increased. The expulsion rate is lower 8 weeks after delivery. Lactation may increase the risk of perforation but does not increase the risk of expulsion.

After therapeutic abortion   There is no evidence of increased rates of failure, expulsion or removal when an IUD is inserted immediately after termination of first trimester pregnancy. However, expulsion rates are higher after second trimester termination.

After spontaneous miscarriage IUD insertion after miscarriage is not associated with higher risk of complications. If not inserted immediately, wait for 2 weeks after therapeutic abortion or miscarriage.

General advice about technique

As the method of insertion is different for each device, *insertion is safest if the manufacturer's instructions are followed meticulously.*

1. Throughout the whole procedure a no-touch technique is employed so that only clean gloves need be worn. However, if manipulation of the sterile IUD in its holder is needed then sterile gloves should be worn.
2. Following bimanual examination of the pelvis, the cervix is exposed with a speculum while the patient lies in a modified lithotomy position. The left lateral position may be preferred.
3. The cervix is cleansed with antiseptic solution and grasped with 12-inch atraumatic forceps (Allis's forceps are often used). This stabilizes the cervix, and gentle traction straightens the uterocervical canal, allowing controlled IUD insertion while helping to achieve correct fundal placement.
4. A fine uterine sound is passed gently to determine the depth and direction of the uterine cavity and the direction and patency of the cervical canal.
5. The device is loaded into the introducer in such a way that it will lie flat in the transverse plane of the uterine cavity when it is released.
6. The device should not remain in the introducer tube for more than a few minutes lest it lose its shape.
7. The introducer tube is carefully inserted through the cervical canal, the IUD released according to the specific instructions for each device, and the introducer withdrawn.
8. Following insertion further sounding of the canal to exclude the low-lying IUD is necessary. Good fundal placement is essential to achieve a low incidence of expulsion and pregnancy.
9. The thread(s) of the tail of the IUD should be trimmed with long scissors to about 3 cm from the external os.

NB:
   a. Some experienced fitters do not use a sound to determine the size of the uterine cavity. Some do not use forceps to stabilize the cervix, with no increase in complication rates in experienced hands. However, application of Allis's forceps is

not particularly uncomfortable for most women and the use
of a tenaculum is recommended for inexperienced doctors.
  b. The skill and attitude of the fitter may influence the incidence
     of unwanted effects more than the type of device fitted.
  c. Doctors who wish to insert IUDs are recommended to
     undergo the appropriate training (Ch. 1).

Problems at insertion

Pain: vasovagal syncope   Severe pain associated with
vasovagal syncope – 'cervical shock' – is rare, but may be caused by
distension of the internal cervical os with the sound or the introducer. It has become less common since smaller devices and
narrower introducer tubes have become available. The majority of
cases are mild and after an interval the operator can continue, using
1% local analgesic gel or a local analgesic injection applied to the
cervical canal. In severe cases the insertion procedure should be
stopped, the patient placed head down and the airway maintained.
If shock occurs as the IUD insertion is being completed the IUD can
be left in place and the patient allowed to recover.

The incidence of cervical shock may be reduced by inserting the
IUD during menstruation or, in the anxious patient, by applying 1%
local analgesic gel to the cervical canal.

Epileptic attacks   These are sometimes precipitated by IUD
insertion. They are not necessarily associated with pain and usually
occur 2–3 minutes after the stimulus.

Perforation   This occurs in about 1 in 1000 insertions: rates
may be slightly lower with copper-bearing devices.

Perforation may cause sudden pain or bleeding but often goes
unrecognized. If suspected, immediate gynaecological opinion is
required. Laparoscopy or laparotomy may be necessary.

Failure to insert   This may be due to anatomical abnormality,
patient anxiety or poor operator technique. If unusual difficulty is
encountered, the fitting should be abandoned and the patient asked
to return at a later date to see a more experienced doctor or referred
to a gynaecologist or IUD problem clinic.

Resuscitation measures in IUD clinics

1. IUD insertion should always be carried out in a calm, relaxed,
   unhurried atmosphere and with a gentle reassuring approach to
   the patient at all times.

2. At the earliest sign of vasovagal attack, insertion may need to be abandoned or the device removed. The patient should be kept supine, the head lowered and the legs elevated to the vertical position if necessary in order to restore blood flow.
3. A clear airway must be maintained – probably no more than supporting the chin will be necessary. Any tight clothing, especially around the neck, should be loosened.
4. A Brook airway size 900, or other appropriate appliance such as a Laerdal pocket mask, should always be at hand. The latter is disposable but may be reused by replacing the detachable one-way valve.
5. Overtreatment should be avoided, but simple procedures should be instigated at the first sign of trouble.
6. Correct positioning should always take precedence over more heroic procedures.
7. Where a persistent bradycardia is in evidence, atropine may be given intravenously in a dose of 0.6 mg. It should be borne in mind always that the injudicious use of drugs may do more harm than good.
8. If oxygen is available it may be administered using an Ambu bag.
9. In the very rare situation where the patient fails to regain consciousness she should be transferred by ambulance to an accident and emergency department or the nearest intensive care unit.

Instructions to patients

These are not complicated and refer to checking that the IUD is in place and to coping with side-effects.

Feeling for the IUD thread   Instruct the woman how to feel for the thread(s) coming through the cervical os. This can cause problems since the thread(s) of modern devices are soft and not easily felt and the woman becomes anxious when she fails to locate them.

It is much more important to instruct her to feel the cervix each month after the end of her period and to ensure than no firm plastic is protruding. If she can feel the plastic end of the device, it means that it is partially expelled and she should consult her doctor.

After insertion   Bleeding is of no consequence in the first 24 hours and reassurance is all that is required. Pain, similar to menstrual cramps, can be controlled by simple analgesics, e.g. aspirin or paracetamol.

Pain and discharge A severe attack of acute, or any continuous, lower abdominal pain should be reported to the doctor. So too should excessive vaginal discharge, particularly if it is offensive.

Intercurrent therapy Medical treatment, e.g. with antibiotics, has no adverse effect on IUDs. It has been suggested that patients with copper IUDs should not have short-wave diathermy, which might induce heating in the copper coil, but this risk is theoretical. Reports that the use of anti-inflammatory drugs such as cortico-steroids and aspirin increases the failure rate with IUDs have not been confirmed.

Follow-up

1. The patient should be seen 6–8 weeks after insertion and annually thereafter, unless symptoms develop necessitating an earlier appointment.
2. At each visit she should be asked about her menstrual pattern, pelvic pain and vaginal discharge.
3. Pelvic examination should be carried out to exclude any abnormality, to confirm that the IUD is in position and to take a cervical smear if screening guidelines dictate.

Removal

An IUD may be removed to allow a patient to become pregnant, because contraception is no longer needed, or because a change of contraceptive method is desired. Complications, especially bleeding and pain, pregnancy or partial expulsion may also necessitate removal.

Unless pregnancy is desired, IUDs should not be removed in the latter half of the menstrual cycle if intercourse has occurred within the preceding seven days.

The recommended lifespans of different types of IUD are given earlier in this chapter.

At the menopause, the IUD should be removed 12 months after the last menstrual period.

Most studies indicate that after IUD removal fertility is unimpaired and the conception rate is similar to that after cessation of other methods of contraception.

Technique

Visible threads   This is most easily carried out during a menstrual period but may be undertaken at any time in the cycle, provided continuing contraceptive cover is not required (see above).

1. Check the size and position of the uterus by bimanual examination.
2. Expose the cervix with a speculum.
3. Grasp the retrieval thread(s) firmly near the cervical canal with a pair of straight artery forceps.
4. Apply gentle downward traction.
   Usually the IUD will be withdrawn without difficulty and with minimal pain. If resistance to removal is encountered, or if the patient experiences pain, stop traction and then:
   a. Grasp the cervix with tissue forceps and apply gentle traction to straighten out the uterocervical canal.
   b. Continue traction on the threads and remove in the usual way.
   c. Sometimes it may be necessary to dilate the cervical canal to 3 mm (Hegar 3).
   d. Rarely is it necessary to administer local or general anaesthesia.

Threads that break   If, during removal, a thread or threads break, the stem of the IUD is likely to be in the cervical canal. It may be removed with tissue forceps or a 'hook', but only experienced doctors should attempt to do this in a clinic or practice situation.

1. Apply tissue forceps to stabilize the cervix.
2. If necessary, use a local analgesic gel applied to the cervical canal or an intracervical injection of analgesic.
3. Insert straight artery forceps into the canal and grasp the lower part of the IUD.
4. Remove the IUD with gentle traction.
5. If this fails a small IUD removal hook can be passed into the uterine cavity and locked around the IUD, which is then removed with gentle traction.
6. If all these procedures fail, proceed as for the lost IUD.

Threads not visible   See page 141.

COMPLICATIONS AND THEIR MANAGEMENT

Abnormal bleeding

Menstrual irregularities   For the first few months inter-menstrual bleeding or spotting may occur, but get less with time. Premenstrual spotting for 2–3 days is also common (Table 5.1).

Table 5.1 Abnormal bleeding associated with IUDs

Symptoms	Features	Management
Heavy or prolonged periods	Heavy periods many months after insertion may be due to movement of the IUD in the uterine cavity, partial expulsion or gynaecological pathology. Prolonged bleeding and discomfort may indicate pelvic infection.	With sympathetic reassurance many patients will tolerate such bleeding and keep the IUD. Mefenamic acid (Ponstan) or antifibrinolytic agents may decrease blood loss but if heavy bleeding persists the device should be removed. Heavy bleeding as a new symptom demands vaginal examination and probably removal of the IUD; observation of subsequent period(s); gynaecological referral if necessary. If normal menstrual cycles return another device may be inserted.
Intermenstrual bleeding (IMB)	Especially likely in the luteal phase.	This should be disregarded during the first few months after insertion. If it develops months or years later in an otherwise trouble-free patient, remove the IUD. If it persists, refer for gynaecological investigation.
Intermenstrual spotting (IMS)	May occur at any time in the cycle but most commonly 1–2 days before a period.	Warn patients to expect this and reassure them. If troublesome treat with a nonsteroidal anti-inflammatory agent (NSAI). If persistent examine the cervix to check for disease and partial expulsion of the device.
Amenorrhoea	Any patient presenting with a missed period or more prolonged amenorrhoea should have pregnancy excluded by clinical examination and/or a pregnancy test. NB The pregnancy may be ectopic.	If pregnant (pp. 139–140). If not pregnant and the uterus is of normal size reassure her that her cycle will probably soon return to normal. If amenorrhoea persists for 6 months, appropriate investigation is indicated.
Postcoital bleeding (PCB)	Rarely, if ever, caused by an IUD.	Examine the cervix, take a smear and refer for gynaecological opinion if necessary.

Heavy periods All copper and inert devices cause an increase in the amount and/or duration of bleeding. Although there is great patient variability, the average loss in a normal cycle is 35 ml, with a copper IUD 50–60 ml, and with inert devices 70–80 ml. See also Table 5.1.

Pain

Lower abdominal pain This may occur at insertion, particularly in nulliparous women, and last for a few days.

Cramps These may accompany periods for the first few months and, if severe, may necessitate IUD removal (Table 5.2).

Table 5.2 Pain associated with IUDs

Symptoms	Features	Management
Dysmenorrhoea	Similar to spasmodic dysmenorrhoea.	Simple analgesics may be tried and, if unsuccessful, replaced by NSAI for the first 2–3 days of each period. Unrelieved symptoms may require IUD removal.
Dyspareunia	Although IUDs never cause superficial dyspareunia they are occasionally associated with deep dyspareunia and may sometimes cause the male partner to suffer a sharp pain during intercourse.	Any underlying cause should be treated but if no cause is found the IUD should be removed and the effect of this assessed. When the male partner complains of pain during intercourse the patient should be examined to exclude a partially expelled device or a sharp thread protruding from the os. In both cases the IUD should be removed and replaced, or a different IUD may be tried later.
Lower abdominal pain	Dull ache not related to periods. Often no cause is found.	Exclude pelvic infection and partial expulsion of the IUD. If it persists and no cause is found the device may have to be removed.

Vaginal discharge

Watery or mucoid discharge is common in women wearing an IUD, particularly a copper device. It is usually only of nuisance value.

In the presence of a low-grade anaerobic infection the discharge may become offensive and unpleasant. If profuse or persistent, cervical or vaginal swabs should be taken to exclude infection. Bacterial vaginosis is more common among IUD users than among women not using an IUD. If no infecting organism is identified or if treatment is not successful then, as a last resort, replacement with a similar IUD but with the threads cut off may cure the problem. Subsequent removal of this IUD will obviously be more difficult.

Pelvic infection

The incidence of pelvic inflammatory disease (PID) associated with IUDs has been difficult to establish as the diagnosis is usually based on clinical criteria. Patients with vaginal discharge and/or uterine pain are commonly labelled as suffering from PID – particularly if they have an IUD in place – yet these symptoms do not by themselves signify infection.

In the 1970s studies showed an increase in the risk of pelvic infection in IUD users, the rates being about 3.8–5.2 per 100 women. In the 1980s there was a general impression that the risk of PID was doubled in IUD users. Recently, however, analysis of a large database collected by WHO (Farley et al 1992) has shown that there is only a slight risk of PID during the first 20 days after insertion and thereafter infection rates are not increased over that in the general population (about 1% per year). Infection rates were much lower among women who had devices inserted after 1980 and were inversely related to age (Leading Article 1992). The Oxford FPA study showed that married women over 25 using IUDs have a rate of PID of 2 per 1000 woman years.

The most important factor in the risk of PID is the lifestyle of the woman. Although infection can be introduced at the time of IUD insertion, the uterine cavity is free of bacteria 1 month later; pelvic infection developing more than 4 months after IUD insertion is due to other factors such as sexually transmissible disease. The risk of PID is therefore increased if the woman has many sexual partners. In stable, monogamous relationships, IUD use carries no risk of PID.

The levonorgestrel IUD reduces the risk of pelvic infection.

Minimizing the risk of infection   To keep risks to a mini-mum, IUDs should be removed and replaced as infrequently as possible.

It has also been suggested that:

1. Prophylactic antibiotics might be given at the time of insertion, but so far studies have provided little justification for this.
2. Tailless devices should be used or the tails inserted within the uterine cavity. The evidence for this is not convincing and problems with removal would occur.

Policies on screening for infection before IUD insertion should be determined by local incidence rates. (Bromham 1993).

Infertility   This can result from PID and is an important consideration in the young nulliparous woman; the risk should be fully discussed before an IUD is inserted. The risk of infertility after laparoscopically verified PID is 6% after 1 episode of mild disease, 30% after 1 episode of severe disease and over 50% after 3 or more episodes. The risk of tubal infertility is not increased among IUD users who have only one sexual partner; it is higher among women with more than one sexual partner, whether or not an IUD is used.

Pelvic actinomycosis   This has been reported but is rare. Actinomycosis-like organisms are often identified on Papanicolaou smears from IUD users, but if the patient is symptom-free the IUD may be left in place and no treatment is required. The smear should be repeated at 6 and 12 months. If the woman has any relevant symptoms, the device should be carefully removed trying to avoid vaginal contamination, the tails cut off and the device sent for culture. Appropriate treatment should be instituted as required.

Diagnosis

1. Clinical features range from virtually none to those of acute sepsis. Essential symptoms and signs of acute PID are lower abdominal pain, purulent vaginal discharge, and tenderness on moving the cervix: if all three are present there is a 50% probability of PID. The probability is increased by finding a fever in excess of 38°C, a palpable pelvic adnexal mass, or elevation of the white blood count, erythrocyte sedimentation rate, or C-reactive protein.
2. High vaginal and cervical swab culture may identify aerobic or anaerobic organisms or both.

3. The possibility of pregnancy should be excluded with a sensitive hCG assay as ectopic pregnancy is one of the differential diagnoses.
4. Laparoscopy can confirm the diagnosis in doubtful cases.
5. If in doubt, it is better to treat suspected PID than not to treat at all.

Management

In mild cases the diagnosis should be established and treatment with antibiotics started (Ch. 13). If there is no response after 24 hours the IUD should be removed. In moderate cases with more definite clinical signs the IUD should be removed before starting antibiotic therapy and the patient referred for a gynaecological opinion. Severe cases associated with marked lower abdominal pain and fever should be admitted to hospital.

Any patient with a past history of PID and who is suspected of developing pelvic infection should be treated. Most cases are mild and respond successfully to antibiotics such as metronidazole (Flagyl), amoxycillin (Amoxil), or tetracycline, for a full 7 days. If *Actinomyces israelii* is identified on culture, the IUD should be removed and treatment with penicillin instituted.

Pregnancy

If pregnancy is suspected, the possibility of ectopic pregnancy should always be borne in mind. Nevertheless, over 90% of pregnancies with an IUD in place are intrauterine.

Intrauterine pregnancy

The pregnancy may progress successfully to term. However, the incidence of spontaneous mid-trimester abortion, bleeding, amnionitis, premature labour and perinatal mortality are all increased if the IUD is left in place. Studies have shown no evidence that the presence of an IUD in pregnancy increases the risk of congenital abnormality.

Management Up to 12 weeks' gestation, if threads are visible and the device moves easily, remove it gently. Ultrasound may aid removal of devices when the threads are not visible.

Beyond 12 weeks, or in most cases when no threads are visible, or if the device does not move easily, leave it in place. Refer early for antenatal care. Advise the patient to seek immediate medical attention if she develops bleeding, fever, amniotic fluid leak, etc.

If left in place throughout pregnancy, the IUD is usually expelled with the placenta and membranes. If not, X-ray or ultrasound should be used early in the puerperium to locate it.

Extrauterine or ectopic pregnancy

The incidence of ectopic pregnancy in non-IUD users has been increasing in developed countries including Britain, and is now around 1 in 200 pregnancies. IUDs provide more protection against intrauterine than extrauterine pregnancy.

If pregnancy occurs in an IUD user, the risk of its being ectopic is between 1 in 35 and 1 in 11. An analysis of randomized trials of different IUDs has concluded that the risk of ectopic pregnancy depended on the type of IUD. Copper-bearing devices with 200 mm² of copper reduced the risk of ectopic pregnancy compared to non-contraceptors, and for devices with 350 mm² of copper ectopic pregnancy rates were one-tenth those of non-contraceptors. A similar effect was seen with medicated devices: those releasing 20 µg/day of levonorgestrel had ectopic pregnancy rates estimated at one-tenth those of non-contraceptors. The risk of ectopic pregnancy is higher in older women (Sivin 1991).

Management The symptoms of ectopic pregnancy – pain and menstrual irregularity – may be mistakenly attributed to pelvic inflammatory disease or even to the IUD itself. A high index of suspicion of ectopic pregnancy is important and any suspected case requires an immediate gynaecological opinion.

Classical symptoms of pregnancy such as amenorrhoea may be missing. The diagnosis should be suspected if there is any unexplained pelvic pain or lower abdominal cramps or any irregular bleeding, especially if a period is scanty, late or missed. Older pregnancy tests were often negative because hCG levels are low, but the newer ultra-sensitive hCG tests are likely to be accurate.

LOST THREADS AND LOST DEVICES

Threads which are too long can be a nuisance to the patient. They can cause irritation to the user, discomfort to her partner and if pulled on can partially remove the device. Threads which are too short can lead to difficulty in finding the IUD and, unless they have become visible after the next menstrual period, become numbered among 'lost' threads. To avoid both these problems threads should be cut, at the time of insertion, 3cm from the external os. Nevertheless, in prospective studies 7–9% of users had absent threads at their follow-up visits.

Lost threads

When threads are not visible at the external os, the device may be in the uterine cavity, embedded in the uterine wall, in the peritoneal cavity, or expelled altogether from the body. Before looking for threads, pregnancy should be excluded by a sensitive pregnancy test.

To look for threads in the clinic or surgery   Follow the procedure below.

1. Carefully expose the cervix, in a good light, as this will allow short threads in the cervical canal to be seen.
2. If no threads are seen, clean the cervix and explore the endocervical canal (up to the level of the internal os) with Spencer Wells forceps, opening and closing the instrument within the canal. In about one-third of cases the threads will be brought down.
3. Gently sound the uterine cavity, when necessary applying an Allis tissue forceps to the cervix to straighten out the canal. Any device in the canal or uterus will usually be felt by the sound.
4. A notched plastic sound, such as the Emmett or Retrievette Thread Retriever, should be passed into the uterine cavity. This will retrieve the threads in about 50% of cases (Bounds et al 1992). However, this procedure may displace the device itself; if it does, the device should be removed and a new one fitted.
5. One or more of a variety of IUD retrievers, such as an IUD hook or Patterson alligator forceps, may be used to retrieve the device itself. This may, however, be best performed in a specialist IUD clinic.
6. If these procedures fail, the IUD should be presumed lost and the patient referred for ultrasonography (p. 143). The patient should be advised that she is at risk of pregnancy and should use another reliable contraceptive while doubt exists about the presence of the IUD.
7. In a specialist IUD clinic a further attempt may be made after pretreatment of the cervix, for example with ethinyloestradiol or mifepristone, and using premedication with mefenamic acid and possibly local anaesthetic. Only 4% of women with lost threads will ultimately require uterine exploration under general anaesthesia (Bounds et al 1992).

Expulsion of an IUD

This problem may occur with all types of IUD, but the risk is lowest with copper-bearing devices. The risk is greatest in the first 3 months after insertion, when 50% of expulsions occur. Multiparous women have lower expulsion rates than women who have never been pregnant. Most expulsions occur during menstruation and the patient is often unaware of what has happened.

The skill of the fitter in ensuring correct fundal placement is an important factor in reducing expulsion rates.

Complete expulsion

Although expulsion of the whole device into the vagina is uncommon, patients should be told to examine towels and tampons, especially in the first three months, to check this.

They should also report unexplained pelvic pain or intermenstrual bleeding as these may signify expulsion. If the patient wishes, another IUD may be inserted. Second insertions, even of the same type of IUD, are associated with lower expulsion rates than first insertions.

Partial expulsion

This is much more common than complete expulsion. Part of the device, usually the end of the vertical stem, is found protruding from the cervical canal. The patient or doctor may notice this or it may present as unexplained pain or intermenstrual bleeding. The device should be removed, and if the patient wishes, another inserted.

The lost IUD

Lost inert devices have remained in the peritoneal cavity for years without producing problems. However, they do tend to migrate and may be found anywhere in the abdomen. Open or linear devices theoretically cause few problems but closed devices could cause intestinal obstruction. Copper devices cause a sterile inflammatory reaction and rapidly become adherent to the omentum or bowel. Abdominal pain may be present, or the patient may be otherwise asymptomatic.

All devices should be removed from the peritoneal cavity as soon as possible, although some authorities believe there is less urgency to remove inert linear devices in asymptomatic patients. That decision, however, will be made by the gynaecologist to whom the patient is referred. The flow diagram (Fig. 5.5) shows the management sequence.

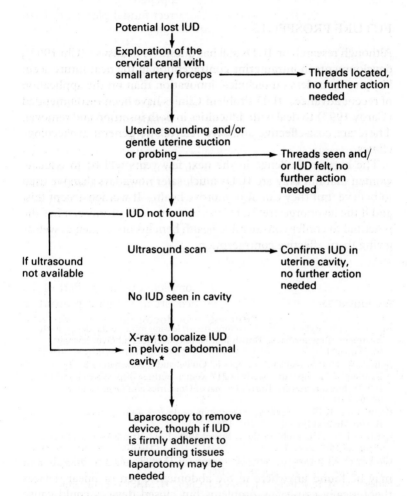

*Since there is no scientific evidence that the delivery of ionising radiation in the first 2 weeks of gestation in humans is teratogenic the need to observe the 10-day rule is being questioned.

Fig. 5.5   Flow diagram for lost IUDs.

Displaced IUD within the uterine cavity

Occasionally, rotation of the IUD within the uterine cavity can occur. This will cause pain and bleeding and will necessitate removal of the device. Rarely, downward displacement may lead to cervical perforation. In both cases referral to a gynaecologist for removal is advised as general anaesthesia may be necessary.

FUTURE PROSPECTS

Although research on IUDs still has questions to answer (Chi 1993), developments in intrauterine contraception in the near future seem likely to focus less on technical innovation than on the application of recent advances. IUD Problem Clinics have been recommended (Cardy 1993) to deal with difficulties in both insertion and removal. These are cost-effective and save referrals to general gynaecology clinics.

The biggest challenge in the next few years will be to educate women that not only are IUDs much safer nowadays than we used to believe, but they can also improve health. If women accept this, and if the levonorgestrel IUD lives up to its early promise, it has the potential to confer considerable health benefits on women as well as giving them effective contraception.

REFERENCES

Andersson J K, Rybo G 1990 Levonorgestrel-releasing intrauterine device in the treatment of menorrhagia. British Journal of Obstetrics and Gynaecology 97: 690–694

Bounds W, Hutt S, Kubba A, Cooper K, Guillebaud J, Newman G B 1992 Randomised comparative study in 217 women of three disposable plastic IUCD thread retrievers. British Journal of Obstetrics and Gynaecology 99: 915–919

Bromham D R 1993 Intrauterine contraceptive devices – a reappraisal. British Medical Bulletin 49: 100–123

Cardy G 1993 IUD problem clinic, Bristol 1988–1992. British Journal of Family Planning 19: 229–231

Chi I 1993 What have we learned from recent IUD studies: a researcher's perspective. Contraception 48: 81–108

Farley T M M, Rosenberg M J, Rowe P J, Chen J H, Meirik O Intrauterine devices and pelvic inflammatory disease: an international perspective. Lancet 1992; 339: 785–788

Leading Article 1992 Does infection occur with modern intrauterine devices? Lancet 339: 783–4

Luukkainen T 1993 The levonorgestrel-releasing IUD. British Journal of Family Planning 19: 221–224

Mestman J H, Schmidt-Sarosi C 1993 Diabetes mellitus and fertility control: contraception management issues
American Journal of Obstetrics and Gynecology 168: 2012–2020
Sivin I 1991 Dose- and age-dependent ectopic pregnancy risks with intrauterine contraception. Obstetrics and Gynecology 78: 291–297
Wildemeersch D, Van Kets H, Van der Pas H, Vrijens M, VanTrappen Y, Temmerman M, Batar I, Barri P, Martinez F, Iglesias-Craft L, Thiery M 1994 IUD tolerance in nulligravid and parous women: optimal acceptance with the frameless CuFix implant system (GyneFix). Long-term results with a new inserter. British Journal of Family Planning 20: 2–5

6. Barrier methods

Ailsa Gebbie

Occlusive pessaries (Caps)
  Diaphragm
  Cervical cap
  Vault cap
  Vimule
  Damage to occlusive pessaries

Female condom

Home-made barriers

Condoms

Spermicides
  Creams and jellies

Vaginal suppositories
Foaming tablets
Aerosol foam
C-film
The vaginal contraceptive sponge
New spermicides and delivery systems

Adaptations of coital technique
  Coitus interruptus
  Coitus reservatus
  Coitus designed to avoid the vagina

Risks/Benefits

A barrier method of contraception is the most logical approach to the interruption of the process of human reproduction. Fertilization is prevented by arresting the progress of sperm as they make their rapid journey from the male partner to the female. From earliest times, an extensive array of barrier methods has been used by couples attempting to control their fertility. Nowadays, such methods continue to offer considerable advantages in terms of safety and reversibility. The efficacy of barrier methods depends critically on quality of use. Their relatively high failure rates are reduced significantly when they are used consistently and correctly by well-motivated couples.

A marked decline in the use of barrier methods occurred following the widespread availability of oral contraceptives in the 1960s and 1970s. Subsequent adverse publicity about the risks of the pill increased their popularity again.

The AIDS virus and the spread of HIV infection into the heterosexual population have focused attention on barrier methods. The 'Safer Sex' campaign in the United Kingdom, promoting use of condoms to combat spread of the virus, has attempted to break down many traditional taboos concerning the openness with which sexuality and contraception may be discussed and dealt with.

147

Barrier methods comprise:

1. Occlusive pessaries and condoms for use by the female.
2. Condoms for use by the male.
3. Spermicides.
4. Adaptations of coital technique.

OCCLUSIVE PESSARIES (CAPS)

For thousands of years women have attempted to avoid pregnancy by blocking the access of sperm to the cervix. Various materials such as sponges and pads of cotton were used, but occlusive pessaries did not appear until the 19th century. The German gynaecologist Hasse (using the pseudonym Mensinga) is credited with introducing the diaphragm in 1882. Wilde described the use of a rubber check pessary made to a wax model of the patient's cervix almost 50 years earlier. This type of cervical cap was used in Britain before the diaphragm, but its use was not approved by the American Food and Drug Administration until 1988. Since the 1950s the diaphragm or 'Dutch cap' has been by far the most commonly used type of occlusive pessary. Female barrier methods remain an unpopular method of contraception and are currently used by only 1–2% of sexually active women (OPCS 1991).

Types   Four occlusive pessaries are in current use – the diaphragm, cervical cap, vault cap and the vimule.

Diaphragm

A diaphragm consists of a thin, latex rubber hemisphere, the rim of which is reinforced by a flexible flat or coiled metal spring. Sizes of the external diameter range from 55 to 95 mm, in 5 mm increments, but in practice most women use the 70–80 mm sizes (Fig. 6.1).

Variations

1. The flat-spring diaphragm has a firm watch-spring
   (Fig. 6.2A), is easily fitted and remains in the horizontal
   plane on compression. It is suitable for the normal vagina
   and is often tried first.
2. The coil-spring diaphragm has a spiral coiled spring
   (Fig. 6.2B), is considerably softer than the flat-spring, and is
   particularly suitable for a patient who has strong muscles or
   who is sensitive to the pressure of the flat-spring type. With the

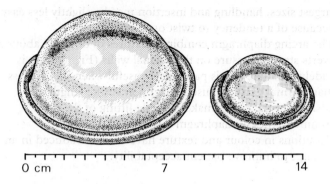

Fig. 6.1 Large and small diaphragms.

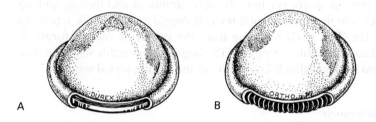

Fig. 6.2 **A**. Flat-spring Durex diaphragm to show rim in cross-section;
B. Coil-spring Ortho diaphragm to show rim in cross section.

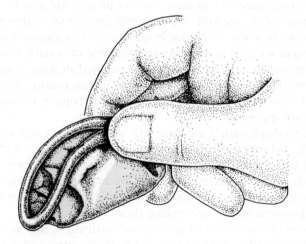

Fig. 6.3 Arcing diaphragm.

largest sizes, handling and insertion may be slightly less easy because of a tendency to twist on compression.
3. The arcing diaphragm combines features of both the above and exerts strong pressure on the vaginal walls (Fig. 6.3). It is widely available and is particularly useful when there is less than normal vaginal muscular support or the length and position of the cervix makes reliable fitting of the more common types of diaphragm difficult.
4. Variations in colour and texture have been introduced in an attempt to improve patient acceptability.

Mode of action

The diaphragm acts as a physical barrier during sexual intercourse to prevent sperm reaching the cervical mucus and thereby gaining access to the upper genital tract. It should lie diagonally across the cervix (Fig. 6.7), reaching from the posterior vaginal fornix to behind the pubic symphysis. The largest comfortable size should be used as the vagina is known to expand during sexual arousal.

Effectiveness

Because a sperm-tight seal between the rim of the diaphragm and the vaginal walls is quite impossible to achieve, the use of a spermicide in conjunction with all caps is recommended in order to provide maximum effectiveness. As spermicides add greatly to the 'messiness' of the method, a few patients may decide to depend on the barrier function of the diaphragm alone. Continuous use of a diaphragm without spermicide and removal on a daily basis for washing and immediate reinsertion is advised in some countries overseas. This cannot be recommended in this country although there is a distinct lack of scientific evidence to support the value of adjunctive spermicides.

When a diaphragm is used correctly in conjunction with spermicide, the failure rate (FR) is 4–8 per 100 woman years. With less careful use, the FR is quoted as high as 10–18 per woman years (Bounds 1994). A decline in FRs is found when diaphragms are used by experienced users who have completed their families rather than those women who are spacing their pregnancies.

Causes of failure, apart from poor motivation, are incorrect insertion or fitting, displacement during intercourse, and defect in the cap due to careless handling.

Indications

1. When a couple wish the woman to use a barrier method of contraception and find other contraceptive methods unacceptable.
2. When there are medical reasons which exclude the woman from taking hormonal contraception.
3. When a couple need intermittent, or infrequent, yet predictable contraception.

Contraindications

1. Poor vaginal muscular support or prolapse, although this may be overcome by careful assessment of the size and type of diaphragm fitted. Fitting should be delayed until at least 6 weeks postpartum to allow muscle tone to return.
2. Psychological aversion, or inability to touch the genital area.
3. Inability to learn insertion technique.
4. Lack of hygiene or privacy for insertion, removal and care of the diaphragm.

Advantages

1. No systemic side-effects.
2. Effective when fitted and used correctly.
3. Does not interfere with lactation.
4. Spermicide provides extra lubrication if vaginal dryness is a problem.
5. Reduction in the risk of most non-viral sexually transmissible diseases and pelvic inflammatory disease, thereby significantly reducing the risk of tubal infertility.
6. Reduction in the risk of pre-malignant disease and carcinoma of the cervix. The use of spermicidal agents may be the actual protective factor for cervical cancer.

Disadvantages

1. Requires premeditation, and thereby there is loss of spontaneity with intercourse.
2. Spermicide makes the method rather 'messy'.
3. May cause:
   a. Discomfort to the wearer or her partner during intercourse.
   b. Loss of cervical and some vaginal sensation.

4. Has to be fitted and checked regularly by a trained doctor or nurse.
5. Does not provide protection against the transmission of HIV and other viral infections.
6. Sensitization to rubber or spermicide may develop.
7. Increased incidence of symptomatic urinary infection. This is thought to be the result of altered bladder neck angle and increased vaginal carriage of coliforms in diaphragm users. Women with recurrent urinary infections should be advised to use an alternative method of contraception.
8. Toxic shock syndrome has been reported following prolonged retention of a diaphragm in a very small number of cases.
9. Efficacy depends on correct use and sustained motivation.

Fitting a diaphragm requires time and patience on the part of trained personnel. Models and diagrams of the female anatomy will often improve understanding. An initial examination should be performed to assess the following:

1. Position and condition of the uterus and cervix.
2. Length of vagina and muscle tone.
3. Measurement of the distance between the posterior fornix and the posterior aspect of the pubic symphysis.

Screening procedures should be carried out according to routine practice.

Selection and fitting

1. A diaphragm, corresponding roughly in size to the distance between the posterior fornix and the symphysis pubis, is chosen (Figs 6.4 and 6.5).
2. With the patient supine, the labia are separated, the diaphragm is compressed and inserted into the vagina, downwards and backwards into the posterior fornix, before being released (Fig. 6.6).
3. The anterior rim is tucked behind the pubic symphysis and the position of the cervix checked (Fig. 6.7).
4. Secure fitting is checked. When the patient strains down, the anterior rim of the diaphragm should not project or slip.
5. Too large a diaphragm may project anteriorly, be immediately uncomfortable, or become uncomfortable or distorted after being worn (Fig. 6.8A).

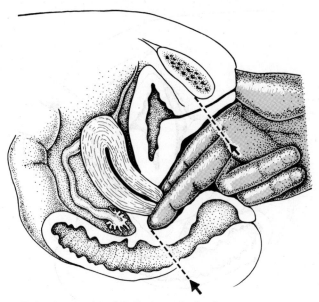

Fig. 6.4 Estimating the size of diaphragm to be fitted.

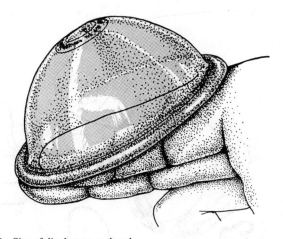

Fig. 6.5 Size of diaphragm on hand.

6. If the diaphragm is too small, a gap will be felt between the anterior rim and the posterior surface of the symphysis pubis, or it may even be inserted in front of the cervix (Fig. 6.8B).

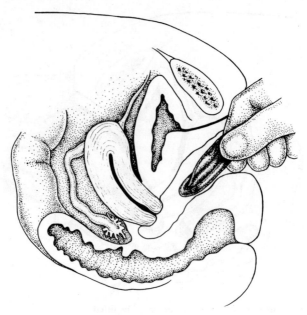

Fig. 6.6   Diaphragm being inserted.

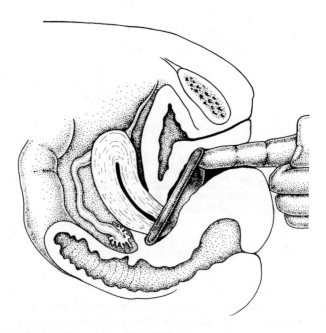

Fig. 6.7   Checking the position of the diaphragm.

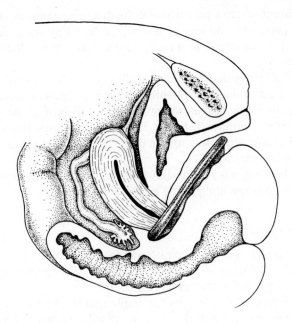

Fig. 6.8A   Diaphragm too large.

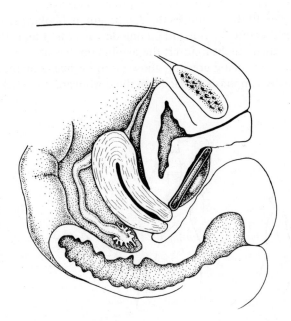

Fig. 6.8B   Diaphragm too small.

7. Persistent anterior protrusion of the diaphragm may be due to a mild cystocele, and may be discovered only after the patient strains or stands up. In this case, a cap other than a diaphragm is required.
8. The flat-spring diaphragm is usually used dome-upwards and, if reversed (to increase retention behind the pubic symphysis), is slightly more difficult to remove. The coil-spring type is normally recommended for use dome-downwards. However the decision which way up the diaphragm is fitted is crucial in only a few patients.
9. The diaphragm is removed by hooking the index finger under the anterior rim and pulling gently downwards.

Teaching the patient

1. The woman squatting, or with one foot on a chair, or occasionally lying on her back, according to her preference, is first taught to feel the cervix (Fig. 6.9).
2. The instructor then inserts the diaphragm for the patient, allowing her to feel the cervix covered with the thin rubber. This is extremely important since correct placement of the diaphragm over the cervix is vital to its success.
3. The patient then removes the diaphragm by hooking her finger under the anterior rim and pulling downwards (Fig. 6.10).
4. She is then taught to insert the diaphragm herself, the instructions being precisely those given for fitting by the doctor or nurse. Emphasis is placed on the downward and backward

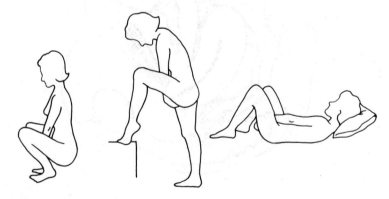

Fig. 6.9 Positions for inserting a diaphragm.

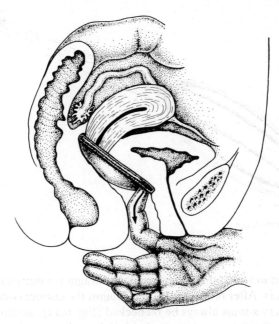

Fig. 6.10 Patient removing a diaphragm (standing position).

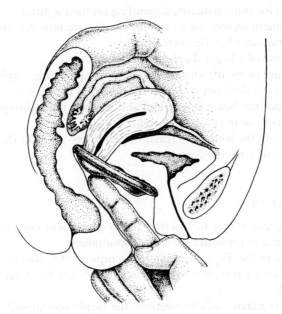

Fig. 6.11 Checking a diaphragm covering the cervix (standing position).

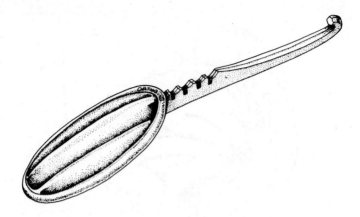

Fig. 6.12   Introducer.

direction in which the compressed diaphragm is inserted into the vagina. After releasing the diaphragm, the correct covering of the cervix must always be rechecked (Fig. 6.11), as should the snug fit of the anterior rim behind the pubic symphysis.
5. Variation in the order of teaching these techniques may be required for some patients, depending on their aptitude.
6. If the patient repeatedly inserts the diaphragm into the anterior fornix this can often be overcome by:
   a. The use of a larger diaphragm.
   b. The use of an introducer (Fig. 6.12), or an arcing diaphragm where the difficulty is due to the length of the cervix.
   c. The partner being willing and able to learn the technique of insertion on the patient's behalf.
   d. Allowing the woman to teach herself in privacy with the aid of a hand cassette instructor.

Instructions for use

1. The diaphragm may be inserted at any convenient time prior to intercourse to minimize the loss of spontaneity.
2. Insertion of the diaphragm can be incorporated as part of the woman's regular nightly routine, whether or not intercourse is planned.
3. To ensure maximum effectiveness, the diaphragm should always be used with spermicidal cream or jelly. Use of the

spermicidal agent C-film in conjunction with a diaphragm is less messy and appears as effective as other spermicides particularly for older women.

4. A ribbon of cream or jelly approximately 5 cm long, or a moistened C-film is placed on the upper side of the diaphragm prior to insertion.
5. If the diaphragm has been in place for more than 2 hours prior to intercourse, additional spermicide should be inserted into the vagina.
6. The diaphragm should be left in position for at least 6 hours after the last act of coitus.
7. Care of the diaphragm is essential, and after removal it should be washed in warm, soapy water and dried carefully. It should be restored to its normal rounded shape and stored in its container in a cool place. It should never be boiled. Perfumed soap, disinfectants or detergents should never be used to clean it nor talcum powder to dry it.

Follow-up

It is customary, but not mandatory, to provide a woman with a practice diaphragm for 1 week. This allows her to gain confidence in the technique of insertion, removal and care of the diaphragm and to assess whether it is comfortable, especially during micturition and defaecation. Practice caps were formerly sterilized and used over and over again. This is no longer recommended, and practice caps should be for single-patient use only.

The second visit allows rechecking of the size and fitting. The diaphragm should not be used for contraceptive purposes during this practice week. The woman should be reviewed after 3 months, and yearly thereafter.

A diaphragm should be replaced annually, or immediately if any defect develops. The size and fitting should be reviewed if the woman loses or gains 4 kg in weight, and after pregnancy or vaginal surgery.

Cervical cap

This cap is shaped like a thimble and is designed to fit closely over the cervix. It is held in place by precise fitting onto the cervix and by suction, not by spring tension as in the diaphragm.

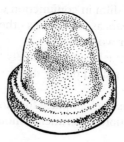

Fig. 6.13   Cervical cap.

Variations

1. The Prentif cavity-rim cap, made of firm pink rubber with an integral thickened rim incorporating a small groove, is the most commonly used. This groove is intended to increase suction to the sides of the cervix. Sizes, measured from the internal diameter of the rim, range from 21 to 31 mm (Fig. 6.13).
2. Other one-size rubber or polythene caps are available but not widely used.
3. Intracervical caps and stem pessaries are not recommended.

Mode of action

By covering the cervix, the cap acts as a physical barrier to the entrance of sperm into the cervical canal.

Effectiveness

Recent studies found pregnancy rates varying from 8 to 20 per 100 woman years. Approximately half the pregnancies were due to user failure, and the other major contributor was accidental dislodgement of the cap during intercourse.

Indications

When there is a request for an occlusive pessary by a woman who is unsuitable for a diaphragm, provided the cervix is normal and healthy with parallel (not conical) sides, pointing down the axis of the vagina and not acutely backwards.

Contraindications

1. Short, damaged, conical or unhealthy cervix.
2. Purulent cervical discharge suggesting infection.
3. Inability to reach the cervix with the fingers.

Advantages

1. Suitable for patients with poor muscle tone and some cases of uterovaginal prolapse.
2. Not felt by the male partner.
3. No reduction in vaginal sensation.
4. Fitting unaffected by changes in the size of the vagina, either during intercourse or as a result of changes in body weight.
5. Unlike a diaphragm, a cervical cap may be kept in place for several days. Some have proposed leaving it in situ for as long as the intervals between menses, *although this is not recommended*. In the UK the standard practice is to advise patients not to wear it for longer than 24 hours at a time.
6. Unlikely to produce urinary symptoms.

Disadvantages

1. Requires accurate selection of cap size and fitting to avoid displacement during intercourse.
2. Self-insertion and removal of a cervical cap are more difficult than with a diaphragm.
3. An unpleasant odour may develop if the cap is left in place for more than a day or two.

Selection and fitting

1. The correct size is that which allows the rim to touch the vaginal fornices easily without a gap, comfortably accommodates the cervix, and is not displaced when the patient bears down.
2. With the patient in the supine position, the labia are separated, the rim of the cap is compressed and then guided along the posterior vaginal wall until the posterior rim is just behind the cervix. The thumb and first two fingers are used as illustrated in Figure 6.14.
3. The cap is allowed to open by removing the thumb and then it is pushed upwards onto the cervix with the fingertips (Fig. 6.15). A final check is made to ensure that the cervix is palpable through the bowl and that no gap is left above the rim.

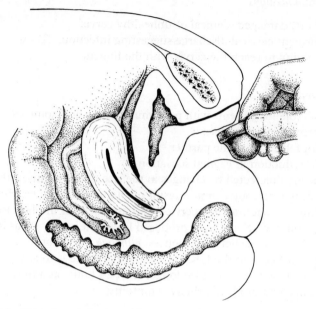

Fig. 6.14   Cervical cap being inserted.

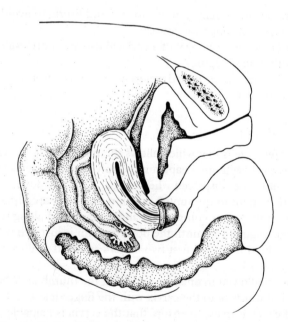

Fig. 6.15   Cervical cap in situ.

4. The cervical cap is removed by inserting a fingertip between the rim of the cap and the cervix, easing the cap downwards and withdrawing it with the index and middle fingers.

Teaching the patient

The woman is taught to feel her cervix, and to insert and remove the cap, according to the instructions given above for fitting. In time, an experienced user will often develop her own technique for inserting and removing a cervical cap and, provided it is effective, this is quite acceptable.

Instructions for use and follow-up

The instructions for use of the diaphragm also apply to the cervical cap.

1. Spermicidal cream or jelly is strongly advised and should be used to fill one-third of the bowl of the cap.
2. Further spermicide should be inserted into the vagina immediately prior to intercourse.
3. The position of the cervical cap should always be rechecked prior to each act of coitus to ensure that accidental dislodgement has not occurred.
4. The schedule of follow-up visits is the same as for the diaphragm.

Vault cap

This cap, made of rubber, is an almost hemispherical bowl with a thinner dome through which the cervix can be palpated (Fig. 6.16).

It is designed to fit into the vaginal vault, stays in place by suction, and covers, but does not fit closely to, the cervix. Five sizes are available ranging from 55 to 75 mm, in 5 mm steps.

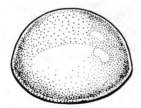

Fig. 6.16   Vault cap (Dumas).

Indications

1. Wish to use an occlusive cap.
2. Unsuitability for, or inability to use a diaphragm.
3. Unsuitability of the cervix because of its shape, position or condition for a well-fitting cervical cap.

Selection, fitting and teaching

These instructions are precisely the same as for the cervical cap, with modifications only in the siting of the upper rim. The correct size should cover the cervix without exerting pressure on it, and fit snugly into the vaginal vault (Fig. 6.17).

Instructions for use and follow-up

These are identical to those of the cervical cap, with a spermicidal agent being used to fill one-third of the bowl of the vault cap prior to insertion.

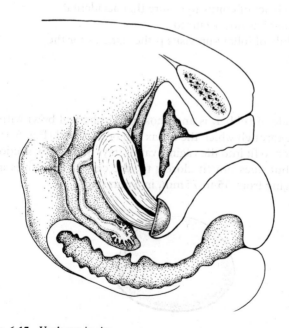

Fig. 6.17 Vault cap in situ.

Vimule

This is a variation of the vault cap with a thimble-shaped prolongation of the dome (Fig. 6.18). There are three sizes – small (45 mm), medium (48 mm) and large (51 mm). The vimule has fallen into some disrepute because of its association with vaginal abrasions and lacerations, possibly because of the relatively sharp-edged rim.

Indications

It is used specifically for the patient requiring a vault cap to accommodate a cervix which is so long that it prevents suction being exerted by a Dumas cap on the vaginal vault.

Selection, fitting and teaching

Again, this is identical to that of the cervical cap apart from the exact siting of the upper rim (Fig. 6.19). A vimule may often provide the solution for a patient who proves difficult to fit with an occlusive

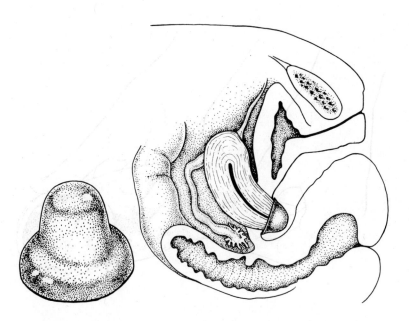

Fig. 6.18 Vimule.   **Fig. 6.19** Vimule in situ.

pessary. A string attached to the vimule facilitates removal while learning, but should be removed once the user is confident.

Instructions for use and follow-up

These are identical to those for the cervical cap, using a spermicide in the same manner.

Damage to occlusive pessaries

Some oil-based vaginal or rectal suppositories, pessaries, ointments, creams and gels can damage these barriers. Patients should be warned routinely against relying on them during treatment with such preparations and advised about alternative methods.

FEMALE CONDOM

The female condom is a polyurethane sheath, 15 cm long by 7 cm in diameter, its open end attached to a flexible polyurethane ring (Fig 6.20). A removable polyurethane ring inside the condom serves as an introducer and anchors the device in the vagina.

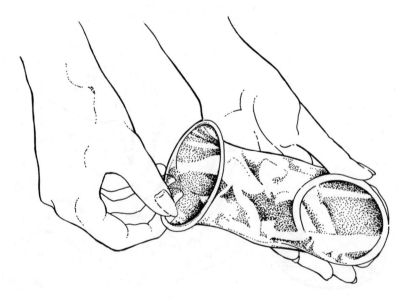

Fig. 6.20   Female condom.

The condom comes in a single size, has a silicone based, non-spermicidal lubricant and is for single use only. It has been commercially available in the UK since 1992 and is available over the counter under the trade name Femidom (Reality in North America and Femy in Spain). Initial adverse responses to female condoms will undoubtedly become less when couples become familiar with their use.

Mode of action

In common with all barrier methods, female condoms prevent spermatozoa gaining access to the female upper genital tract.

Effectiveness

As yet, there are no large scale studies of use–failure rates but rates equal to those with the male condom seem likely. Bounds et al (1992) in a small study found a use–effectiveness failure rate of 15% at 12 months. Motivated women who use female condoms consistently and correctly would be expected to have very low pregnancy rates.

Indications

1. When a couple wish the woman to use a reversible method of contraception.
2. For greater protection against sexually transmissible diseases than all other methods.

Contraindications

Some couples find female condoms psychologically unacceptable.

Advantages

1. An effective method of contraception when used correctly and consistently.
2. Available over the counter for purchase in most pharmacies and free from some family planning clinics.
3. Affords very high protection against sexually transmissible diseases including viral infections by protecting the vulva and urethra.

4. Stronger than latex male condoms with less risk of splitting and not weakened by oils.
5. Less diminution of sensation for the man than with latex condoms.
6. Can be inserted a long time (i.e. hours) in advance of intercourse thereby allowing less disruption of the sexual act.

Disadvantages

1. Unattractive appearance.
2. Altered sensation and a 'rustling' noise during intercourse.
3. Some initial difficulty with insertion may be experienced but this tends to improve rapidly with repeated use.
4. Can occasionally be pushed completely into the vagina or penetration can take place outside it.
5. Expensive.

Instructions for use

1. Insert the female condom squatting, with one foot on a chair, or lying down.
2. Squeeze the sheath covered inner ring between thumb and other fingers and slide the condom into the vagina similar to inserting a tampon.
3. Once the condom is in the vagina, push the inner ring as high as possible so that it will remain there during intercourse.
4. The outer ring should lie closely against the vulva.
5. Immediately after intercourse, hold the outer ring together and gently pull the condom out.
6. Discard in a bin and not down the toilet.

HOME-MADE BARRIERS

These cannot be advocated in any way, but their use is widespread, particularly in developing countries. For centuries women have used pads or sponges as barriers to conception, and when soaked in household substances such as vinegar, lemon juice, butter, cooking oil, Coca-Cola or even fluoride toothpaste there will be a mild spermicidal effect. Detergents or caustic substances must never be used as they will damage the vaginal mucosa.

Postcoital douching should be discouraged.

CONDOMS

The condoms first described historically were used for decoration, and thereafter for protection against disease. Fallopio, the Italian anatomist, described the use of a linen sheath in 1544 to protect the wearer from syphilis. With the development of vulcanized rubber and then liquid latex, condoms could be inexpensively mass-produced resulting in worldwide availability and an effective, reversible male method of contraception.

The condom is recognized by such familiar names as French letter, Johnny, sheath, rubber, protective etc. They may be purchased from chemists, supermarkets and vending machines, by mail order and 11% are provided free by family planning clinics. General practitioners are currently unable to prescribe condoms free on prescription but may have access to providing them free through an HIV prevention budget. Condoms have been extensively promoted in the 'Safer Sex' campaign as an effective barrier against the spread of the AIDS virus. Prominent advertising has attempted to increase the public's awareness of the risks of unprotected intercourse and to encourage condom use. New trends in marketing and packaging condoms aim to increase consumer appeal and to escape from their association with clandestine sex.

Types   A large range of types is now available:

1. Most condoms are now made of fine latex rubber and consist of a circular cylinder (3.0–3.5 cm diameter, 15–20 cm long, 0.03–0.08 mm thick) with one closed, plain or teat-shaped end and an integral rim at the open end. They are packaged individually, rolled to the rim and hermetically sealed in foil. Until recently, only one size was available but the need for both larger and smaller sizes has been recognized and these can now be purchased.
2. Lubricated, spermicide-incorporating, coloured and textured variations have been introduced in an effort to improve acceptability.
3. Allergy condoms are available for the small number of people who develop hypersensitivity.
4. Condoms which are longer and exceed the British Standards are being marketed specifically to offer added protection against infection with the AIDS virus.
5. Sheaths made from sheep's intestine (Fourex) are being actively marketed. Despite their unaesthetic appearance, they have improved sensitivity compared with latex condoms but their efficacy against sexually transmissible infections is unknown.

Mode of action

Like all barrier methods, condoms prevent spermatozoa from reaching the female upper genital tract.

Effectiveness

In the UK, condoms are required to meet stringent specifications set down by the British Standards Institute (BSI) and should carry the Kite Mark sign as an indicator of quality. However, recent doubts have been cast on the relevance of laboratory quality control testing to breakage rates during human use. Studies suggest breakage rates of condoms may be as high as 12% (Steiner 1993). Users become technically more competent with experience and have fewer accidents. Tightness of condoms may be a factor in their failure and larger condoms may be needed by some individuals.

When motivated couples use condoms correctly, pregnancy rarely occurs, but the use–failure rate overall is around 4 per 100 woman years. If the condom is not used at the beginning of intercourse or is applied only just before ejaculation, pre-ejaculatory secretions may contain sufficient sperm to cause pregnancy.

Indications

1. When a couple wish the man to use a reversible method of contraception.
2. During the period of instruction in the use of a cap.
3. Following childbirth or therapeutic abortion, before another method is adopted.
4. Condoms may be used for personal protection against sexually transmissible disease, even when a hormonal method is used to prevent conception.
5. When other methods are unacceptable or additional contraception is required.

Contraindications

1. When they are psychologically unacceptable.
2. Any malformation of the penis.
3. Where allergy to rubber develops in either partner.

Advantages

1. Effective when used correctly and consistently.
2. Widely available, inexpensive and often provided free.

3. Simple to use with no local or systemic side-effects.
4. Protection, although not absolute, against sexually transmissible disease including the AIDS virus. Undamaged latex condoms are impermeable to sexually transmissible organisms including viruses when tested in vitro. As yet there is little solid scientific evidence to confirm these findings in vivo.
5. Protection against carcinoma and pre-malignant disease of the cervix.
6. Improvement of performance in some patients with premature ejaculation.

Disadvantages

1. Unattractive appearance.
2. Loss of pleasurable sensation particularly transmission of body heat.
3. Requires application prior to coitus and prompt removal thereafter, which couples may find an unacceptable interruption.
4. Erectile difficulty may be increased, though some men in later years find the use of a condoms helps to maintain an erection.

Instructions for use

1. If the condom is not prelubricated with a spermicide, the woman should insert a spermicidal cream, jelly or pessary into the vagina before intercourse. Some condoms come packaged with spermicidal pessaries.
2. The condom is unrolled onto the erect penis before any contact with the vulva is made, leaving the tip of the condom empty to accommodate the ejaculate.
3. During withdrawal, the condom should be held firmly at the base of the penis so that it remains in place until after the penis has been withdrawn.
4. The penis should be washed before any further contact with the woman occurs.
5. Disposable condoms should not be re-used.
6. Condoms should not be used after the expiry date marked on the packet. The older the condom, the more likely it is to break during use (Steiner et al 1992).
7. Oil-based lubricants such as Vaseline, baby oil and petroleum jelly drastically reduce the tensile strength of condoms. Other vaginal creams and pessaries such as antifungal and oestrogen

preparations can be oil-based and could theoretically affect the strength of latex condoms.

8. Condom users should always be informed about the availability of postcoital contraception should the condom burst or slip off.

SPERMICIDES

These contraceptive agents comprise a chemical capable of destroying sperm, incorporated into an inert base. The commonly used spermicides contain non-ionic surfactants which alter sperm surface membrane permeability, causing osmotic changes which result in sperm death. Nonoxynol-9 was the original agent to be developed and is still the active constituent of most products.

It is emphasized that the use of spermicides as a contraceptive measure alone is not recommended and their main role is to improve the contraceptive effect of other barrier methods. They may be purchased from chemists and by mail order. They are available free from family planning clinics and free on prescription from general practitioners. Spermicidal products are available in a variety of different forms; most are suitable for all purposes (Table 6.1).

Creams and jellies

The chemical is incorporated in a stearate soap base in a cream, or in a water-soluble base in a jelly. Both liquefy at body temperature and disperse rapidly throughout the vagina.

Vaginal suppositories

The base consists of gelatin, glycerine or wax. They are foil-packed and easy to handle. Since they spread less easily throughout the vagina, weight for weight they are probably less effective than creams and jellies.

Foaming tablets

These are hard white discs which effervesce on contact with moisture, releasing the spermicide and forming CO_2 foam.

Aerosol foams

The spermicide is incorporated in an emulsion of oil and water and is stored under gas pressure in a rigid container. It is released into an applicator as required, by pressure on a valve on top of the container.

Table 6.1 Commonly used spermicides

Product	Manufacturer	pH	Chemical constituent	Storage	Shelf-life	Reapplication if intercourse delayed
Jellies						
Duragel	LRC Products Ltd	6.0–7.0	Nonoxynol-11 2%	30°C	3 years	3 hours
Ortho-gynol	Ortho	4.5	p-di-isobutylphenoxy polyethoxyethanol	Room temp.	3 years	Any subsequent coitus or delay of a few hours
Gynol II	Ortho	4.5–4.7	Nonoxynol-9 2%	Cool place	2 years	Any subsequent coitus or delay of a few hours
Staycept	Syntex	4.25–4.75	Octoxynol 1%	Cool place	2 years	1 hour
Creams						
Duracreme	LRC Procucts Ltd	6.0–7.0	Nonoxynol-11 2%	30°C	3 years	3 hours
Orthocreme	Ortho	6.0	Nonoxynol-9 2%	Room temp.	3 years	Any subsequent coitus or delay of a few hours
Pessaries						
Orthoforms	Ortho	4.5–5.0	Nonoxynol-9 5%	Cool place	3 years	1 hour
Staycept	Syntex	4.25–5.25	Nonoxynol-9 6%	Cool place	2 years	1 hour
Double check	FP Sales Ltd	5.0	Nonoxynol-9 6%	Cool place	2 years	1 hour
Foams						
Delfen	Ortho	4.5–5.0	Nonoxynol-9 12.5%	Room temp.	3 years	1 hour
C-film	Arun Products Ltd	5.0–7.0	Nonoxynol-9 28%	Room temp.	5 years	Each act of coitus, active for 2 hours
Sponge	FP Sales Ltd	4.7	Nonoxynol-9 1g	Room temp.	3 years	Effective for 24 hours

C-film

This consists of squares of water-soluble, semi-transparent film which dissolve rapidly in the vagina to release nonoxynol-9.

Mode of action of spermicides

The action of spermicides is twofold:

1. The base material of the preparation physically blocks sperm progression.
2. An active chemical kills sperm without damaging other body tissues.

Effectiveness

Nonoxynol-9 and its derivatives are unable to diffuse into cervical mucus and retain spermicidal action therein. Sperm, which enter the cervical mucus before being immobilized by spermicide within the vagina, can survive and ascend the genital tract. Therefore, when used in isolation, spermicides are ineffective contraceptives. Failure rates have been reported as low as 3 per 100 woman years and as high as 28 per 100 woman years.

Indications

1. Spermicides are used in conjunction with diaphragms, condoms, IUDs (Ch. 5) and coitus interruptus to increase the effectiveness of these methods.
2. To give some measure of protection against sexually transmissible diseases. They have been known for some time to give significant protection against bacterial infections, but also appear to inactivate HIV rapidly in vitro. To date, no data exist to show that spermicides are active against HIV in vivo.

Contraindications

1. Allergy in either partner.
2. Aerosol foam should not be used with the diaphragm because, if pressure builds up in the vagina, the cap could possibly be displaced.

Advantages

1. Provide extra lubrication if dryness is a problem.
2. Readily available without a prescription.
3. No evidence of topical vaginal toxicity and very limited, if any, systemic absorption.
4. Protection against carcinoma of the cervix.

Disadvantages

1. Unacceptably high failure rate when used alone.
2. Require premeditation prior to intercourse.
3. Varying degrees of 'messiness' according to the preparation.
4. Vaginal pessaries are unsuitable for use in tropical countries, as they melt. However, melted pessaries will solidify if cooled in the pack, and still retain their activity.
5. Aerosol preparations may be difficult to use if the container is not shaken properly. They are also expensive.
6. Occasional complaints of an unpleasant odour, stinging or discomfort in the vagina.
7. Usage of spermicides greatly in excess of normal doses can cause lesions and ulceration within the vagina as a dose-related effect. The damaged vaginal epithelium could enhance the entry of sexually transmissible organisms.
8. There is no apparent increase in spontaneous abortion or fetal abnormality associated with spermicide use in the periconceptional phase despite past anxiety over this issue.

Instructions to patients

1. Creams and jellies may be inserted into the vagina with an applicator 2–3 minutes before intercourse, or on an occlusive pessary (pp. 158–159). A dose of 2 g is adequate.
2. Foaming tablets are slightly moistened and inserted high into the vagina 3–10 minutes before intercourse.
3. Pessaries are inserted about 15 minutes before intercourse.
4. One applicatorful of foam should be inserted into the vagina just before intercourse (Fig. 6.21). The aerosol can is shaken well to ensure adequate mixture of the spermicide and the foam.
5. C-film is inserted with the finger high into the vagina, ideally over the cervix 3–5 minutes before intercourse. Alternatively, it may be placed over the glans penis and transferred into the

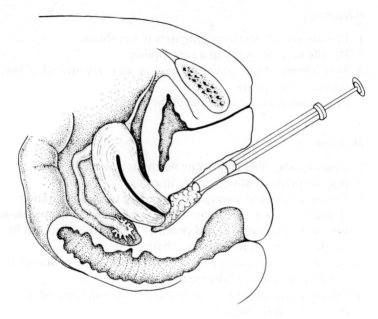

Fig. 6.21   Foam insertion.

vagina in this way. It may be applied to the upper surface of the diaphragm instead of cream or jelly by those who find the latter too messy.
6. If spermicide is inserted more than 2 hours before intercourse takes place a second dose of spermicide should be used.

The vaginal contraceptive sponge

The contraceptive sponge has been researched and marketed extensively in the United States, but has achieved less popularity in the UK. Under the brand name Today it can be purchased over the counter and is available free from some family planning clinics. It consists of a soft, white circular sponge 5.5 cm in diameter, made of polyurethane foam and impregnated with 1 g nonoxynol-9. A polyester loop is attached to facilitate removal (Fig. 6.22). It should be inserted high into the vagina, with the indented surface positioned over the cervix. The spermicide is activated when the sponge is moistened prior to insertion. A new sponge called Protectaid (p. 179) may offer particularly effective anti-HIV action.

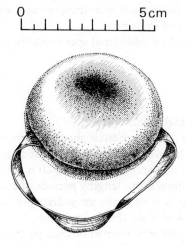

Fig. 6.22   Today vaginal contraceptive sponge.

Mode of action

The Today sponge prevents pregnancy in three ways: as a barrier, as a mechanism for absorbing semen and as a carrier for spermicide.

Effectiveness

Studies in the UK comparing the sponge and diaphragm found the sponge to be much less reliable. However, in the United States the failure rates were found to be similar, particularly in nulliparous women. Generally, women have found it to be a very acceptable addition to the range of barrier methods of contraception.

Indications

1. Women who want to use a vaginal method of contraception but do not wish to seek medical advice or fitting.
2. Women of lower fertility, such as lactating mothers or perimenopausal women, and those spacing pregnancies.

Advantages

1. One size is suitable for most women, although it has been suggested that a larger size of sponge may reduce the risk of pregnancy in parous women. It can be purchased across the counter without the need for fitting or prescription.

2. Women find it convenient and simple to use, and particularly like the absence of messiness.
3. There is no need for additional spermicide before each act of intercourse.

Disadvantages

1. The relatively high failure rate.
2. Small numbers of cases of toxic shock syndrome have been reported, but the overall risk appears to be in the region of 1 case per 2 million sponges used, which is reassuring. Traumatic manipulation, lengthy periods of insertion and use during menstruation or in the immediate postpartum period increase the risk of toxic shock syndrome.
3. A very small number of women or their partners may be sensitive to the spermicide.
4. Expensive.

Instructions for use

1. The sponge must be moistened thoroughly and inserted high into the vagina (Fig. 6.23).

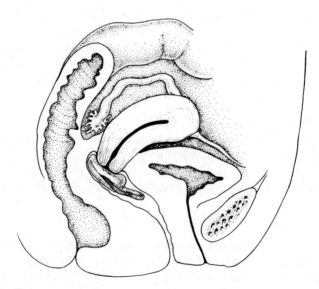

Fig 6.23   Today sponge in situ.

2. It may be left in situ for up to 24 hours.
3. Intercourse may be repeated as often as desired during this time.
4. The sponge should be kept in place for at least 6 hours after the last intercourse, removed and then thrown away.
5. Use during menstruation should be avoided.
6. It may be kept in place whilst swimming or bathing.

New spermicides and delivery systems

Chlorhexidine   This broad-spectrum antiseptic is being actively investigated as a vaginal contraceptive. It has spermicidal action comparable to nonoxynol-9 but can permeate cervical mucus and retains undiminished spermicidal action therein (Chantler 1992). In addition it appears active against sexually transmissible infections including HIV.

Cholic acid   This exerts strong spermicidal and antiviral activity. It is combined with low concentrations of nonoxynol-9 and the surfactant benzalkonium chloride in the new Protectaid sponge. This new combination is being evaluated to offer contraception with particularly effective anti-HIV action.

Gramicidin   This antibacterial agent appears to exert marked HIV inactivation in vitro and is being considered for clinical application as a spermicide with antiviral activity.

Propranolol   Currently being evaluated as a vaginal contraceptive, this appears to be as effective as conventional spermicides. It acts by inhibition of sperm motility but is unlikely to offer protection against sexually transmissible diseases.

ADAPTATIONS OF COITAL TECHNIQUE

Coitus interruptus

This is the oldest method of birth control, widely used in Christian and Muslim communities but less so in Oriental countries. It was first described in the Bible (Genesis 38, verse 9) when Onan spilled his seed on the ground to prevent conception when forced to sleep with his brother's wife. St Augustine based his condemnation of contraception on this, leading eventually to the doctrine set out in *Humanae Vitae* which still today condemns the practice of coitus interruptus.

Description

Coitus interruptus is the withdrawal of the erect penis from the vagina before ejaculation. It is described by users as 'being careful', 'withdrawal' and by local euphemisms implying stopping before the effective 'end of the line'. When questioned, users often claim not to use contraception, and unless asked specifically about coitus interruptus a false history of infertility may be assumed. The method requires discipline on the part of the male and is practised most successfully by those able to recognize the imminence of orgasm and to withdraw quickly prior to ejaculation. Unfortunately, it is often the method practised unsuccessfully by young inexperienced males.

It has been estimated that 4% of the sexually active population in the UK rely on coitus interruptus as their method of contraception.

Mode of action

Since ejaculation occurs outside the vagina, semen is not deposited within the vagina and pregnancy should not ensue. However, pre-ejaculatory secretions containing thousands of sperm may escape from the urethra during penetration, resulting in pregnancy.

Effectiveness

Failure rates vary with the age and experience of the couple and range from 5 to 20 per 100 woman years.

Advantages

1. No equipment, preparation or medical supervision required.
2. Costs nothing.
3. No serious side-effects.
4. Allows total privacy about the couple's sexual relationship.

Disadvantages

1. High failure rate.
2. No protection from sexually transmissible diseases.
3. Limits full enjoyment of sexual intercourse.

Coitus reservatus

This involves vaginal penetration but restriction of movement, so that intravaginal stimulation does not lead to ejaculation either within or outside the vagina.

Coitus designed to avoid the vagina

Coitus interfemora This practice involves the stimulation of the erect penis and ejaculation between the thighs of the woman.

Oral and anal sex These variations are practised increasingly. Contraceptive counsellors should expect the possibility of their discussion, especially in relation to sexually transmissible diseases.

RISKS/BENEFITS

Selection of a barrier method of contraception is often a matter of compromise between advantages and disadvantages. Any method of contraception is always better than none, and the most effective method is the one the patient chooses to use. Medical advisers can ensure that barrier methods are used effectively and happily. Failures with occlusive methods do occur. Patients may be at risk of pregnancy following dislodgement of a diaphragm or a burst sheath. In these situations, couples should be aware of the widespread availability of postcoital contraception (Ch. 9).

REFERENCES.

Bounds W, Guillebaud J, Newman G B 1992 Female condom (Femidom). A clinical study of its use-effectiveness and patient acceptability. British Journal of Family Planning 18: 36–41

Bounds W 1994 Contraceptive efficacy of the diaphragm and cervical caps used in conjunction with a spermicide – a fresh look at the evidence. British Journal of Family Planning 20: 84–87

Chantler E 1992 Vaginal spermicides: some current concerns. British Journal of Family Planning 17: 118–119

Office of Population Censuses and Surveys 1991 General Household Survey 1989. HMSO, London

Steiner M, Foldesy R, Cole D, Carter E 1992 Study to determine the correlation between condom breakage in human use and laboratory test results. Contraception 46: 279–288

Steiner M, Piedrahita C, Glover L, Joanis C 1993 Can condom users likely to experience condom failure be identified? Family Planning Perspectives. 25: 220223 and 226

7. Natural regulation of fertility

Margaret Foxwell
Peter Howie

Scientific basis of natural family planning methods

Methods
  Calendar method
  Basal body temperature (BBT) method
    Instructions
    Interpretation
  Ovulation (mucus: Billings) method
    Instructions
    Interpretation
    Ovulation method during breastfeeding
  Cervical palpation method
  Sympto-thermal method
  Multiple index method
    (double check)

Effectiveness
  Variable effectiveness of BBT

Advantages

Disadvantages

Training of natural family planning teachers

Future prospects
  Intelligent thermometers
  Cervical mucus
  Hormone measurements

NFP choice

Family planning after childbirth
  Breastfeeding and fertility
  Clinical events after delivery
  Lactational amenorrhoea method (LAM)
  Complementary family planning options
    for breastfeeding women
    Barriers and spermicides
    Hormonal methods
    IUDs
    Natural methods
    Sterilization

Appendix

Natural family planning (NFP) is defined as voluntary avoidance of intercourse during the fertile phase of the menstrual cycle in order to avoid pregnancy. NFP thus involves a continual awareness of fertility status including the day of ovulation (Flynn 1988).

Fertility awareness can be used either to achieve or postpone pregnancy and provides a method for those who do not wish to use other methods of contraception. If it is intended to postpone pregnancy, then abstinence is mandatory during the fertile period.

The first method of NFP to be developed was the Rhythm or Calendar method. It is based on the fact that ovulation occurs about 2 weeks before menstruation, regardless of the length of the woman's cycle and on the belief that the life span of the sperm was once thought to be 3 days and of the ovum 2 days. Using this information it is then possible to calculate the time in the cycle when the woman is most likely to be fertile (fertile period) and to avoid intercourse during that time. The method is not very effective and has been virtually abandoned in NFP clinics.

Improved understanding of reproductive physiology has led to the development of more reliable methods of NFP, based on biological indicators rather than on mathematical calculations of the fertile period. These include basal body temperature (BBT), ovulation method (mucus: Billings) and multiple index methods.

SCIENTIFIC BASIS OF NFP METHODS

The ovarian or menstrual cycle lasts an average of 28 days with a normal range of 21–35 days. The cycle is divided into:

1. The first 'half' or follicular phase, when the egg is developing inside the graafian follicle within the ovary.
2. The second 'half' or luteal phase when, following ovulation (the actual release of the egg from the ovary), the cells within the follicle change character to become the corpus luteum.

Whatever the duration of the cycle, and provided ovulation occurs, it is the luteal phase of the cycle which is constant in length (around 14 days), and the follicular phase which changes. In a 35-day cycle ovulation will occur around day 21, and in a 23-day cycle around day 9; thus ovulation occurs not 14 days from the start of the cycle but 14 days before the end of one cycle and the beginning of the next. This point is fundamental to the understanding of the calendar method of NFP.

The developing ovarian follicle secretes increasing concentrations of oestrogen as the egg matures. Oestrogen concentrations reach a peak 24 hours or so before ovulation, triggering the release of a surge of luteinizing hormone (LH) from the pituitary, which stimulates ovulation itself. After ovulation, the corpus luteum secretes increasing amounts of progesterone, concentrations of which reach a maximum at around the mid-luteal phase. Changes in cervical mucus are a result of the cyclical fluctuations in oestrogen and progesterone (Fig. 7.1).

The signs and symptoms produced by hormonal fluctuation during the menstrual cycle can be observed by the woman. They are known as *clinical indicators* and form the basis of NFP methods. The life span of the ovum is not more than 24 hours after its release from the ovary. Under optimal conditions, the life span of the sperm is now recognized to be not more than 6 days.

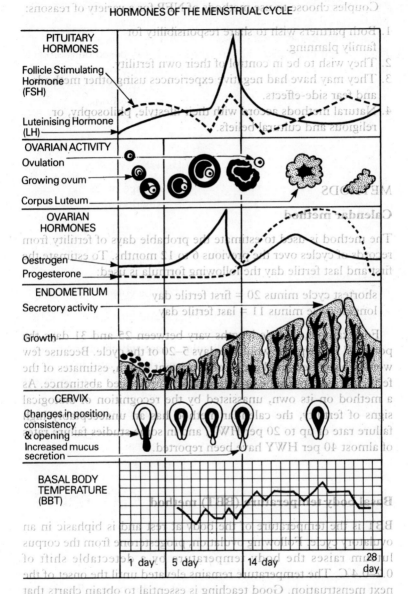

Fig. 7.1 Hormones of the menstrual cycle (reproduced with kind permission of Dr Anna Flynn).

Couples choose to use methods of NFP for a variety of reasons:

1. Both partners wish to share responsibility for family planning.
2. They wish to be in control of their own fertility.
3. They may have had negative experiences using other methods and fear side-effects.
4. Natural methods accord with their lifestyle, philosophy, or religious and cultural beliefs.

METHODS

Calendar method

The method is used to estimate the probable days of fertility from records of cycles over the previous 6 to 12 months. To estimate the first and last fertile day the following formula is used:

shortest cycle minus 20 = first fertile day
longest cycle minus 11 = last fertile day

For example, if cycle lengths vary between 25 and 31 days the potential fertile phase would be days 5–20 of the cycle. Because few women have menstrual cycles of consistent length, estimates of the fertile period have to be broad, requiring prolonged abstinence. As a method on its own, unassisted by the recognition of biological signs of fertility, the calendar method has an unacceptably high failure rate of up to 20 per HWY, and in some studies failure rates of almost 40 per HWY have been reported.

Basal body temperature (BBT) method (at rest)

BBT is the temperature of the body at rest and is biphasic in an ovulatory cycle. Following ovulation, progesterone from the corpus luteum raises the body temperature by a detectable shift of 0.2–0.4°C. The temperature remains elevated until the onset of the next menstruation. Good teaching is essential to obtain charts that are easy to interpret. 10% of charts are difficult to interpret but users improve with experience. The thermal shift due to ovulation is small but easily identifiable if the temperature is recorded under standard conditions, and if a properly designed chart is used (not a standard clinical temperature chart).

Instructions

1. Record the temperature at approximately the same time each morning, immediately on waking, before getting out of bed, drinking tea or any other activity.
2. Use an ovulation thermometer, as its expanded scale 36–38°C makes it easier to read, or use a digital thermometer which reduces the recording time to 45 seconds, and gives an easy and reliable reading.
3. Record the temperature orally for 5 minutes, or vaginally or rectally for 3 minutes. Whichever route is chosen it must be used consistently throughout the cycle.
4. Record the temperature as a dot in the centre of the square on the line. If the mercury stops between two marks record the lower reading.
5. Record any disturbances such as cold, 'flu, any alteration to normal time of waking, or a late night especially when alcohol is consumed.
6. Start a new chart on the first day of menstruation. This enables the temperature shift in relation to the cycle length to be seen at a glance.

Interpretation

The postovulatory infertile phase begins once three consecutive daily temperatures have been recorded which are at a higher level than the previous six consecutive daily readings. (Days 1–4 of the cycle, and any disturbances as described above are excluded.)

The three-over-six rule can be easily identified if a cross is drawn on the chart with the three high temperatures in the top right segment and the previous six low temperatures in the bottom left segment (Fig. 7.2). Intercourse can take place safely from the third morning of the elevated temperature until the onset of the next menstruation.

A 'spike' temperature may occur. This is defined as a temperature which is usually more than 0.2°C above the previous recordings. It may be caused by disturbances previously discussed. One spike among the six consecutive lower temperatures may be ignored. A rise in temperature due to an illness such as 'flu is quite different; the temperature rises to fever level and can be easily distinguished.

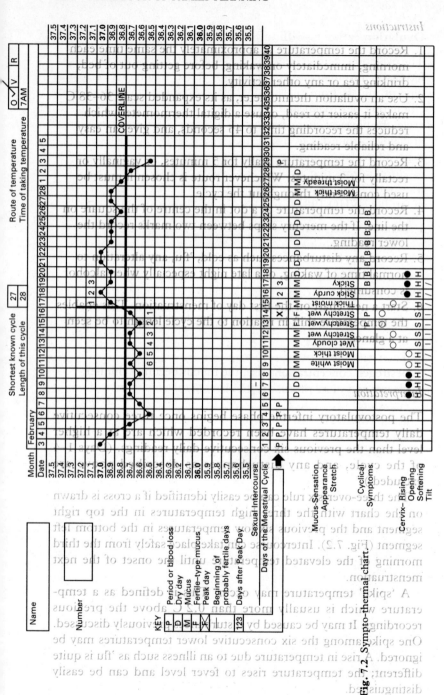

Fig. 7.2 Sympto-thermal chart.

Ovulation (mucus: Billings) method

The ovulation method depends upon the fact that the occurrence of fertility in a woman is accompanied by the secretion of a particular type of mucus from the cervical glands. Under the influence of circulating oestrogen and progesterone at different times of the cycle, the physical characteristics of the mucus undergo a sequence of changes from day to day. *Fertile type mucus* indicates the imminence of ovulation and facilitates the passage of sperm. *Infertile type mucus* confirms that ovulation has occurred and inhibits sperm transport. The woman can be taught to recognize her outward signs of fertility (WHO 1981a).

1. Following menstruation 'dry days' may be experienced (Fig. 7.3). A positive sensation of dryness is felt at the vulva and no mucus is seen. The number of dry days may vary in each cycle – many in a long cycle, few if any, in a short cycle.
2. The change of sensation from dryness to moistness at the vulva will occur at the first appearance of mucus, which may be observed as cloudy, yellowy white in colour and of a sticky, tacky consistency.
3. Then with the approach of ovulation and the peak of fertility as oestrogen concentrations rise, the mucus becomes thinner, clearer and more profuse (often having the consistency of raw egg white) which produces a smooth and lubricated sensation at the vulva. The last day of any lubricated sensation, or appearance of fertile mucus is described as the 'peak day'. The peak can be recognized as such only in retrospect (WHO 1983).

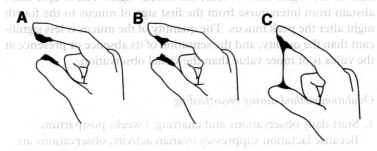

Fig. 7.3 Changes in cervical mucus. **A.** Infertile mucus – cloudy, white and sticky. **B.** Intermediate mucus – less cloudy but not stretchy. **C.** Fertile mucus – clear, slippery and stretchy.

4. Following the peak and with the onset of progesterone secretion by the corpus luteum the mucus changes abruptly to a sticky, flaky type, or disappears altogether. There is a definite sensation of dryness at the vulva. This phase continues until the onset of the next menstruation.

Instructions

A charting system is used to record daily observations (Fig. 7.4). To enable couples to recognize the mucus signs, they are advised to abstain during the first learning cycle.

1. Start charting on the first day of menstruation.
2. Record each day's observation at night.
3. Make observations throughout the day when going to the toilet. Use toilet tissue to wipe the vulva before and after micturition.
4. Mucus, when present, can be picked up between thumb and first finger to test its capacity to stretch (Spinnbarkeit).
5. If a combination of different types of mucus is observed the most fertile characteristics of the mucus over the entire day are recorded at night.
6. Record the 'peak day' with an X.
7. Record the following three days 1.2.3.

Interpretation

To aid interpretation, intercourse should be avoided during days of menstrual loss because during a short cycle bleeding may mask the onset of mucus. During dry days following menstruation intercourse should take place on alternate nights only, as the presence of seminal fluid in the vagina may obscure the mucus signs. The couple must abstain from intercourse from the first sign of mucus to the fourth night after the peak mucus. The quantity of the mucus is less significant than the quality, and the sensation of its absence or presence at the vulva is of more value than the visual observation.

Ovulation method during breastfeeding

1. Start daily observations and charting 3 weeks postpartum. Because lactation suppresses ovarian activity, observations are made for 2 weeks to find the basic infertile pattern (BIP) which may be characterized by continuous dry days; continuous mucus without change from day to day – sticky and opaque or

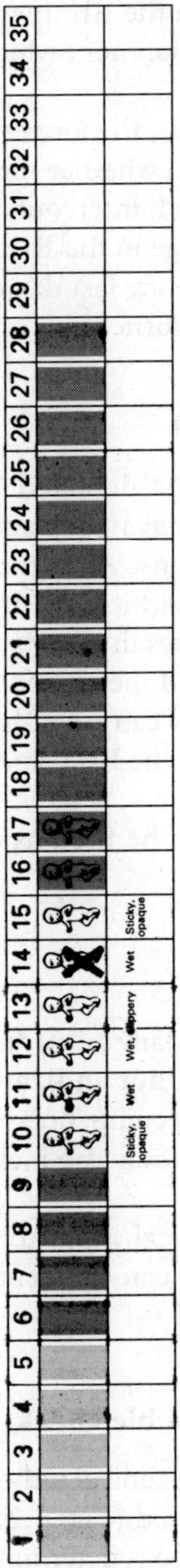

Fig. 7.4 Ovulation method.

watery or of a milky character; or a combination of dry days and mucus. Any change in the BIP may indicate ovarian activity and follicular development which signals a possible return of fertility.

2. Record the number of feeds, the longest interval between feeds, the use of supplements and whether the baby is fed at night.

3. When the BIP is recognized, intercourse may take place on alternate nights. Any change in the BIP requires abstinence until the fourth night from the last day of the change, i.e. 4 nights after the BIP has returned.

Cervical palpation method

Changes in the cervix can be detected by daily palpation by a woman or her partner. This may not be acceptable to some women for cultural or aesthetic reasons. After menstruation, the cervix is low in the pelvis and easily felt; it feels firm and dry and the os is closed. As ovulation approaches the cervix rises upwards by 1–2 cm, feels soft and wet to touch and the os opens.

Self palpation of the cervix can be of help during breastfeeding and the perimenopause when the BBT and cervical mucus changes may be difficult to interpret.

Cervical palpation can also be used as part of a multiple index method.

Sympto-thermal method

This method combines the daily recording of the BBT, cervical mucus observations and minor indicators of fertility such as mid-cycle pain, spotting or bleeding, breast symptoms, bloatedness and mood changes. Some women also include daily changes in the cervix.

Using more than one clinical indicator increases the accuracy with which the fertile period can be identified, thus reducing the length of abstinence required.

Multiple index method (double check)

This method combines all the clinical indicators to detect the fertile period with the calendar method (Fig. 7.2).

The onset of the fertile period is determined by cross-checking the first day of the mucus signs with the calendar calculation (i.e. the shortest cycle minus 20) – whichever indicator comes first marks the onset of the fertile period. The fourth day of peak mucus is cross-checked against the morning of the third day after the BBT shift – whichever indicator comes last marks the end of the fertile period.

EFFECTIVENESS

In theory, NFP methods are very effective but because of the abstinence required during the fertile phase they are all open to user failure, as couples often break the rules. The theoretical failure rate is 1–5 per HWY depending on the method used. However, since effectiveness depends so much on motivation the actual failure rate may be as high as 30 per HWY; or as low as 2.2 per HWY when used meticulously (WHO 1981b). Motivation also varies according to whether the methods are being used to avoid or delay pregnancy. The WHO prospective trial of 725 couples using the ovulation (mucus) method, found the failure rate for couples wishing to avoid pregnancy was 17.1 per HWY, compared with 22.2 per HWY for those wanting simply to delay the next pregnancy.

Variable effectiveness of BBT

1. When intercourse is confined to the postovulatory part of the cycle only, the failure rate is only 1.2–6.6 per HWY.
2. When using BBT plus the calendar method to indicate infertile days in the preovulatory phase so as to allow intercourse then, the failure rate is 5.0–19.3 per HWY.

Studies on NFP effectiveness have shown that a single index method is less efficient than the multiple index method.

Motivation is essential for the successful use of any method of family planning and this is particularly true of NFP. A couple's motivation is increased if they have a knowledge and understanding of the basic principles of reproduction and of the woman's signs of fertility. They should know what they are doing and why. Both need to be committed, and each must cooperate with one another, especially where, in the use of periodic abstinence to postpone pregnancy, adjustments to their sexual behaviour are required.

Periodic abstinence may not be acceptable particularly if one partner is less motivated than the other. Couples may then decide to use barrier methods during the fertile period. For this combination to be effective, the woman must observe her signs of fertility with the same care as she would if abstaining during the fertile phase and appreciate the fact that barrier methods can fail. It should be noted that the use of the diaphragm and spermicides make the recognition of the mucus signs difficult if not impossible.

ADVANTAGES

1. No deleterious physical side-effects.
2. No follow-up required (after proper instruction) once efficient use is achieved.
3. Morally and culturally acceptable in any society where a period of abstinence is accepted and other methods of contraception are not.
4. Many couples value their increased self-awareness and the knowledge of their own fertility.
5. Promotes involvement of the man and enhances a couple's relationship, being dependent as it is upon mutual respect, understanding and communication.
6. Can be taught to most women regardless of culture and level of education. Effective use of most methods can be learned within 3 months (WHO 1981b).
7. The methods are applicable to all phases of a woman's life whether her periods are regular or not; during adolescence; when breastfeeding or approaching the menopause.
8. NFP can be used either to achieve or postpone pregnancy.

DISADVANTAGES

1. The learning period of about 3 months is relatively long.
2. Keeping daily records of signs and symptoms of fertility, particularly for the multiple index method, may be irksome.
3. The commitment and cooperation of both partners is essential because if one is not motivated the method is likely to be discontinued.
4. Periodic abstinence (6–16 days depending on the method used) is essential, possibly requiring an adjustment of sexual behaviour. This may cause emotional stress for some couples.
5. Not a suitable method for those not in a stable relationship.
6. Mucus changes may be difficult to observe or interpret in the presence of vaginal infection or after treatment to the cervix e.g. cautery, conization, or laser.

7. Since failure of NFP may result from acts of intercourse occurring when sperm and egg are 'ageing', it was thought that there might be a possible increased risk of spontaneous abortion or congenital malformation. However, the WHO study (WHO 1984) concludes that these risks are no greater than those expected in the general community, or following failure of any other method of family planning.

TRAINING OF NFP TEACHERS

The successful use of NFP depends on adequate initial teaching by a competent instructor. To acquire the necessary skills to teach NFP, attendance at a recognized course is necessary. The National Associations for Natural Family Planning run courses for health professionals and non-medically qualified personnel combining theory and supervised practical sessions (see useful addresses).

FUTURE PROSPECTS

All NFP methods rely on the couple abstaining from intercourse during the fertile period. The longer the period of abstinence required, the more difficult it is to obey the rules. Most research initiatives are aimed at developing ways of detecting more accurately the start and end of the fertile period, allowing a shorter period of abstinence.

Intelligent thermometers

In an effort to improve and simplify the measurement of BBT, electronic digital readout thermometers have been developed. The simplest display the temperature and calculate whether there has been a significant rise compared with the temperature recorded on the preceding days. Others combine the BBT reading with the calendar method and indicate by means of red or green lights whether or not it is safe to have intercourse. The most sophisticated device 'The Rabbit' (Rabbit Computer Company, Los Angeles, USA) uses BBT measurements for up to 12 preceding cycles to predict the beginning of the fertile period and not just the end.

All these devices are relatively expensive and require some degree of sophistication on the part of the user.

In future, skin patches containing heat sensors may become available, eliminating the need for thermometers. It is possible that such novel and accurate measuring devices might increase the acceptability of the use of BBT measurements for detecting ovulation.

Cervical mucus

The mucus method relies on the detection of qualitative changes in the character of cervical mucus. The quantity of mucus also alters during the cycle. Disposable calibrated syringes have been developed to allow women to aspirate cervicovaginal fluid and record daily volumes. An increase in fluid volume occurs 1 to 8 days before ovulation and reaches a maximum 24 to 48 hours before the peak.

Other approaches involve the measurement of cervical mucus conductivity, uteroglobin content, guaiacol peroxidase, and mucus peroxidase. At present these measurements require complicated laboratory procedures but it is not inconceivable that a litmus paper test for some constituents of cervical mucus may some day become available.

Hormone measurements

Measurement of oestrogen and progesterone in saliva, urine and breast milk would allow couples to use home kits to determine the fertile period. Over-the-counter kits are available for detecting the LH surge (and thus impending ovulation). They are expensive and are mainly used by couples wishing to achieve rather than to avoid a pregnancy. Kits designed to measure urinary oestrogen or pregnanediol or the ratio between them are being tested.

NFP CHOICE

NFP methods are often not mentioned unless a specific request is made. Individuals or couples may not be aware of this choice and that it may be an acceptable, even preferable, alternative for them at that time.

Health professionals should know about modern methods of NFP, be prepared to discuss them with those seeking contraceptive advice, and if not been trained to teach NFP methods, should be ready to refer those who are interested to a qualified teacher.

FAMILY PLANNING AFTER CHILDBIRTH

After having a baby, the great majority of mothers wish to postpone the next pregnancy until they are physically and socially ready to have another child. If a mother bottle-feeds from birth or fails to establish breastfeeding, normal ovulatory menstrual cycles will usually return between 5 and 12 weeks postpartum so that contraception should be started around 4 weeks after delivery (Howie & McNeilly 1982).

In breastfeeding mothers, there is a variable period of ovarian suppression which can last for a year or more. This contraceptive effect of breastfeeding is particularly important in those developing countries where contraception is not readily available or not culturally acceptable during lactational amenorrhoea. New guidelines describing the lactational amenorrhoea method (LAM) have been devised for mothers who wish to use breastfeeding either to space their pregnancies or delay starting alternative contraception.

Breastfeeding and fertility

Evidence that successful breastfeeding delays the return of fertility comes from a number of sources:

1. Delayed return of menstrual cycles – the phase of lactational amenorrhoea.
2. Lower pregnancy rates in breastfeeding mothers than in bottle-feeding mothers when contraception is not used.
3. Hormonal and ultrasound studies showing absent or impaired ovarian function during breastfeeding, especially during the phase of lactational amenorrhoea.

The key to the inhibition of fertility during lactation is the sucking of the infant which disrupts the hypothalamo-pituitary-ovarian axis. Nipple stimulation during sucking sends neural impulses to the maternal hypothalamus and interferes with the normal pulsatile secretion of pituitary hormones. As the intensity of infant sucking reduces, the ovarian activity of the breast feeding mother progressively returns to normal.

Clinical events after delivery

The breastfeeding mother passes through a series of different phases associated with her returning fertility (Fig. 7.5).

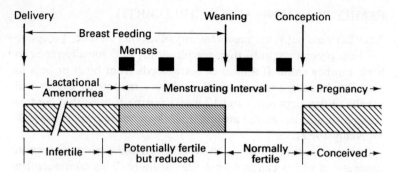

Fig. 7.5 Fertility during the interbirth interval, involving the phases of lactational amenorrhoea, the menstruating interval and pregnancy.

During the greatest part of lactational amenorrhoea, the mother is infertile because ovulation is inhibited and there is no endometrial growth. The first menstrual bleed is a sign of returning ovarian activity. The cycle before first menstruation may be ovulatory *so that the mother may conceive at this stage*. The chances of this happening increase with time after delivery and become more likely in those mothers who abruptly reduce sucking frequency and duration.

After the end of lactational amenorrhoea, the majority of breast-feeding mothers notice a progressive return to normal menstrual cycles. As the infant's sucking reduces, there is only limited ovarian follicle development and endometrial growth, and at this stage the mother may have light, anovular bleeds, but remain infertile. When breastfeeding occurs less frequently, inhibition from the sucking becomes minimal, ovulation and normal menstruation will occur and the mother is potentially fertile, although her fertility may still be reduced compared to her own non-lactating cycles.

After weaning, all inhibition is removed and the mother returns to normal fertility.

The lactational amenorrhoea method (LAM)

The frequency of breastfeeding, presence or absence of artificial feeds, the baby's age (i.e. time since delivery) and the return of menses can all be used to give some indication of the return of ovulation and, therefore, fertility.

The times at which menstruation and ovulation resume in breastfeeding mothers varies widely between populations and

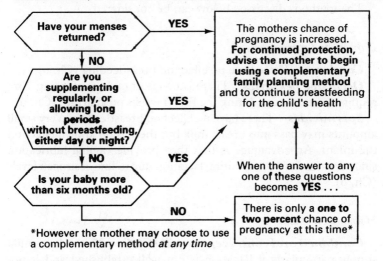

Fig. 7.6 The algorithm of the lactational amenorrhoea method
(after Labbok et al 1994).

between mothers within the same population. LAM represents a
series of consensus guidelines based on an algorithm with a set of
defined rules to work from (Fig. 7.6). It was designed to be in an
easy format to teach to health workers and their clients and should
be regarded as an introductory family planning method. Mothers
should still be encouraged to introduce complementary methods at
an appropriate time during breastfeeding. LAM is a method
acceptable to most religious and cultural groups. If used correctly,
it provides highly effective protection during the period defined by
the rules. At the present time, the guidelines are *only valid for the first
6 months postpartum.*

If optimal breastfeeding is encouraged, maternal and child health
will improve and effective child spacing be promoted. Optimal
breastfeeding behaviours are described in Appendix 7.1.

Complementary family planning options for breastfeeding women

All breastfeeding women should be counselled on complementary
family planning methods. The use–effectiveness of all methods will

be higher during breastfeeding than in the non-lactating state because of the inhibition of fertility during lactation.

The methods discussed below can be considered.

Barriers and spermicides

Condoms   These have no effect on breastfeeding (Ch. 6).

Occlusive pessaries   There is no effect on breastfeeding. Size requirements change during the first 6 weeks postpartum (Ch. 6).

Spermicides   These have no effect on breastfeeding. Very small amounts may pass into breast milk but there is no known effect on the infant. An advantage is that they provide vaginal lubrication since dryness may occur during lactation due to low oestrogen levels (Ch. 6).

Hormonal methods

Combined oral contraceptive pill (COC)   This reduces milk supply particularly if lactation is not well established and is not recommended for use during the early months. The progestogen-only pill (POP) is always preferable as COC adds nothing to the efficacy of POP combined with full lactation if menstruation has not been re-established.

POPs: injectables: implants   These are generally thought to have either no effect on milk volume or possibly to slightly enhance it. Some hormone passes into breast milk but there is no evidence of adverse effects on the infant. Their use may be associated with irregular menses towards the end of lactation.

IUDs

These have no effect on breastfeeding. An IUD may be expelled if inserted before day 30 postpartum and insertion requires the skill of a trained health care worker. There is increased risk of perforation. The new levonorgestrel-releasing IUD is suitable during lactation (Ch. 5).

Natural methods

These have no effect on breastfeeding and may be the only method acceptable to some mothers. Fertility signs are more difficult to interpret during lactation and, therefore, extended abstinence is required (p. 190).

Sterilization

Vasectomy   The period of lactational amenorrhoea may give contraceptive cover while waiting for her partner's vasectomy to become effective.

Tubal occlusion   This has no effect on breastfeeding. Short-term mother/infant separation occurs although this is unlikely to jeopardize the success of breastfeeding if it is already established.

Sterilization within the first 3 days of childbirth, although perhaps convenient, is not usually recommended as it is more likely to be regretted, increases the risk of postpartum thromboembolism (p. 210) and may, in theory, interfere with the successful establishment of lactation if mother and baby are separated for a long time.

REFERENCES

Flynn A M, Brooks M 1988 A manual of Natural Family Planning. Unwin Hyman Ltd, London
Howie P W, McNeilly A S 1982 Effect of breast feeding patterns on human birth intervals. Journal of Reproduction and Fertility 65: 545–557
WHO 1981a A prospective multicentre trial of the ovulation method of natural family planning. 1. The teaching phase. Fertility and Sterility 36: 152–158
WHO 1981b A prospective multicentre trial of the ovulation method of natural family planning. 2. The effectiveness phase. Fertility and Sterility 36: 591–598
WHO 1983 A prospective multicentre trial of the ovulation method of natural family planning. 3. Characteristics of the menstrual cycle and the fertile phase. Fertility and Sterility 40: 773–778
WHO 1984 A prospective multicentre trial of the ovulation method of natural family planning. 4. The outcome of pregnancy. Fertility and Sterility 40: 593–59

Appendix 7.1

EIGHT OPTIMAL BREASTFEEDING BEHAVIOURS WHICH ARE COMPATIBLE WITH THE LACTATIONAL AMENORRHOEA METHOD (LAM)

1. Allow new-born to breastfeed as soon as possible after birth, and to remain with the mother for several hours following delivery.
2. Breastfeed frequently, whenever the infant is hungry, both day and night.
3. Breastfeed exclusively for the first 6 months.
4. After the first 6 months when supplemental foods are introduced, breastfeeding should precede each supplemental feeding.
5. Continue to breastfeed for up to 2 years and beyond.
6. Continue breastfeeding even if the mother or the baby becomes ill.
7. Avoid using a bottle, pacifiers (dummies), or other artificial nipples.
8. Mothers should eat and drink sufficient quantities to satisfy their hunger and thirst.

8. Sterilization

Anna Glasier

Female sterilization
  Laparoscopy
  Minilaparotomy
  Techniques
    Diathermy
    Falope ring
    Clips
    Laser
    Non-surgical methods
  Clinical management
    Examination
    Timing of operation and preoperative advice
    Postoperative advice
    Follow-up
  Complications
    Immediate
    Late
Vasectomy
  Techniques
    Division and ligation
    Variations in technique

Clinical management
  Assessment
  Examination
  Timing of operation
  Preoperative and postoperative advice:
    follow-up
  Complications
    Immediate
    Late

Indications

Contraindications

Advantages

Disadvantages

Counselling

Effectiveness

Reversibility

Risks/benefits

Appendices

It has been estimated that worldwide more than 138 million women of reproductive age have chosen sterilization as their method of contraception – a 45% increase over the last decade. Vasectomy too is becoming an increasingly acceptable method of contraception and is used by over 42 million couples throughout the world, the majority of whom live in developing countries.

In Britain almost 50% of couples aged 35–44 are using either female or male sterilization as their method of contraception.

FEMALE STERILIZATION

Female sterilization usually involves the blocking of both fallopian tubes which can be reached either by laparotomy or minilaparotomy or more commonly laparoscopy. Sterilization may also be achieved by the removal of both tubes (salpingectomy) or by hysterectomy, if either procedure is indicated by the presence of gynaecological disease such as hydrosalpinx or fibroids. Although there is probably nothing to choose between minilaparotomy and laparoscopic female sterilization in terms of safety and efficacy, the latter is now the technique of choice, because it allows sterilization to be done as a day case procedure.

Laparoscopy

General anaesthesia (GA) is normally used, although spinal or local anaesthesia (LA) may be employed, particularly in developing countries where skilled anaesthetists may not be available. In the United Kingdom (UK) laparoscopic sterilization is usually performed as a day case procedure.

A pneumoperitoneum is created by the insufflation of nitrous oxide or carbon dioxide into the peritoneal cavity. Through a small subumbilical incision, a trochar and cannula are introduced into the gas-filled abdomen and the trochar replaced by the laparoscope (Fig. 8.1). With a fibre-optic light source connected, the pelvic

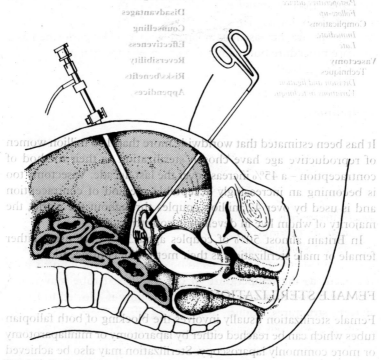

Fig. 8.1 Laparoscopy.

organs are inspected. Operating forceps are introduced through a second cannula inserted either suprapubically or in the iliac fossa. Sterilization is performed either by diathermy or the application of clips or rings to both tubes (see below). After the release of gas from the peritoneal cavity the instruments are withdrawn and the skin incisions closed with sutures (absorbable or non-absorbable), clips or staples.

Minilaparotomy

Laparotomy using a small (3–5 cm) suprapubic incision avoids the need for sophisticated equipment and can be done almost as quickly as laparoscopic sterilization. The uterus is manipulated vaginally to bring the fallopian tubes to the level of the incision. The tubes are delivered through the incision and rings or clips applied. Alternatively the tubes may be ligated using a variety of methods, including the Madlener and Pomeroy techniques, most of which involve excision of a small portion of tube.

In the UK, minilaparotomy is most commonly used when sterilization is performed immediately postpartum; as at that time the uterus is large, the pelvis very vascular, and the risks of laparoscopy are increased. Minilaparotomy may be performed as a day case procedure but many surgeons prefer the patient to stay in hospital for 24–48 hours.

Techniques

Whatever the approach, the fallopian tubes may be blocked or divided in a number of ways.

Diathermy

One or more areas of the tube are cauterized by diathermy (Fig. 8.2) Unipolar diathermy has been replaced by the potentially safer technique of bipolar diathermy which allows only the tissue held between the jaws of the forceps to be cauterized. Local burns may still occur as the temperature of the cauterized tube may reach 300–400°C and thus can cause thermal injury if allowed to touch adjacent structures. Failure to cauterize all the layers of the tube results in a relatively high failure rate and cautery near the cornual portion of the tube is thought to increase the risk of ectopic pregnancy.

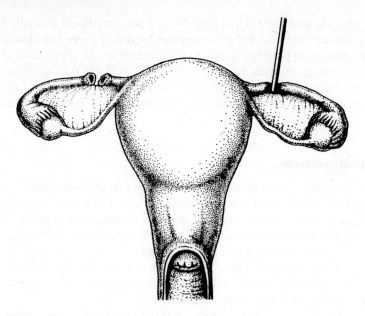

Fig. 8.2 Diathermy coagulation of fallopian tubes.

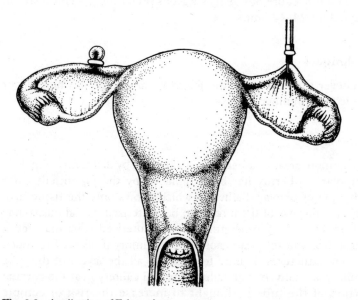

Fig. 8.3 Application of Falope rings.

Falope ring

The ring is made of silicone rubber and, using a specially designed applicator, is placed over a loop of tube (Fig. 8.3). It destroys 2–3 cm of tube and may be difficult to apply if the tube is wide or fibrotic. Ischaemia of the loop causes significant postoperative pain.

Clips

A variety of clips have been designed for tubal occlusion. The clips destroy a much smaller length of tube (Fig. 8.4) and thus allow easier reversal, but special care must be taken to ensure that the whole width of the tube is occluded – some surgeons routinely apply two clips to each tube. Those most commonly used in the UK are probably the Hulka–Clemens clip (Fig. 8.5A) made of stainless steel and a polycarbonate, and the smaller Filshie clip (Fig. 8.5B) made of titanium lined with silicone rubber.

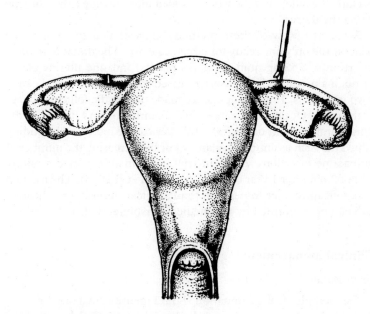

Fig. 8.4 Application of clips.

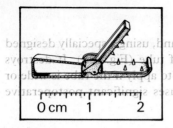 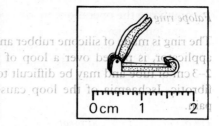

Fig. 8.5   A. Hulka–Clemens clip; **B**. Filshie clip.

Laser

Recent advances in laser technology have led to attempts at division of the tubes by laser vaporization. The carbon dioxide laser divides the tube very cleanly, which ironically may allow a high incidence of spontaneous tubal recanalization, and therefore failure. The Nd:Yag laser, although probably more effective, is extremely expensive.

Non-surgical methods

A number of chemical agents have been tested for their ability to occlude the fallopian tube when instilled into the tube either directly or via the uterus.

A recent review of these methods suggests that the quinacrine pellet is the only one ready for large-scale use. The method involves insertion of 252mg quinacrine (as pellets) into the uterine cavity through a modified IUD inserter passed through the cervical canal. Two insertions, 1 month apart, are made during the follicular phase of the cycle. Occlusion is caused by inflammation and fibrosis of the intramural segment of the tube. Efficacy can be increased by adding adjuvants such as antiprostaglandins or by increasing the number of quinacrine insertions. A recent trial in Vietnam reported a failure rate of 2.6% after 1 year of follow-up (Hieu et al 1993). The method is significantly safer to perform than surgical sterilization, cheaper, and can be performed by nonmedical personnel (Ch. 17).

Clinical management

Examination

1. General physical examination should identify any risks for anaesthesia and any factors which might contraindicate or

complicate the operation, such as previous abdominal operations or gross obesity.
2. Pelvic examination, in order to exclude existing pathology such as ovarian cyst or fibroids, is mandatory and a cervical smear should be taken if indicated.

Timing of operation and preoperative advice

1. It is not usually practical to arrange sterilization for a particular time of the cycle and women should be told to continue using their current method of contraception until their operation. It is not necessary to stop the combined pill before sterilization as the risk of thromboembolic complications is negligible.
2. If an IUD is in situ it should be removed at operation, unless the operation is being done at midcycle and intercourse has taken place within the previous few days.
3. Immediate postpartum or postabortion sterilization is more likely to be regretted and, as discussed earlier (Ch. 2), carries more risks.
4. It is not necessary to shave the pubic area or abdomen before laparoscopy or mini-laparotomy.

Postoperative advice

1. Skin incisions closed with absorbable sutures require no further treatment. If clips or non-absorbable sutures are used they will be removed before leaving hospital, or arrangements made to have this done at home. The wounds will usually heal within 10 days.
2. Slight bruising and discomfort may sometimes be experienced around the wounds for a few days.
3. Gas remaining in the peritoneal cavity often causes abdominal discomfort or shoulder pain for 24–48 hours.
4. Most women return to work within 48 hours of sterilization.
5. A minilaparotomy wound takes a few days longer to heal and heavy lifting should be avoided for about 3 weeks.
6. Female sterilization is effective immediately and sexual activity may be resumed when the couple feel like it.

It may be helpful to provide a leaflet containing a summary of this information (Appendix 8.1).

Follow-up

The patient is usually seen after 6 weeks by her general practitioner (GP), the referring doctor, or the gynaecologist who did the operation. The resumption of menses may be delayed in women who have stopped using the combined pill. However, if the patient is amenorrhoeic pregnancy should always be excluded as she may have already been pregnant at the time of sterilization. If she was previously using an IUD, check that it has been removed.

Complications

Immediate

1. The operation carries a small operative mortality – less than 8 per 100 000 operations.
2. Vascular damage or damage to bowel or other internal organs may occur during the procedure and is usually recognized at the time of operation. Patients should therefore be made aware of the rare need for a laparotomy and consequent longer stay in hospital. Unrecognized bowel damage should be suspected in any patient with unexplained pain, pyrexia and abdominal rigidity occurring within the first 2 weeks of sterilization. Such cases should be referred to hospital urgently.
3. Thromboembolic disease is rare, but is more likely if the procedure is done immediately postpartum.
4. Infection or oozing from the wound does occasionally occur and can be managed symptomatically.

Late

Menstrual cycle   Female sterilization does not alter ovarian activity or menstruation. Kasonde and Bonnar (1976) demonstrated no measurable change in menstrual blood loss following sterilization in women who had been using barrier methods of contraception. Women who stop using the combined pill will almost certainly notice that their periods become heavier, perhaps more painful and less predictable, and should be warned of this. In contrast, women whose previous method of contraception was an IUD, will notice an improvement in their bleeding patterns. Despite this, there have been a number of studies which have demonstrated an increased incidence of hysterectomy among women who have been sterilized (Templeton & Cole 1982, Rulin et al 1993). Bearing in mind the inevitable changes in menstrual bleeding patterns associated with advancing age and with stopping the combined pill (the most commonly used method of reversible contraception) it may be that women who have been sterilized are more likely to seek hysterectomy, or more willing to accept it, if they are already incapable of further childbearing.

Abdominal pain and dyspareunia These may occur after sterilization and are said to be more common after cautery. Repeat laparoscopy usually fails to demonstrate any pathology and the symptoms may sometimes be a manifestation of regret.

Psychological and psychosexual problems These are rare and when they do arise tend to do so in those who have had problems before sterilization. Many studies in fact report a better mental state after sterilization.

Bowel obstruction Resulting from adhesions, this is a very rare complication.

Ectopic pregnancy This has been reported in up to 50% of failures following cautery and in 4% following mechanical occlusive methods (Filshie 1989). Women should be advised that *if they miss a period and have symptoms of pregnancy they should seek medical advice urgently.*

VASECTOMY

Techniques

Vasectomy involves the division or occlusion of the vas deferens to prevent the passage of sperm. It can be performed under LA or GA. A variety of techniques for vas occlusion is available but the principle is the same in all of them.

Division and ligation

The vas is palpated through the skin of the upper scrotum and fixed either instrumentally or between the fingers and thumb. The vas within its fascial sheath is exposed through a small skin incision, the fascia is opened longitudinally and the vas ligated and divided (Figs 8.6 and 8.7) or occluded with clips or by diathermy. Interposing the fascial sheath between the cut ends of the vas is thought to increase the effectiveness of the procedure. The sheath and scrotal skin are closed separately. The vas may be approached either by a single midline incision or by two incisions, one on each side.

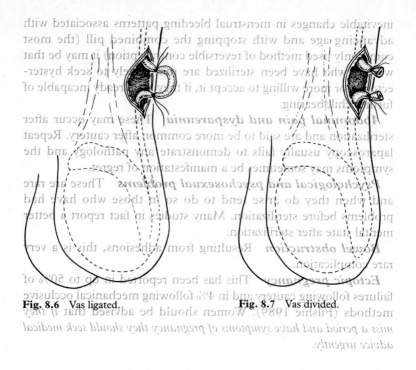

Fig. 8.6 Vas ligated. **Fig. 8.7** Vas divided.

Variations in technique

Excision Excising a small portion of vas is unlikely to increase effectiveness unless at least 4cm of vas is excised and excision makes reversal more difficult. It does, however, allow the portion of vas to be examined histologically which may help in subsequent cases of litigation but also increases the expense of the procedure.

Looping Loop each cut end of vas back on itself.

Clips Occlusion using a small silver clip.

Diathermy Occlusion using unipolar diathermy with a specifically designed probe which is passed one centimetre proximally and distally down the divided vas coagulating the tissue for 3–4 seconds until the muscle becomes opaque.

No-scalpel vasectomy (NSV) Developed in China in 1974 and now quite widely used, this technique makes use of specially designed instruments for isolating and delivering the vas through the scrotal skin and substitutes a small puncture for the skin incision. Any of the standard methods of occlusion may be used. NSV is quick and is associated with a lower incidence of infection and haematoma. A comparison between NSV and conventional vasectomy in Thailand reported a complication rate of 0.4% compared with 3.1% (Nirapathpongporn et al 1990). Training in the technique can be arranged through the Association for Voluntary Surgical Contraception in New York.

Open-ended vasectomy The vas can simply be divided and the cut ends left open. This technique is seldom used as it almost certainly increases failure rates but it does facilitate reversal.

Non-surgical techniques Percutaneous injection of sclerosing agents such as polyurethane elastomers or occlusive substances such as silicone is being used in China. The technique avoids any skin incision and furthermore the silicone plug is said to be easily removed and pregnancy rates of 100% up to 5 years after vasectomy reversal have been claimed (Hargreave 1992).

No large randomized controlled studies have been done to determine whether any one method is more effective than another and efficacy probably depends most on the experience of the surgeon.

Clinical management

Assessment

In addition to the points covered in counselling (p. 218) a history should be taken to exclude any factors which may complicate the operation and which may determine whether LA or GA should be used. These should include:

1. A history of previous genital or inguinal surgery
   e.g. orchidopexy.
2. A history of reaction to LA or contraindications to GA
   (including fear or extreme anxiety).

Examination

In some family planning clinics where vasectomy is done under LA, the man is counselled by a nurse or doctor and not seen by the surgeon until the time of operation. In this case it is good practice to examine the man prior to recommending him for vasectomy. It is annoying for the patient and a waste of operating time if a problem which precludes vasectomy under LA is not discovered until the patient is being prepared for surgery.

Timing of operation

Some surgeons refuse to perform a vasectomy on men whose wives are pregnant and insist that the operation is delayed until after the safe delivery of a healthy baby. While this would seem sensible to most clinicians, some couples see pregnancy as an extremely convenient time during which the vasectomy can become effective. Each couple should be considered individually in respect of the timing of the operation.

Preoperative and postoperative advice: follow-up

The patient is usually asked to shave the upper scrotum himself before he presents for operation – this saves both time and embarrassment.

He is advised to wear underpants which give good scrotal support for a few days after the procedure.

Most men return to work the following day but the risk of haematoma formation is probably reduced if strenuous physical exercise is avoided for 3 or 4 days.

It *must* be made clear that it takes some time for remaining sperm to disappear from the distal portion of the vas and that an alternative method of contraception *must* be used until there is azoospermia. The rate at which azoospermia is achieved depends on the frequency of ejaculation. In developing countries where laboratory facilities for examining seminal fluid do not exist, couples are advised to use other contraception until after 20 ejaculations. In the UK seminal fluid is examined after 12 and 16 weeks and, if sperm are still present, usually monthly thereafter. Not until two consecutive negative samples have been confirmed can the vasectomy be considered to be complete. Instructions for the collection of specimens and their delivery to the laboratory should be given to the patient who should be informed once the vasectomy is complete.

Men who experience complications or in whom vasectomy fails seem to be particularly ready to sue. In order to avoid successful litigation it is imperative that counselling for vasectomy is clear and detailed and covers every eventuality. We have a check list which counsellors tick as they cover all the points in the discussion with the couple. Recently, we have introduced a detailed information leaflet (Appendix 8.2) which is sent out with the first appointment informing the couple about complications and the failure rate before they attend for counselling. They are asked to sign a form stating that they have read and understood the information sheet in addition to the standard form consenting to operation.

Complications

Immediate

Bruising and haematoma Almost everyone will experience scrotal bruising but in 1–2% of men postoperative bleeding will be sufficient to cause a haematoma. Local support and analgesia are usually adequate treatment but a small number of men will require admission to hospital for drainage of the haematoma.

Wound infection This occurs in up to 5% of men and may need treatment with antibiotics.

Failure Up to 2% of men fail to achieve azoospermia. If sperm continue to appear in the ejaculate for months the vasectomy can be re-done. The timing of a 're-do' or exploration is a matter for discussion between the patient and surgeon. The continued presence of sperm may be due to infrequent ejaculation but if this does not appear to be the case and if many sperm are present, it seems a little hard to ask the patient to provide specimens month after month before admitting defeat.

Late

Sperm granulomas Small lumps may form at the cut ends of the vas as a result of a local inflammatory response to leaked sperm. These may be painful and palpable and pain can persist for years. Excision usually solves the problem. Sperm granulomas may also physically unite the cut ends of the vas and increase the chance of failure.

Late recanalization Failure can occur up to 10 years after vasectomy despite two negative samples of seminal fluid following the procedure. It is rare (1 in 1000) but pregnancy as a result of late recanalization is always a sensitive issue. It is not tactful to cast any doubt on the paternity of the pregnancy. Seminal analysis can be offered but if no sperm are seen in the ejaculate this may cause major domestic problems for the couple concerned. Every case must be handled individually but it is sometimes best simply to offer a re-do without semen analysis.

Antisperm antibodies After vasectomy most men develop detectable concentrations of auto-antibodies presumably in response to leakage of sperm. Their presence may compromise fertility if reversal is sought.

Cardiovascular, endocrine and auto-immune disease Concerns about a possible link between vasectomy and cardiovascular disease were raised in the 1970s following the observation that vasectomy increased atherosclerosis in rhesus monkeys. It was suggested that this may be attributable to increased levels of auto-antibodies which might alter the risk of auto-immune disease in general, including joint disease and multiple sclerosis. Several large studies, including a cohort study in the USA of over 10000 vasectomized men, have failed to substantiate increased rates of 98 diseases and in fact suggested that vasectomy was associated with a lower death rate (Massey et al 1984).

Cancer Two epidemiological studies from the USA and Scotland (Strader et al 1988, Cale et al 1990) suggested an increased risk of testicular cancer following vasectomy. This observation has not been substantiated by later research. A large study of over 73000 Danish men (Moller et al 1994) concluded that testicular cancer is no more common in men who have been vasectomized than in other men. A number of large epidemiological studies from the USA have also suggested an increased risk of prostate cancer following vasectomy (Lancet Editorial 1991). The World Health Organization (WHO) convened a meeting in 1991 to review biological and epidemiological evidence and concluded that there was no known biological mechanism to account for any association, and that any causal relationship between vasectomy and prostate cancer was unlikely. A meeting of the National Institute of Health in the USA in 1993 endorsed the WHO conclusions and recommended that there was insufficient basis to change policies regarding vasectomy. More studies are in progress.

At present we advise men that the question of a link between vasectomy and prostate cancer has been raised but not substantiated. We further point out that prostate cancer is a common disease which affects old men and that most of them do not die from it.

INDICATIONS

1. Couples who are absolutely certain that their family is complete.
2. Individuals or couples who choose to have no children.
3. When one partner:
   a. Carries a significant risk of transmitting an inherited disorder.
   b. Suffers from chronic ill-health which would (in the case of the woman) contraindicate pregnancy or affect the couple's ability to bring up children.

In the last two instances it is sensible to sterilize the affected partner.

CONTRAINDICATIONS

Unless the couple is absolutely certain that, for whatever reason, they want no or no more children, sterilization should not be performed. It is not unusual for a woman to request sterilization because no other method of contraception suits her, or because she believes that the procedure will enhance her libido, or improve her pattern of menstruation. Rarely, the referring doctor implies the same misconception.

Up to 10% of couples regret the decision to undergo sterilization and 1% of these will seek reversal. Factors which are known to increase the risk of regret include:

1. Marital/relationship problems.
2. Young age.
3. Timing of sterilization – women who are sterilized immediately postpartum or postabortion are more likely to seek reversal.
4. Psychiatric illness in either partner.

ADVANTAGES

Both *male and female* sterilization provide highly effective long-term contraception without the need for continued motivation or compliance.

The advantages of *male* as opposed to *female* sterilization are:

1. It is a simpler procedure.
2. It can be performed under local anaesthetic as an outpatient procedure.
3. It requires no sophisticated equipment and is much cheaper to perform.
4. Mortality and significant operative morbidity are virtually non-existent.
5. Its efficacy can be checked.

The advantages of *female* as opposed to *male* sterilization are:

1. It is immediately effective.
2. A woman's reproductive life is finite; a man retains his fertility for many years and has potentially more opportunity to regret the decision to be sterilized.

DISADVANTAGES

1. Female sterilization carries a risk of operative mortality and morbidity (p. 210).

2. Sterilization cannot always be reversed (p. 219).
3. Sterilization is more complicated than alternative methods of contraception requiring the provision of specialized facilities and trained personnel.
4. Vasectomy is not effective immediately, and other contraception must be used until two consecutive negative sperm counts are obtained.

COUNSELLING

In her study of counselling services for sterilization and vasectomy, Isobel Allan (1985) points out that most couples seeking sterilization have been thinking about the operation for some considerable time. The counselling session should provide opportunities for information, explanation, discussion and advice and should enable a couple to decide what is in their own best interests. Many couples are quite certain of their wishes and the consultation should not be unduly prolonged unless doubt is expressed or perceived. The couple should be prepared to provide details about themselves, their circumstances, and the reason for requesting sterilization. The counsellor should provide information about the procedure, and its implications, and should cover:

1. Description of operation and associated myths/misconceptions.
2. Failure rate.
3. Risks/side-effects.
4. Issue of reversibility.
5. Possibility of wanting more children.
6. Which partner should be sterilized.

Information sought from the couple should include:

1. Reason for the request.
2. Relevant medical, gynaecological and obstetric histories.
3. Ages, occupations and social circumstances.
4. Numbers, ages and health of their children.
5. Previous and current contraception and any problems experienced.
6. Stability of the marriage and the possibility of its breakdown.
7. Quality of their sexual life.

In Isobel Allan's study many couples were unable to recall much of the consultation and a leaflet which covers the same points should be available for the couple to take away.

Counselling for female sterilization is usually done by the GP or family planning doctor who refers the woman to a gynaecologist who covers many of the points a second time. In the UK, female sterilization is usually performed under GA in hospital and the surgeon who does the operation prefers to see the woman in the outpatient department before arranging the operation. Vasectomy undertaken in hospital is usually organized in a similar way with an outpatient consultation prior to the procedure. Vasectomy under LA is often done in a clinic setting or in the GP surgery. Sessionally employed surgeons often operate on men who have been counselled by someone else. In some large family planning clinics specially trained nurses do the counselling and only seek a medical opinion if there are contraindications, doubts, or clinical problems.

EFFECTIVENESS

Failure of female sterilization varies according to both the method used and the experience of the surgeon. Failure rates for the various methods have been reported as follows:

    diathermy 2–5/1000
    clips and rings 1–3/1000
    tubal ligation 1/1000

Vasectomy is generally accepted as being more effective than female sterilization. In the Oxford/FPA study, Vessey and colleagues (1982) reported:

1. A failure rate of 0.02 per hundred woman years (HWY) after vasectomy and 0.13 per HWY for female sterilization
2. That after 7 years follow-up, 1% of all women who had been sterilized (by a variety of techniques) had become pregnant.

REVERSIBILITY

Despite careful counselling, it is inevitable that a few couples will request reversal of their sterilization. This is most likely to happen when the marriage breaks down and one or other partner starts a new relationship. Although as many as 10% of couples regret being sterilized only 1% of these will request reversal.

Reversal of female sterilization is more likely to be successful after occlusion with clips which have been applied to the isthmic portion of the tube since only a small section of tube will have been damaged. Patients should realize that reversal involves laparotomy, does not always work (microsurgical techniques are associated with around 70% success) and carries a significant risk of ectopic pregnancy (up to 5%). Reversal is unlikely to be available on the NHS in many parts of the UK.

Reversal of vasectomy is technically feasible in many cases with patency rates of almost 90% being reported in some series. Pregnancy rates are much less (up to 60%) perhaps as a result of the presence of antisperm antibodies.

Some laboratories now offer a sperm banking service to men prior to vasectomy. The availability of such services complicates counselling since the concept seems to contradict the advice that a couple should not consider vasectomy unless they are absolutely certain they want no more children.

RISKS/BENEFITS

Although sterilization operations do carry small but significant risks, the overall benefits in terms of effectiveness and convenience tend to outweigh these in well motivated and adequately counselled couples.

In a couple who have completed their family, the procedure avoids the need for continued motivation in contraceptive usage and the long-term side-effects of effective reversible methods, such as the combined pill and IUD.

REFERENCES

Allen I 1985 Counselling services for sterilisation, vasectomy and termination of pregnancy. Policy Studies Institute no 641. London

Cale A R J, Farouk M, Prescott R J, Wallace I W J 1990 Does vasectomy accelerate testicular tumour? Importance of testicular examinations before and after vasectomy. British Medical Journal 300: 370

Filshie G M 1989 Laparoscopic female sterilization. Baillieres Clinical Obstetrics and Gynaecology 3: 609–624

Hargreave T B 1992 Towards reversible vasectomy. International Journal of Andrology 15: 455–459

Hieu D T, Tran T T, Tan D N, Nguyet P T, Than P, Vinh D Q 1993 31,781 cases of non-surgical female sterilization with quinacrine pellets in Vietnam. Lancet 342: 213–217

Kasonde J M, Bonnar J 1976 Effect of sterilization on menstrual blood loss. British Journal of Obstetrics and Gynaecology 83: 572–575

Lancet Editorial 1991 Vasectomy and Prostate Cancer 337: 1445–6

Massey F J, Bernstein G S, O'Fallon W M et al 1984 Vasectomy and Health: results from a large cohort study. Journal of the American Medical Association 252: 1023–1029

Moller H, Knudsen L B, Lynge E 1994 Risk of testicular cancer after vasectomy: a cohort study of over 73 000 men. British Medical Journal 309: 295–299

Nirapathpongporn A, Huber D, Kieger J N 1990 No-scalpel vasectomy at the King's birthday vasectomy festival. Lancet 335: 894–895

Rulin M C, Davidson A R, Philliber S G, Graves W L, Cushman L F 1993 Long-term effect of tubal sterilization on menstrual indices and pelvic pain. Obstetrics and Gynecology 82: 118–121

Strader C H, Weiss N S, Daling J R 1988 Vasectomy and the incidence of testicular cancer. American Journal of Epidemiology 128: 56–63

Templeton A A, Cole S 1982 Hysterectomy following sterilization. British Journal of Obstetrics and Gynaecology 89: 845–848

Vessey M P, Lawless M, Yeates D 1982 Efficacy of different contraceptive methods. Lancet i: 841–842

Appendix 8.1

STERILIZATION OF THE FEMALE BY LAPAROSCOPY

For a pregnancy to start, an egg must combine with a sperm. This usually takes place in one of the fallopian tubes which join the ovaries to the womb. All methods of female sterilization block the tubes.

The operation we intend to carry out is called laparoscopy. A short general anaesthetic is required. Through a one-inch long cut below the navel (tummy button) an instrument is passed through the abdominal wall. This allows careful inspection of the womb, tubes and ovaries, etc. If they appear normal, another small instrument is passed through a separate, even smaller incision. This allows the tubes to be blocked with small clips or rings or by means of a very small electric current.

Complications are rare and recovery rapid so that you will usually be allowed home the same day as your operation. Some patients experience pain in the region of the shoulders or vaginal bleeding for some days after the operation, but this need not cause any concern. Very rarely, some unsuspected abnormality will be seen or will occur at the time of operation so that a more major operation is necessary, but it must be emphasized that this is very unusual.

You will be sterile from the time of the operation and it is safe to resume intercourse as soon as you have completely recovered from the operation. Apart from the fact that you can no longer conceive, neither your periods nor your desire for sex will be affected. Once sterilization has been performed it is permanent and does not require to be repeated after a number of years. Reversal of the operation, which is occasionally requested, is difficult.

Failure of the operation permitting further pregnancy is rare but does occasionally occur. Therefore, if at any time after operation your period is more than 2 weeks late you should consult your family doctor as soon as possible.

Appendix 8.2

MALE STERILIZATION

You have expressed an interest in having a vasectomy. You and your partner will be given an appointment to find out more about the procedure before a date is arranged for your operation. This information leaflet tells you about the operation, the effectiveness and side-effects. It is designed to give you the facts and to help you decide whether this is to be your chosen method of contraception. It is not meant to sound off-putting but it tells you about the possible complications. You will have the opportunity to discuss the information and to ask questions when you come to the clinic for your vasectomy counselling appointment. All methods of contraception carry some risk and it is up to you to decide which method is most acceptable. We hope that this information sheet will help you in making your decision.

What is a vasectomy?

A tube called the vas deferens carries sperm from each testis into the penis. Vasectomy is the cutting or blocking of both these tubes to prevent the passage of sperm. The vas are cut just above the testis. Vasectomy does not interfere with the production of seminal fluid so you will not notice any difference in the amount of fluid you produce when you ejaculate – the fluid simply will not contain sperm. The operation is done under local anaesthetic and takes less than half an hour. A small cut is made in the skin in the middle or on each side of the scrotum and the vas which lies just beneath the skin can then be cut or blocked. The skin may be closed with a stitch or tape or simply left to heal without any closure.

How effective is vasectomy?

Vasectomy is not 100% effective but one of the advantages of the procedure is that its efficacy can be tested. It takes some weeks for all the sperm that the remain in the vas (tube) to disappear and the rate a which this happens depends on how often you have intercourse. You will be asked to send a specimen of seminal fluid to the laboratory 12 weeks after your operation and again at 16 weeks. In most cases both samples will be

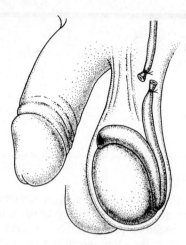

Fig. 8.8   Vasectomy.

free of sperm and we will let you know that your operation is complete. In some cases it takes more than 16 weeks for the sperm to clear and you will be asked to continue to send samples every 4 weeks until two consecutive samples are free of sperm. In up to 2% of cases (2 in 100 men) sperm continue to appear and you will be advised to have the vasectomy explored, usually under general anaesthetic in hospital. **Until you have been told that your operation is complete, you or your partner should continue to use another method of contraception.**

In 1 in 1000 cases the vasectomy fails at a later date – the two ends of the vas heal with time and rarely the canal re-opens (so called 'late recanalization'). If this happens your partner may become pregnant despite you having had two sperm-free samples and being told that your operation was complete. Late re-canalization may happen some years after you have had your vasectomy. By comparison, sterilization in the female fails in around 3 per 1000 cases.

Are there any problems?

Complications can be divided into those which might occur immediately after the vasectomy and those which do not occur for some years.

Immediate complications

All surgical operations carry some risk and vasectomy is no exception but the problems are usually minor.

Between 5 and 10% of men experience minor local problems after the procedure. Once the local anaesthetic has worn off (after about 2 hours) you will probably feel some discomfort which is usually helped by taking a mild painkiller (paracetamol or aspirin). Most men notice a certain amount of swelling and bruising around the operation site which lasts a few days. Sometimes the site can become infected and you may require antibiotics. If you notice persisting pain, swelling or redness you should contact your GP. Occasionally a moderate amount of bleeding occurs and the blood slowly collects at the base of the scrotum causing a large swelling or haematoma. 1 in 100 men require hospital treatment for this complication and although this can be a rather frightening event, it does not cause any long-term problems.

Long-term consequences

In 10–15% of men, leakage of sperm from the cut end of the vas causes some inflammation and occasionally small painful lumps (sperm granulomas) may appear. Very rarely the pain may last for years after a vasectomy but further surgery usually cures the problem.

A large amount of research has been carried out on the long-term effects of vasectomy in order to establish whether the procedure has any effect on general health. While there seems to be no good evidence for any serious long term effects, a number of studies have raised the possibility of there being a link between prostate cancer and vasectomy.

Cancer of the prostate is relatively common in men although rare below the age of 65. In Scotland about 650 men die from the disease each year compared with about 2700 men dying from lung cancer and about 1300 women who die from breast cancer. The cause of prostate cancer is not known but it is in some way dependent on the male hormone testosterone.

Most cancers are associated with certain risk factors; for example men who have worked with some chemicals are much more likely to develop bladder cancer than usual. We do not know what risk factors are related to prostate cancer.

Does having a vasectomy increase your change of later developing cancer of the prostate? A lot of medical research has investigated the possibility of a relationship between vasectomy and prostate cancer. A number of large studies in China and in the United States of America have suggested that there is no link between vasectomy and the risk of prostate cancer. Indeed, in the Chinese study, men who had a vasectomy were healthier than those who had not but prostate cancer is rare in Chinese men. Recently, however, two more studies from America have suggested that there may be a link and that 20 years after a vasectomy your risk of developing prostate cancer may be almost double that of men of the same age who have not had a vasectomy. The risk of a man in Scotland developing prostate cancer is around 1 in 2000. If the American studies are correct this means that if you have a vasectomy your risk increases to 1 in 1000. Cancer of the prostate is a relatively benign condition and although 1 in 25 men aged 74 years will have a tumour of the prostate, the vast majority will live to a ripe old age and die of other causes.

The World Health Organization (WHO) held a meeting of experts in 1991 to discuss the issue. The experts decided that, despite many years of research, there is no known biological reason for vasectomy causing prostate cancer. It is hard to see how vasectomy might affect the risk of prostate cancer. It is more likely that for some reason men who decide to have a vasectomy have some characteristics which also make them more likely to develop prostate cancer although we do not know what these characteristics might be. WHO recommends that more research should be done but that family planning policies should not be changed.

One or two small studies have also suggested a link between vasectomy and testicular cancer. Again there is no obvious physiological basis for such a link and it is possible that men who have recently had a vasectomy may be more likely to examine themselves and so find a lump in the testis.

What does this mean for you? All methods of contraception carry some risk. When you decide on a family planning method you weigh up the risks and benefits for you and your partner. Long-term use of the contraceptive pill carries a small risk for women as does female sterilization. On the whole, whatever the method, using contraception is probably safer than either having a baby or having an abortion. Moreover, apart from the health risks involved, individual couples must consider what an unplanned pregnancy would mean to their lives. While you and your partner have to decide for yourselves whether or not to choose a vasectomy, many couples may consider that the small risk of problems is acceptable when balanced with the benefits of an extremely effective method of contraception.

Can vasectomy be reversed?

Yes, but reversal is not always successful. It requires a intricate operation and even if the cut ends of the vas are successfully united and sperm can get through, fertility may not be normal. The operation may not be available from the National Health Service so if you were to request reversal you might have to pay for it. You should not have a vasectomy if you think that you might at some time want to have the operation reversed.

Practical details

This information leaflet is being sent to you before your appointment for counselling. You should expect to be in the clinic for about half an hour for this consultation. It is helpful if your partner accompanies you as she may also have some questions. Unfortunately, we do not have crèche facilities and you may find it difficult to concentrate if you are being distracted by your children so we strongly recommend a baby-sitter if you can find one!

If you decide to go ahead with vasectomy you will be given a date for the operation. You should remember to shave the scrotum and the skin around the base of the penis before you come to the clinic. This is best done in the bath the night before the operation.

After the operation you will have a short rest before going home. You will probably be in the clinic for less than one hour. You should rest at home for the remainder of the day and will probably find it comfortable to wear either an athletic support (jock strap) or a pair of well-supporting under-pants for a couple of days.

Most men return to work the following day but you should avoid lifting heavy weights or doing other heavy manual work for 3 or 4 days. It is not sensible to arrange unavoidable commitments or energetic holidays immediately following the operation.

We hope that you have found this information leaflet helpful. When you come to the clinic you will be asked to sign a copy saying that you have read and understood the information and been given the opportunity to ask questions. The signed copy will be kept in your record; this copy is for you to keep.

I have read the information leaflet and have had the opportunity to ask questions.

I understand that we should continue to use some other method of contraception until I have been informed that the vasectomy is complete.

I understand that the operation does not work in a small number of cases and therefore must be re-done, and that very rarely the procedure may fail some time after having apparently been successful initially.

I understand that vasectomy cannot always be successfully reversed and that should I wish a reversal the operation may not be available from the National Health Service.

I understand that up to 10% of men experience minor complications such as bleeding, haematoma formation and infection, and that such complications occasionally require treatment in hospital.

I understand that there have been some concerns raised about the long-term effects of vasectomy but that present knowledge suggests that these are not significant.

Signature...........................

Date.........................

9. Emergency postcoital contraception

Anna Glasier

Risk of pregnancy

Methods
  Oestrogens
  Ethinyloestradiol and levonorgestrel
  Intrauterine devices (IUDs)

Mode of action
  Combined oestrogen–progestogen regimen
  Intrauterine devices

Effectiveness

Indications

Contraindications

Side-effects
  Combined oestrogen–progestogen regimen
  Intrauterine devices

New prospects
  Levonorgestrel
  Danazol
  Antiprogesterones

Clinical management
  Assessment
    History
    Examination
  Information
  Follow-up

Use and availability

Appendix

For centuries women have adopted measures or used devices or preparations to try to prevent pregnancy after intercourse has taken place. Violent physical exercise in an attempt to dislodge semen from the genital tract; potions, seeds or herbs taken orally or placed in the vagina; and postcoital douching have all been known to have been used as long ago as 1500BC. Modern approaches to emergency or postcoital contraception (PCC) using steroid hormones and the IUD date back only some 30 years.

RISK OF PREGNANCY

Pregnancy can occur as a result of intercourse taking place at any time during the fertile period, usually regarded as being 3 days before and 1 day after the estimated day of ovulation. During this period, the risk of pregnancy following a single act of intercourse is around 28%. Sperm survive in the reproductive tract capable of fertilization for at least 4 days after intercourse and perhaps longer. Most women find it difficult to recall exactly the date of their last menstrual period (LMP). Cycle length varies from month to month and ovulation does not always reliably occur on the same day each cycle. While it may be tempting to take physiology into account and withhold emergency contraception when there is no genuine risk of conception (e.g. after intercourse on day 24 in a cycle which is usually 28 days in length) this is probably not in the patient's best interests unless she has real contraindications to, or is too late for, hormonal emergency contraception.

METHODS

Oestrogens

High-dose oestrogens were used in early trials of hormonal emergency contraception and proved very effective but must be given over 5 days and are thus associated with a high incidence of side-effects particularly nausea and vomiting. When an association between high-dose oestrogens and vaginal adenosis and malignancy was recognized the approach was abandoned. Although it is still used occasionally in Holland (ethinyloestradiol 5 mg daily for 5 days), there is really no place for oestrogen alone today.

Ethinyloestradiol and levonorgestrel

In the UK the standard method of postcoital contraception, first described by Yuzpe and Lancee in 1977, consists of a combination of 100 μg ethinyloestradiol and 500 μg levonorgestrel given *twice*, with the second dose taken 12 hours after the first – the combined oestrogen–progestogen (CEP) regimen. The Committee on Safety of Medicines gave approval for the use of this regimen in the UK in 1984. One proprietary preparation of CEP is available (Schering PC4). It is expensive and only four tablets are supplied. Many doctors make up their own supplies using packets of the combined oral contraceptive pill (COC) Ovran which contains the same type and dose of hormones. This is considerably cheaper and extra pills can be given to be taken should vomiting occur. Although Ovran is not licensed for this purpose, the practice is so widespread that provided the pills are placed in a container with instructions for use, this would appear to be perfectly acceptable practice medicolegally.

Intrauterine devices (IUDs)

Postcoital IUD insertion is sometimes used as an alternative to CEP if there are contraindications to high-dose steroids or if a woman presents more than 72 hours after intercourse. IUD insertion may be used for up to 5 days after the calculated earliest day of ovulation (i.e. up to day 19 in a woman with a 28-day cycle). Thus, if intercourse occurs before ovulation, the IUD may be inserted more than 5 days after intercourse and may be used for multiple exposure (repeated episodes of intercourse). It may well be effective beyond 5 days after ovulation, although most clinicians are reluctant to extend the time limits for fear of contravening the 1967 Abortion Act. IUD insertion is an invasive procedure not always acceptable to women requesting PCC. It is particularly useful for women who wish to continue with the method for long-term contraception.

MODE OF ACTION

Combined oestrogen–progestogen regimen

The exact mode of action of the CEP regimen is not known. However, there is some evidence that it:

1. Interferes with corpus luteum function and possibly inhibits ovulation if given in the follicular phase of the cycle.
2. May have a direct effect on the endometrium in which both histological and biochemical changes have been described, suggesting that CEP may inhibit or disrupt implantation.

The observation in early studies that high-dose oestrogen was associated with increased risk of ectopic pregnancy led to the suggestion that tubal motility may be altered but this is not supported by any experimental evidence (see Glasier 1993a for review).

Intrauterine devices

There is evidence that the IUD diminishes the viability of ova, the number of sperm reaching the fallopian tube and their ability to fertilize the egg. However, since it is so often used effectively days after the act of intercourse, postcoital IUD insertion almost certainly acts by inhibiting implantation.

EFFECTIVENESS

The efficacy of emergency contraception is difficult to measure accurately. Women present for treatment at every stage of the cycle and, even with accurate cycle data, the genuine risk of pregnancy is hard to estimate. Moreover, in many of the published studies significant numbers of subjects have been lost to follow-up. Failure rates of between 0.2 and 7.4% have been reported for the standard CEP regimen used in the fertile phase of the cycle. In our own study (Glasier et al 1992) 4 women out of a total of 398 became pregnant after using CEP giving an overall failure rate of 1%.

The IUD is an extremely effective PCC. In a review (Fasoli et al 1989) of a total of 879 postcoital IUD insertions only one pregnancy was reported and this ended in a spontaneous abortion.

INDICATIONS

Adhering to the rules for the time limits as described above, emergency postcoital contraception may be used in the following circumstances:

1. After unprotected intercourse.
2. After 'accidents' with a barrier method e.g. burst condom or diaphragm removed within 6 hours of intercourse.
3. If one or more COC pills have been missed at the beginning or end of a packet so that the pill-free interval is prolonged beyond 7 days, it is appropriate to give hormonal emergency contraception.
   It is not usually appropriate to prescribe emergency contraception for women who have forgotten to take one or more COC pills at other times – the risk of conception occurs some days after the missed pills when ovarian follicular development, freed from inhibition by the oral contraceptive, is sufficient to allow ovulation to occur. Pregnancy should be prevented if the rules for missed pills are followed (pp. 61, 62).
4. It may be appropriate to use emergency contraception after missed progestogen-only pills (POP) since ovulation is not inhibited by the POP in many women (Ch. 4).
5. Occasionally women are so insistent that they need emergency contraception that even if it is unnecessary (e.g. after one missed pill) it is sometimes easier to give it than to withhold it. The CEP regimen will not do them any harm and under these circumstances serves to relieve anxiety.

CONTRAINDICATIONS

1. Pregnancy.
2. Multiple exposure. If there has been unprotected intercourse more than once in a cycle, conception may have already

occurred by the time emergency contraception is given. Obviously if a woman has already conceived, emergency contraception will not work. If she has not and is refused emergency contraception, then she runs the risk of conceiving from the act of intercourse which has just occurred.

As always there is room for a pragmatic approach. If a woman would opt for termination of pregnancy, then there is no reason not to give her emergency contraception. If she is uncertain, or would definitely continue with the pregnancy should one occur, then the risks of teratogenicity – such as they are – should be discussed.

3. Contraindications to oestrogen therapy. In reality, an acute exposure to oestrogens, albeit in high doses, is highly unlikely to be dangerous even for women in whom COC would be contraindicated. Pregnancy, particularly if unwanted, is usually even more strongly contraindicated for them – if such a woman is genuinely at risk of conception, there are very few instances in which CEP need be refused, provided she understands the risks.

A very recent thromboembolic event or an attack of classical migraine with neurological disturbance at the time of presenting for emergency contraception might be regarded as genuine contraindications; diabetes or hypercholesterolaemia would not.

4. A history of ectopic pregnancy is sometimes considered to be a contraindication but provided the patient is advised of the theoretical risk, hormonal emergency contraception should not be withheld and is preferable to IUD insertion.

5. The IUD is not recommended for women with a history of recent pelvic inflammatory disease (although these histories can often be rather vague). Nor is it recommended for someone who is HIV positive.

SIDE-EFFECTS

Combined oestrogen–progestogen regimen

1. Nausea and vomiting are due to the high dose of oestrogen. In our own study, when patients were specifically asked to record this event, 59% of women complained of nausea on the day of treatment and 16% vomited. In our routine clinics spontaneous complaints of side-effects are much less frequent.

Nausea and vomiting may decrease compliance and some doctors routinely prescribe an anti-emetic such as cyclizine along with the CEP. Others supply two spare tablets (six in all) and one family planning clinic advises patients that if they vomit, the spare tablets should be placed in the vagina. No data are available, but it is possible that a higher dose should be used for vaginal administration.
2. Breast tenderness.
3. Disturbance of menstruation is often complained of in that the subsequent period is heavier and sometimes more painful than normal. It may also be early or late but patients should be advised that it is most likely to arrive at the expected time.

Intrauterine devices

1. Insertion may be difficult and painful, particularly in nulliparous women.
2. Women should be counselled about the risk of infection as for routine IUD insertion.

NEW PROSPECTS

Levonorgestrel

Levonorgestrel alone has been shown to prevent pregnancy when administered postcoitally. It probably works by rendering the endometrium unsuitable for implantation. It is sold over the counter (as Postinor) in some Eastern European and Asian countries. A recent study (Ho 1992) reported a failure rate of 1.5% when 750 µg levonorgestrel was taken twice, 12 hours apart within 48 hours of intercourse, and side-effects were less common than with the CEP regimen. 'Home-made' preparations for women in whom both oestrogen and the IUD are contraindicated would require 25 tablets of a levonorgestrel-only pill such as Microval to be given twice!

Danazol

Danazol is a semi-synthetic steroid preparation which is strongly gestogenic and widely used for the treatment of endometriosis. It has been tested as a postcoital agent. However there is some doubt about its efficacy (Webb et al 1992) and further work needs to be done.

Antiprogesterones

Progesterone is a pre-requisite for implantation and antiprogest-ational hormones given in early pregnancy induce menstrual bleeding and abortion. Preliminary studies suggest that the anti-progesterone mifepristone (RU 486) may be a highly effective emergency postcoital contraceptive with significantly fewer side effects than CEP. There were no pregnancies among almost 600 women treated with a single dose of 600 mg RU 486. However, up to 42% of women experienced a delay in the onset of menstruation of more than 3 days (Glasier et al 1992, Webb et al 1992). The dose of RU 486 used was that recommended for termination of pregnancy and is almost certainly far more than is required. Further studies – including dose-finding studies and an extension of the time limit to 120 hours – are being undertaken by the World Health Organization.

CLINICAL MANAGEMENT

Assessment

History

While it is of interest to take a careful history and record the points listed below, in practice it is only mandatory to exclude ongoing pregnancy and to determine whether the 72-hour limit has been exceeded. Of interest for the records are:

1. Age and parity.
2. Relevant past medical history.
3. Contraindications to hormonal contraception and the IUD.
4. Details of the woman's normal cycle.
5. Date and normality of LMP.
6. Timing of intercourse in relation to both the stage of the cycle and the time elapsed since intercourse took place.
7. Method of contraception, if any, being used and the reason for presentation e.g. burst condom.

In accident and emergency departments and busy clinics this information can be collected by self-administered questionnaire.

Examination

1. Record the blood pressure.
2. Pelvic examination. Routine pelvic examination is not necessary and may deter women – particularly young

women – from returning. It is, however, essential if there is any
suspicion that the patient may already be pregnant e.g. if the
LMP was abnormal in timing or character. If pregnancy is
suspected and if the uterus is not enlarged a pregnancy test
should be done before treatment is given.

Information

Many clinics give standard information sheets which outline the
points covered below and advise the timing of the second dose of
pills (Appendix 9.1).

1. Patients should be informed about the way in which emergency
   contraception acts. It should be stressed that it may inhibit
   implantation since to some women this may be morally
   unacceptable.
2. Patients should be advised of the possibility of failure and asked
   their intentions in the event of this happening. Most women
   opt to have the pregnancy terminated.
3. Information on the risk of teratogenesis if the CEP regimen
   fails is sparse. The increased risk of fetal malformation
   associated with COC use during early pregnancy is, if any,
   extremely small. The Faculty of Family Planning and
   Reproductive Health Care in the UK is currently collecting
   data on the outcome of pregnancies following failed CEP.
   The results of the study should be published soon but it
   would appear that the incidence of malformation is minimal
   (Dr Gill Cardy, personal communication). In our clinic we
   advise women of the data that exist and inform them that
   we do not believe that the continuation of a pregnancy is
   contraindicated.
4. Possible side-effects.
5. Effect on the timing and character of the next menstrual period
   (see below). Since the onset of vaginal bleeding is reassuring to
   women keen to avoid pregnancy it is important to counsel
   patients about this. It should be made clear that emergency
   contraception does not work by 'bringing on a period'.
6. If the need for PCC has arisen as a result of unprotected
   intercourse, a conventional (i.e. non-emergency) method of
   contraception should be discussed and, if appropriate,
   provided. Women who plan to use COC or the POP may be
   advised to start their pills on the first day of menses. There is a
   small risk that the menstrual period may subsequently prove to

be abnormal and only be recognized as such after oral contraception has been started.

7. It is not necessary to ask women to sign a consent form before prescribing emergency contraception; indeed it may deter them from returning, should PCC ever be necessary again.

Follow-up

Not all doctors arrange routine follow-up appointments after prescribing PCC. It is good practice to do so.

Women should be informed that emergency contraception does not always work and that *if their period does not come or if it is lighter or shorter than normal they must return to the clinic so that pregnancy can be excluded.*

Follow-up also permits further discussion about contraception and sexual behaviour which may not have been taken in by the patient at the earlier consultation, faced as she was with the immediate fear of pregnancy and the embarrassment of needing emergency contraception.

Women should be encouraged to return for emergency contraception should the need arise again. Accidents with barrier methods do happen and women sometimes do not take the pill for long or may never even start it. Many women are embarrassed about needing emergency contraception and would not feel able to admit to a second accident. If medical and nursing staff make it clear that some women do need to use emergency contraception more than once in a lifetime, more women would use the method when it was required.

USE AND AVAILABILITY

Although emergency postcoital contraception has been available in the UK for some years, a surprising number of women seem to be unaware of its existence. In 1990, the pharmaceutical company Schering Health Care undertook a survey of women's knowledge of contraception in the UK; 24% of 1007 women surveyed had never heard of postcoital contraception and only 10% had accurate knowledge of the time limits involved.

Women attending family planning clinics or consulting their GP about contraception should be informed about emergency postcoital contraception. Users of barrier methods should be told about it just as women on the pill are advised what to do when they forget to take one.

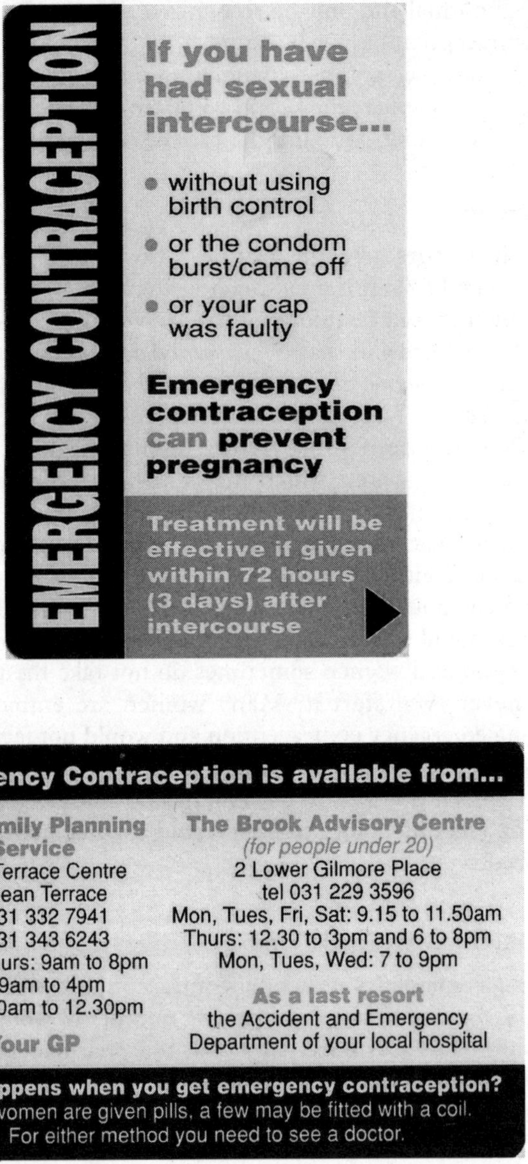

EMERGENCY CONTRACEPTION

If you have had sexual intercourse...

- without using birth control
- or the condom burst/came off
- or your cap was faulty

Emergency contraception can prevent pregnancy

Treatment will be effective if given within 72 hours (3 days) after intercourse

---

Emergency Contraception is available from...

The Family Planning Service
Dean Terrace Centre
18 Dean Terrace
tel 031 332 7941
tel 031 343 6243
Mon - Thurs: 9am to 8pm
Fri: 9am to 4pm
Sat: 9.30am to 12.30pm

Your GP

The Brook Advisory Centre
(for people under 20)
2 Lower Gilmore Place
tel 031 229 3596
Mon, Tues, Fri, Sat: 9.15 to 11.50am
Thurs: 12.30 to 3pm and 6 to 8pm
Mon, Tues, Wed: 7 to 9pm

As a last resort
the Accident and Emergency
Department of your local hospital

What happens when you get emergency contraception?
Most women are given pills, a few may be fitted with a coil.
For either method you need to see a doctor.

Fig. 9.1 Emergency contraception information card.

Women presenting with an unplanned pregnancy should also be informed about emergency contraception for future use. We issue them with a small laminated card, the size of a credit card which fits into a purse (Fig. 9.1). The card gives general information about emergency contraception on one side and details of local availability on the other.

Hormonal emergency contraception must be used within 72 hours of intercourse and can only be prescribed by a doctor. The greatest need for emergency contraception is often at weekends when clinics and GP surgeries are closed and on a Monday morning when they are at their busiest. Many people, particularly the young, often find it difficult to approach their GP for emergency contraception and not all hospital accident and emergency departments will supply it. For these reasons, and recogizing the potential of emergency contraception for reducing unwanted pregnancies, a number of organizations throughout the UK are discussing the proposal to make hormonal emergency contraception available off prescription from pharmacists (Glasier 1993b).

REFERENCES

Fasoli M, Parazzini F, Cecchetti G, Lavecchia C 1989 Postcoital contraception: an overview of published studies. Contraception 39: 459–468
Glasier A 1993a Postcoital contraception. Reproductive Medicine Review 2: 75–84
Glasier A 1993b Emergency contraception: time for de-regulation? British Journal of Obstetrics and Gynaecology 100: 611–612
Glasier A, Thong K J, Dewar M, Mackie M, Baird D T 1992 Randomized trial of mifepristone (RU 486) and high dose oestrogen–progestogen as an emergency contraceptive. New England Journal of Medicine 327: 1041–44
Ho P C 1992 Asian experience with post-coital contraception. Advances in Contraception 8: 216 (Abstract no. 67)
Schering Health Care 1990 Sex and contraception survey. Schering Health Care, The Brow, Burgess Hill, West Sussex, UK.
Webb A M C, Russel J, Elstein M 1992 Comparison of the Yuzpe regime, danazol and mifepristone in oral post-coital contraception. British Medical Journal 305: 927–31
Yuzpee A A, Lancee W J. 1977 Ethinylestradiol and dl-norgestrel as a postcoital contraceptive. Fertility and Sterility 28: 932–6.

Appendix 9.1

EDINBURGH HEALTHCARE NHS TRUST

Postcoital contraception

Hormonal method

The morning-after pill is for emergency use only, to avoid unwanted pregnancy after unprotected intercourse. It is not for routine contraceptive use.

The doctor has prescribed 4 hormone tablets for you. Take 2 tablets now and take the other 2 tablets in 12 hours time at ....

You may feel sick or even vomit after the treatment. If you vomit within 2 hours of taking the tablets, follow the instructions you have been given - take another 2 tablets and contact the clinic for advice at the earliest possible opportunity.

Your next period may come earlier or later than expected. Please keep a note of any bleeding that you have and the dates on which it occurs.

This treatment does not always prevent pregnancy. If it fails, we are still not absolutely certain what effects the hormones would have on the developing fetus but there is no evidence to suggest that the fetus will be damaged.

Follow-up

1. Even if your period comes as normal, it is essential that you return to the clinic for a check up in .... weeks.
2. If you have any severe pain in your lower abdomen, you should contact the clinic or your doctor.
3. If you have intercourse again after taking the tablets, you must use a contraceptive such as the diaphragm or a sheath for the rest of the cycle. You can obtain sheaths from this clinic free of charge.

REMEMBER:

THIS TREATMENT IS ONLY AN EMERGENCY MEASURE TO COPE WITH YOUR CURRENT SITUATION. IT IS VERY IMPORTANT THAT WE SEE YOU AGAIN TO MAKE SURE THAT THE TREATMENT HAS WORKED. YOU WILL ALSO HAVE TO DECIDE WHICH METHOD OF CONTRACEPTION WILL SUIT YOU IN THE FUTURE.

Your next appointment is on: ....

10. Therapeutic Abortion

David Baird

Legal aspects

Counselling

Assessment

Referral

Techniques of Abortion
  Early first trimester (up to 9 weeks)
    Vacuum aspiration (VA)
    Medical abortion
  Late first trimester (9–14 weeks)

Mid-trimester
  Dilatation and evacuation (D & E)
  Medical methods

Complications
  Early
  Late

Follow-up
  Contraception

Conclusion

Appendix

Abortion occurs in every country in the world. The World Health Organization has calculated that approximately 50 million pregnancies are terminated by abortion each year. Even in those countries where abortion is illegal, many women attempt to terminate an unwanted pregnancy illegally (e.g. in Brazil) or travel abroad to a country with more liberal laws (e.g. from the Republic of Ireland to England). Illegal abortions are often performed in unsanitary conditions by unqualified people and as a result are a considerable cause of morbidity and mortality. It is estimated that 100–200000 women die each year due to the complications of abortion (Segal & La Guardia 1990; Fathalla 1992). In contrast, abortion performed using modern methods in optimum conditions is an extremely safe procedure, and legislation of abortion is always followed by a drop in maternal deaths presumed to be due to the reduction in the complications of illegal abortions.

After the Abortion Act was passed in 1967 there was a rapid rise in the number of abortions notified in England and Wales and Scotland (Fig. 10.1) reaching a plateau of 110000 per year in 1988 (Botting, 1991). Since then there has been a gradual rise in the numbers each year but much of this can be explained by demographic changes. The rate of abortion varies according to the woman's age and many of the girls born during the 'baby boom' of

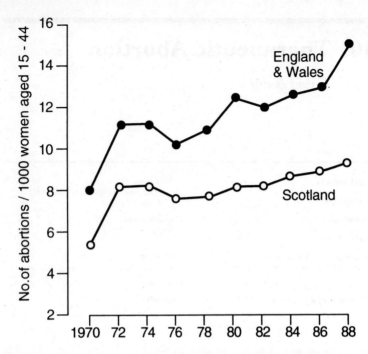

Fig. 10.1 Abortion figures in England & Wales and Scotland 1970–1988.

the mid 1960s have until recently been at the age of maximum risk of abortion. The abortion rate in Britain (9–14 per 1000 women aged 15–45 years) is relatively low compared to many other developed countries and probably reflects a wide acceptance of contraception and a comprehensive network of family planning services.

Women become pregnant without planning to do so either because of lack of forethought or contraceptive failure. Although the timing may be inconvenient, many will choose to have the baby but some will want an abortion. While abortion should never be considered as a method of contraception, failures occur with any method and without access to abortion the ability of women to regulate their fertility and plan their families is impaired. It is important, therefore, that anyone involved in providing contraceptive services should be aware of the legal indications and different methods of therapeutic abortion so that the woman can be helped to come to a sensible decision.

LEGAL ASPECTS

It is illegal in the United Kingdom (UK) to induce an abortion except under specific indications as defined by law. Many couples are under the mistaken belief that there is 'abortion on demand'. The conditions of the 1967 Abortion Act as amended in 1990 state that abortion can be performed if two registered medical practitioners, acting in good faith, agree that the pregnancy should be terminated on one or more of the following grounds:

1. The continuance of the pregnancy would involve risk to the life of the pregnant woman greater than if the pregnancy were terminated.
2. The termination is necessary to prevent grave permanent injury to the physical or mental health of the pregnant woman.
3. The pregnancy has *not* exceeded its 24th week and that the continuance of the pregnancy would involve risk, greater than if the pregnancy were terminated, of injury to the physical or mental health of the pregnant woman.
4. The pregnancy has *not* exceeded its 24th week and that the continuance of the pregnancy would involve risk, greater than if the pregnancy were terminated, of injury to the physical or mental health of the existing child(ren) of the family of the pregnant woman.
5. There is a substantial risk that if the child were born it would suffer from such physical or mental abnormalities as to be seriously handicapped.

Modern methods of inducing abortion are now so effective and safe that almost always it is safer for the woman to have an abortion than to continue with the pregnancy. That is not to say that abortion should be recommended always, but a doctor should think very carefully before refusing to recommend abortion for a woman who is convinced that her mental and/or physical health or the welfare of her children would be better preserved by ending the pregnancy.

There are differences in the law as it applies to abortion between different parts of the UK.

In England and Wales it is illegal to attempt to induce abortion except under the 1967 Abortion Act even if the woman is not pregnant. The *intention* to induce abortion is sufficient.

In Scotland, no criminal charge of inducing abortion can be sustained unless the prosecution can prove that the woman was pregnant.

The 1967 Abortion Act does not apply to Northern Ireland where abortion is only legal under exceptional circumstances e.g. to save the life of the mother.

The law concerning abortion is the subject of continuing debate within the UK. Although a vociferous lobby would wish to make abortion illegal or severely restrict its application, Parliament, reflecting the view of the majority, have repeatedly confirmed their support for the current law. In 1990 the law was amended to reduce the upper limit from 28 to 24 weeks gestation reflecting earlier fetal viability due to advances in neonatal care. An exception was made in the case of a fetus with severe congenital abnormality incompatible with life e.g. anencephaly, when there is no upper limit (Section 5).

COUNSELLING

Faced with the news of an unintended pregnancy many women are emotionally devastated. They may well have conflicting feelings about the pregnancy e.g. to continue with the pregnancy may present insoluble problems and seem quite impractical, whereas to have an abortion may seem abhorrent. It is important to provide a sympathetic hearing in order to allow the woman to explore her own feelings.

Early in the consultation a doctor should indicate that the doctor's role is to provide information and to help the woman decide what is best for her within the constraints of the law. The law recognizes that some doctors have ethical objections to abortion and, hence, no doctor is required to counsel or treat a woman requesting an abortion against his or her moral principles. However, if such a doctor is consulted by a woman requesting an abortion, referal of the woman to another colleague who does not hold similar views is obligatory.

The aim of counselling, therefore, is to help the woman to:

1. Determine her real wishes.
2. Decide on the best course of action.
3. Take responsibility for her own decision.
4. Understand how she came to have an unwanted pregnancy so that she can plan to avoid another.

Information counselling   It is important that the woman be provided with sufficient information so that she can make up her mind. This includes:

1. Alternatives to abortion i.e. keeping the baby or having it adopted. In this respect the following questions are relevant:
   a. Is her husband/partner supportive?
   b. If her partner has deserted her, does she have supportive parents, relatives, or friends?
   c. What are her financial resources?
   Information about maternity grants, leave, social security payments should be made available.
2. Details of the method of abortion (Appendix 10.1).
3. Arrangements by which abortion will be performed. Ideally she should be referred to a National Health Service (NHS) hospital free of charge, but in some parts of the UK it may be necessary for her to pay privately.
4. The likely complications and long term side-effects of the abortion.
5. Future contraception.

The majority of women make up their minds as to what they want within a few days. Some, however, remain ambivalent and may require more extensive professional counselling taking into account the psychological, social and medical factors. Women with severe medical conditions which could worsen in pregnancy e.g. pulmonary hypertension, or with psychiatric disease, require particularly careful assessment of the relative risks of continuing with the pregnancy. Expert medical or psychiatric advice is required in such cases.

ASSESSMENT

After it has been decided that there are grounds for abortion and the woman has been fully counselled, it is important to make a careful assessment.

1. A pregnancy test must always be performed to confirm that the woman is definitely pregnant. Arranging the test, obtaining the result and discussing it with the woman should be achieved with as little delay as possible.
2. The stage of gestation should be determined by pelvic bimanual examination as well as menstrual history. A pelvic ultrasound scan is unnecessary unless there is real doubt about the gestation e.g. irregular menstrual history or obesity making pelvic examination unreliable or if ectopic pregnancy is suspected.

3. A complete medical history is necessary paying particular attention to conditions such as heart or respiratory disease which may influence the choice of method of abortion.

4. Optimally, a high vaginal swab should be taken routinely for bacteriological examination and, if possible, antibiotic therapy started before abortion is performed. There is now good evidence that infection with *Chlamydia trachomatis* is a significant cause of subsequent infertility due to tubal disease. In some populations the incidence of infection with chlamydia, gonorrhoea and other organisms may be so high, e.g. more than 10%, that routine administration to everyone of a broad spectrum antibiotic such as doxycycline or erythromycin before abortion may be a cost-effective way of reducing pelvic infection.

5. Blood should be collected for measurement of haemoglobin concentration and blood group determined.

6. As fetal red cells pass into the maternal circulation during all methods of abortion, women who are rhesus negative should be injected with anti-D immunoglobulin prior to or within 48 hours of the abortion to prevent the development of rhesus isoimmunization.

REFERRAL

Most women seeking an abortion in the UK consult their general practitioner (GP) in the first instance. Others prefer to approach a family planning clinic or pregnancy advisory service directly. Once the decision has been made the woman should be referred to a gynaecologist as quickly as possible.

Provision for abortion varies throughout the UK. In Scotland and North-East England over 90% of abortions are performed in NHS hospitals while in other areas of England, the majority are carried out in private clinics or by charities. The incidence of complications of abortion is directly related to the period of gestation so that an efficient referral system such as exists in Lothian is optimal, although a few days reflection between decision and having the pregnancy terminated is desirable (Glasier & Thong 1991).

TECHNIQUES OF ABORTION

In the last 10 years there have been several advances in the techniques to induce abortion so that safe and effective methods are now available at all stages of gestation. The optimum method depends on gestation, parity, medical history and the woman's wishes. It is usual to divide abortions into first trimester (up to 12 weeks amenorrhoea) when the uterus can be safely evacuated by vacuum aspiration and second trimester (12–24 weeks) when cervical preparation or medical methods are required. However, a more logical classification in keeping with the newer methods is as discussed below.

Early first trimester (up to 9 weeks)

Women seeking abortion at this early stage of pregnancy can be offered a choice of two equally effective methods, vacuum aspiration (VA) and medical abortion. VA has the advantage that the abortion is completed in a single visit and, if general anaesthesia is used, there is no pain or discomfort and the woman is unaware of the events at the time of abortion. Some women choose the medical method because they feel more in control of the situation and it avoids passing instruments into the uterus under general anaesthesia.

Vacuum aspiration

The most frequently used method is VA under local or general anaesthesia. Before 6 weeks gestation it is possible to insert a small (4mm) catheter and, using a hand-held syringe (Fig. 10.2), complete the abortion without dilatation of the cervix because the negative pressure together with the scraping movement of the catheter tip

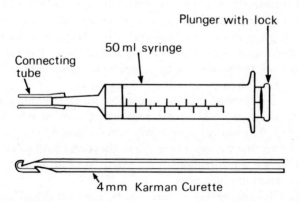

Fig. 10.2 Menstrual extraction kit.

disintegrates the fetus which is tiny at this gestation. This technique is sometimes referred to as 'menstrual extraction'. Beyond 6 weeks it is usually necessary to dilate the cervix in order to insert a larger curette (up to 12mm) through the cervix and the contents of the uterus are usually aspirated using a mechanical pump.

In the UK the operation is mainly performed using general anaesthesia, although in many countries e.g. USA, local paracervical block appears to be sufficient.

VA at this stage of pregnancy is an extremely safe and effective procedure with a very low incidence of complications.

Failure is more likely to occur in very early pregnancy (i.e. within 2 weeks of the missed menstrual period), probably because at this stage it is possible to miss the tiny fetus with the curette. For this reason it may be better to defer the operation until after this time or to use medical methods.

The mortality from VA in the first trimester is less than about 1 per 100 000 i.e. considerably less than the maternal mortality from continuing pregnancy.

Complications which include damage to the cervix, uterine perforation and postabortion infection are rare (Frank 1985).

Medical abortion

Abortion can be induced medically in the first 9 weeks of pregnancy. Although a number of substances which could induce abortion had been known for many years, it was the discovery of the antigestogen mifepristone or RU 486 in 1980 which made medical abortion a practical reality (Baird 1992). Mifepristone (Mifegyne) is a synthetic steroid chemically similar to norethindrone (the gestogen in one of the first combined oral contraceptives) which blocks the biological action of progesterone by binding to its receptor in the uterus and other target organs. Following withdrawal of the effect of progesterone, the uterus contracts and bleeding from the placental bed occurs followed by abortion 2–5 days later.

Initial trials showed that the rate of complete abortion was only 60% necessitating VA on the remaining women who had an incomplete abortion or ongoing pregnancy. However, subsequently it was shown that the rate of complete abortion could be increased to over 95% if a prostaglandin was given 36 or 48 hours after the administration of mifepristone.

In the UK mifepristone is currently licensed for the induction of abortion up to 9 weeks gestation given as a single oral dose of

600 mg (3 × 200 mg tablets) followed 48 hours later by 1 mg vaginal pessary of cervagem (Gemeprost). Cervagem is a synthetic derivative of the naturally occurring prostaglandin E, which causes strong contraction of the uterus. It also causes softening and dilatation of the cervix and is widely used for preparation of the cervix prior to VA and dilatation and evacuation (D & E) in the second trimester.

Contraindications Medical abortion is not a suitable method for all women in early pregnancy, and it is important to take a careful medical history and to counsel the woman accordingly (Table 10.1). Mifepristone binds to the glucocorticoid receptor and blocks the action of cortisol. Thus, any patient on corticosteroids or who has suspected adrenal insufficiency should not be given mifepristone. Prostaglandins can cause bronchospasm – asthma is therefore an absolute contraindication to medical methods.

Side-effects There are very few side-effects following administration of mifepristone (Baird 1993). Although for legal reasons the tablets must be taken in the presence of a doctor or nurse in a hospital or approved place, it is only necessary to observe the woman for about 10 minutes after swallowing the tablets before she goes home. After 48 hours she returns to hospital for insertion of the Gemeprost pessary into the vagina. The fetus is usually aborted in the next 4 hours and this is accompanied by bleeding and pain. The bleeding is usually described as being like a heavy period although rarely (less than 1% of cases) there may be very heavy bleeding requiring resuscitation.

Most women experience period-like pains although there is great variability in degree with some needing no analgesia while others (about 10–20%) may require opiates.

Table 10.1 Contraindications to medical abortion

Absolute	Relative
Adrenal insufficiency	Heavy smoker
Ectopic pregnancy	> 35 years
> 9 weeks gestation	Obesity
Asthma	Hypertension (diastolic > 100 mmHg)
Cardiac disease	
Heavy smoker – older than 35 years	
On anticoagulants or bleeding disorder	

Bleeding usually continues for about 10 days after the abortion although the total amount of blood lost (around 80 ml) is similar to that occurring at the time of VA.

Late first trimester (9–14 weeks)

At this stage of pregnancy the method of choice is VA. Although abortion can be induced by antigestogens and prostaglandins, the incidence of incomplete abortion is high and many women require subsequent surgical evacuation of the uterus. It is necessary to dilate the cervix prior to passing a curette of sufficient diameter to suck out the fetal parts. Forcible dilation of the cervix especially in young nulliparous women may damage the cervix resulting in bleeding or long-term cervical incompetence (Frank et al 1987).

A variety of methods are available to soften and dilate the cervix prior to VA including hygroscopic bougies, prostaglandins and mifepristone.

Bougies   Lamicel or Dilapan are hygroscopic rods which are placed in the cervix several hours prior to surgery and, by taking up water, swell to several times their original diameter and dilate the cervix. Because they require to be inserted by a doctor several hours prior to surgery, they are usually used only in more advanced pregnancies (over 14 weeks) when considerable cervical dilation is required prior to D & E.

Prostaglandin   Gemeprost has a short action and will achieve adequate dilation in only 3 hours.

Mifepristone   This is equally effective at preparing the cervix but takes longer.

Although VA is an extremely safe operation, the blood loss and other complications rise as gestation advances. It is important, therefore, to refer the women for abortion promptly after the decision to terminate the pregnancy has been made.

Mid-trimester

Because termination of pregnancy is more difficult and has more complications after 14 weeks, every effort should be made to reduce the number of mid-trimester abortions. Some gynaecologists are very reluctant to perform mid-trimester abortions except for life-threatening conditions. However, women who are least able to cope with an unwanted pregnancy often first present at this time. In addition, screening for congenital abnormalities such as neural tube defects is usually performed after the 14th week and it may therefore be after the 20th week before severe fetal abnormality is discovered. Thus, it may well be necessary to induce abortion in the mid-trimester. At this stage of pregnancy abortion may be induced either surgically or medically.

Dilatation and evacuation (D & E)

D & E is the method of choice in the USA, but in the UK its use is confined largely to gynaecologists in private practice (Francome & Savage 1992). It may be necessary to dilate the cervix up to a diameter of 20 mm before the fetal parts can be extracted using special instruments.

In skilled hands, D & E is a safe procedure but requires careful training of the operator if complications such as haemorrhage and perforation of the uterus are to be avoided.

D & E has the advantage that the woman is unaware of the procedure which can be performed as a day case. There is evidence from the USA that women prefer D & E although many nurses and doctors find it disturbing.

Medical methods

The alternative medical methods involve inducing uterine contractions so that the fetus is expelled from the uterus.

1. In the past a variety of substances such as hypertonic saline, urea, and Rivanol were injected into the amniotic sac or through the cervix into the extra-amniotic space, e.g. utus paste. Often they were combined with the intravenous infusion of oxytocin or prostaglandins to induce uterine contractions. Such methods were relatively inefficient and the woman underwent a prolonged labour, in some cases of greater than 48 hours, when the risk of infection was increased. Moreover, there was a risk of cardiovascular collapse due to inadvertent injection of prostaglandin or hypertonic solution directly into a vein. For these reasons, although they are still used in some places, they are not to be recommended if more effective methods involving mifepristone and prostaglandins are available.
2. The use of mifepristone as pretreatment has been a major advance in the management of mid-trimester abortion by

shortening the interval between administration of the prostaglandin and abortion of the fetus to 6–8 hours (Rodger & Baird 1990). 600 mg mifepristone is given 36 hours before insertion of a 1 mg Gemeprost pessary into the vagina or infusion of prostaglandin E_2 into the extra-amniotic space. The prostaglandin is repeated at intervals of 3 or 6 hours until expulsion of the fetus occurs. Most women require opiate analgesia to relieve the pains of uterine contractions and in a minority (about 30%) it is necessary to evacuate the uterus of the placenta in whole or in part.

In spite of the disadvantages, induction of abortion by medical means with prostaglandins alone or preferably in combination with mifepristone is a very effective method of abortion associated with a very low incidence of complications. Because it requires less surgical experience, the potential for serious complications are probably less than for D & E and, hence, it will continue to be used in many parts of the world.

COMPLICATIONS

Early

Persistence of placental and/or fetal tissue   This is the commonest complication following abortion. Incomplete or missed abortion is commoner after medically induced abortion in the first trimester and up to 5% of women will require surgical evacuation of the uterus within the first month. However, it should be emphasized that incomplete abortion and ongoing pregnancies also occur after VA with the incidence rising as the gestation increases.

The occurrence of bleeding and presence of residual trophoblastic tissue in the uterus at 2 weeks after a medical or surgical abortion is not in itself an indication to evacuate the uterus. Although an ultrasound scan of the uterus and the measurement of human chorionic gonadotrophin (hCG) in plasma may be helpful in diagnosing an ongoing pregnancy, the decision as to whether evacuation of the uterus is indicated should be made on clinical grounds i.e. continued heavy or persistent bleeding from a bulky uterus in which the cervix is still dilated.

The majority of women with an incomplete or missed abortion will pass the residual tissue with time if they are prepared to be patient. Previous teaching that all women with an incomplete abortion had a high risk of intrauterine infection until the uterus was evacuated, probably stemmed from the time when many incomplete abortions resulted from clandestine attempts to terminate the pregnancy under conditions which were far from optimal. Minor complications such as lower abdominal pain, vaginal bleeding and passage of clots or trophoblastic tissue are relatively common and usually only require reassurance.

Established pelvic infection   Such infection with pyrexia, abdominal pain and offensive vaginal discharge is rare (around 1%) following all methods of abortion particularly if women are screened for pathogens in the vagina e.g. chlamydia and gonorrhoea and treatment with antibiotics started prior to abortion.

Urinary infection, cervical and vaginal lacerations   These are rare complications.

Late

There are very few late complications from abortion if the women have been carefully counselled.

Guilt or regret   Many women feel tearful and emotional in the weeks following the abortion but these feelings usually pass rapidly although occasionally fleeting memories may be triggered by some event.

Psychiatric disease   There is no evidence of an increase in the incidence of serious psychiatric disorder following abortion although relapse can occur in those with pre-existing psychiatric disease. In contrast, the incidence of depression, suicide and child abuse is higher in women who have continued with the pregnancy because abortion was refused (Matejcek et al 1985).

Infertility   Postabortion infection is a significant cause of tubal disease and hence infertility, particularly following illegal abortion. However, as indicated above, with modern methods performed under optimal conditions the incidence of infection is very low.

Pregnancy complications   Damage to the cervix or perfora-tion of the uterus can predispose to cervical incompetence, preterm delivery and/or uterine rupture. However, a large prospective trial carried out by the Royal College of General Practitioners and the Royal College of Obstetricians and Gynaecologists showed that previous induced abortion had no effect on outcome in subsequent pregnancies (Frank et al 1987).

FOLLOW-UP

A follow-up visit at about 2 weeks is desirable for all women irrespective of the timing or method of abortion.

This visit is absolutely essential after administration of prostaglandin for those (about 30%) who have not passed the fetus and/or placental tissue in the few hours after the administration of the Gemeprost. Although the incidence of ongoing pregnancy is low (less than 1%) it will be necessary to evacuate the uterus because of incomplete or missed abortion in about 2–5%. Those women with ongoing pregnancies should be strongly advised to have VA because the development of the fetus could be compromised, although babies born to the few women who have chosen to continue with the pregnancy after medical abortion has failed have been normal.

Follow-up can be undertaken by the GP, family planning clinic, or abortion service. Careful coordination of these services is essential to ensure that any ongoing pregnancies are identified promptly and to treat any complications.

Contraception

The fact that a woman has had an abortion is an indication that she probably requires a review of her method of contraception (if any). It is difficult during the emotionally stressful events surrounding the abortion for a woman to make a reasoned judgement about future methods of fertility control.

A decision about permanent irreversible methods such as sterilization are better left for some months when the events of the abortion can be seen in perspective. However, ovulation returns fairly rapidly after abortion (20–60 days) and contraceptive precautions must be taken early if a further unwanted pregnancy is to be avoided. The method of contraception advised will vary depending on circumstances and needs of the couple.

Hormonal contraception   This can be started immediately following the abortion, although it is probably wise to delay starting it immediately after *medical* abortion if fetal or placental tissue has not been passed following prostaglandin administration. Otherwise, there is always the remote risk that high doses of hormones may be given to a woman who changes her mind and chooses to continue with the pregnancy. This risk must be balanced against the risk of the individual woman's becoming pregnant again in the weeks following abortion due to lack of effective contraception. A reasonable compromise is to advise against intercourse for the 2 weeks between the abortion and the follow-up visit. At the same time, condoms can be supplied in the event of weakening of resolve. All hormonal methods, including injectables and implants, can be started at this time without risk of the woman already being pregnant.

IUDs   An IUD may be inserted immediately following the abortion, under the same anaesthetic if surgical abortion is chosen. Following medical abortion it is probably preferable to wait until the 2-week follow-up before IUD insertion. However, there are no data to suggest that immediate insertion has any additional risks in women in whom products of conception have been identified at the time of prostaglandin administration.

Barrier methods   Any of these may be started immediately but the diaphragm should be checked at follow-up to ensure that the user does not need a different size.

CONCLUSION

Abortion should never be regarded as a method of contraception. Indeed, the request for termination of an unplanned pregnancy is evidence of a lack of knowledge of contraception, failure to use an effective method or failure of the method. Good family planning seeks to reduce the number of unplanned pregnancies and evidence suggests that abortion rates are lowest in those countries with a comprehensive system of sex education and contraceptive services. The occurrence of an abortion is an indication to review the method of contraception and consider whether change to another method which would suit the needs of women better, should be made.

REFERENCES.

Baird D T 1992 Medical Termination of Pregnancy. In: Edwards C R,
    Lincoln D W (eds) Recent Advances in Clinical Endocrinology and Metabolism
    Vol. 14, Churchill Livingstone, Edinburgh, pp. 83–94
Baird D T 1993 The use of antiprogestogens for the termination of pregnancy.
    In: Asch R, Studd J (eds) Annual Progress in Reproductive Medicine.
    Parthenon Publishing, Carnforth, UK, pp. 351–358
Botting B 1991 Trends in Abortion. Population Trends 64. Her Majesty's
    Stationery Office, London, pp. 19–29
Fathalla M F 1992 Reproductive health in the world: two decades of progress and
    the challenge ahead. In: Khanna J, Van Look P F A, Griffin P D (eds)
    Reproductive health: a key to a brighter future. World Health Organization,
    Geneva, pp. 3–31
Francome C, Savage W D 1992 Gynaecologists' abortion practice.
    British Journal of Obstetrics and Gynaecology 99, 153–157

Frank P 1985 Sequelae of induced abortion. In: Porter R, O'Connor M (eds) Abortion: medical progress and social implications. Ciba Foundation Symposium 115, Pitman, London, pp. 67–79

Frank P I, Kay C R, Scott L M, Hannaford P C, Haran D 1987 Pregnancy following induced abortion: Maternal morbidity, congenital abnormalities and neonatal death. British Journal of Obstetrics and Gynaecology 94, 836–842

Glasier A F, Thong K J 1991 The Establishment of a Centralised Referral Service Leads to Earlier Abortion. Health Bulletin 49, 254–259

Matejcek Z, Dytrych Z, Schüller V 1985 Follow up study of children born to women denied abortion. In: Porter R, O'Connor M (eds) Abortion: medical progress and social implications. Ciba Foundation Symposium 115, Pitman, London, pp. 136–146

Rodger M W, Baird D T 1990 Pretreatment with mifepristone (RU 486) reduces interval between prostaglandin administration and expulsion in second trimester abortion. British Journal of Obstetrics and Gynaecology 97, 41–45

Segal S J, La Guardia K D 1990 Termination of pregnancy – a global view. Baillière's Clinical Obstetrics and Gynaecology 4, 235–247

Appendix 10.1

PATIENT INFORMATION SHEET

Abortion has been legal for many years but must be done in an approved place and with the agreement of two doctors who believe that you have good reasons for not wanting to continue with your pregnancy. If you are less than nine weeks pregnant there are two alternative ways of doing the abortion. The following information may help you decide which method you prefer. Remember that you only have a choice if you are less than nine weeks pregnant.

Vacuum aspiration

This is the commonest method and is not normally used in this hospital at more than 12 weeks of pregnancy. Once the gynaecologist has agreed to your request for an abortion you will be given a date to return to hospital usually just for the day.

After being admitted to the Ward you may have a tablet or pessary inserted into the vagina. This, as it dissolves, will soften the cervix (neck of the womb). The abortion procedure itself takes about five minutes and is done under a general anaesthetic i.e. while you are asleep. The cervix is stretched open, a thin plastic tube is inserted into the uterus (womb) and the pregnancy is carefully sucked out. After you wake up from the anaesthetic you may feel a little tearful but this and any period-like discomfort you may have will soon pass and you will be allowed home later the same day. Vacuum aspiration is a very safe procedure but all operations carry a small risk. However, the abortion is over in a single procedure and you are not aware of what is happening.

Medical abortion

Having agreed to your request for an abortion, the doctor will arrange for you to attend the Ward on two separate occasions. At the first visit – which may be immediately after you have seen the doctor today – you will be given tablets of a drug called Mifegyne (RU 486).Once you have swallowed these tablets you can leave the hospital.

Two days later you will come back for the second part of the treatment. During these two days you can behave entirely normally and go to work as usual.

You may have some light bleeding but it is very unlikely that the abortion will take place.

When you go back to the hospital, you will stay on the Ward for about six hours.

You will not be asked to get undressed or to get into bed. A small pessary is put into the vagina which causes the uterus to contract and expel the pregnancy. You will probably have some period-like pains which may be strong enough for you to be given a painkiller and you will have some vaginal bleeding. It is likely that the abortion will occur during the time you are in hospital but the fetus is tiny at this stage of the pregnancy and you will not experience anything much different from your normal period. Medical abortion can only be used if you are less than nine weeks pregnant and is not available to you if you are over 35 years of age and smoke heavily, suffer from asthma or heart disease. Provided that you are suitable for a medical abortion, the main advantage is that you do not need to have an anaesthetic or an operation.

After the abortion

Whichever method is used, you will bleed for up to two weeks, although this will not be heavy. You must see a doctor within a month after the abortion to check that all is well and that you have sorted out some contraception.

You will have an opportunity to discuss any questions you have with the doctors and other staff during the consultation.

11. Legal and ethical aspects of family planning

Mary Anderson

Consent
  Consent to sex
  Consent to medical treatment
  Age of consent
  Mental incapacity and consent
    Minors
    Adults
Confidentiality
  Young people
Abortion
  Conscientious objection to abortion
  Special circumstances
Litigation
  Fertility control
    Barrier methods
    Hormonal contraception
    Emergency contraception
    Intrauterine devices
    Sterilization
  Therapeutic abortion

How to avoid litigation
The process of a claim
Medical defence organizations and
    NHS indemnity

Medical research

**Ethical aspects of acquired
immunodeficency syndrome (AIDS) and
human immunodeficiency virus (HIV)**
  Consent
  Confidentiality

The infertile couple
  In vitro fertilization (IVF)
  Gamete intrafallopian transfer (GIFT)
  Surrogacy

Gender selection

Use of fetal tissue

Appendix

In Western democracies the law remains the final arbiter even on ethical questions. But law and ethics are inextricably linked in many areas of medicine, including family planning.

The law governing medical practice in the United Kingdom (UK) is derived principally from Acts of Parliament and the regulations which follow them and the common law created by decisions made by judges which provide precedents for subsequent cases. Scots law, which is founded on Roman law, differs in many respects from English law.

Medical ethics is difficult to define as an entity (Appendix 11.1). It is an amalgam of philosophy, avoidance of bad practice and moral obligation. Dunstan (1989) describes it as the '...pursuit of ends reckoned altruistic and good and the avoidance of ends reckoned inordinately self regarding and bad'.

A number of ethical and legal issues are relevant to reproductive health care and the family planning consultation.

CONSENT

Consent to sex

While it is generally said that a girl may consent to sexual intercourse once she has reached the age of 16, it is more accurate to say that it is unlawful for a man to have sexual intercourse with a girl who is under 16. A man under the age of 24 who is charged with such an offence may plead a statutory defence of a reasonable belief that the girl had attained the age of consent.

Consent to medical treatment

In all medical practice it is necessary to obtain the patient's consent for every type of procedure and for treatment. Consent can be implicit as well as explicit and although even simply touching a patient may expose a doctor to the charge of assault, it can be assumed that by coming to a clinic and undressing for examination, consent to that examination has, by implication, been given. It is nevertheless good practice always to request permission to examine a patient and certainly if medical students or doctors or nurses in training are present, to request permission both for their presence and for an examination by one of them. In clinics where trainees are present much of the time, it may be helpful to have a notice in the waiting area informing patients of the presence of students and trainees and of their right to refuse to see them. Male doctors and nurses should always examine female patients in the presence of a chaperone.

Consent to investigation or treatment can only properly be given by a patient after the nature and consequences, if any, of the procedure or treatment have been explained. The extent to which the patient should be warned of any risks is still ultimately a matter for the doctor's judgement – the so-called 'therapeutic privilege' – but the greater the likelihood of risk, the greater is the onus on the doctor to disclose it to the patient.

Written consent, although it has no greater legal force than consent given orally, provides the best evidence that the consent was properly obtained from the patient, should any dispute subsequently arise.

Age of consent

Young teenagers often attend family planning clinics or their general practitioner (GP) for advice about contraception and may not wish their parents to know.

In Scotland, the Age of Legal Capacity (Scotland) Act 1991 states that a person under the age of 16 may consent to treatment 'where in the opinion of a qualified medical practitioner...(the child)...is capable of understanding the nature and possible consequences of the procedure or treatment'. In Scotland, the fitting and providing of contraceptives is considered to be covered by the word 'procedure'.

In England and Wales, a child who has attained the age of 16 and is of sound mind is able to give a legally valid consent to any surgical, medical or dental treatment or procedure (Section 8 Family Law Reform Act 1969). Children under 16 who have sufficient under-standing of the purpose, nature, likely effects and risks of a proposed treatment may, as in Scotland, also give their consent. It is for the doctor to decide whether there is sufficient understanding. If not, consent must be sought from the child's parents or the person or body holding parental responsibility.

In 1974 a DHSS circular outlined arrangements for family planning within the National Health Service (NHS). It advised that the provision of contraception to a girl under 16 was a matter for the doctor to decide, and that the girl need not inform her parents. It was stressed that every effort should be made to persuade the girl to discuss matters with her parents but that if she refused the doctor could proceed if he considered it was in the child's best interests. Mrs Victoria Gillick, who herself had four daughters under the age of 16, challenged the DHSS in court in 1982. She lost, but subsequently won her case in the Court of Appeal which considered that under the age of 16 the parents' rights were paramount. The DHSS in turn appealed to the House of Lords which decided that the original DHSS advice was not unlawful and that a child under 16 could give valid consent to contraception or abortion without parental knowledge or agreement provided the child understood what she was doing.

It is, however, still emphasized that every effort must be made to persuade the girl to inform her parents and to explore the reasons if the girl is unwilling to do so.

Mental incapacity and consent

The need to provide contraception for patients who lack full mental capacity is encountered not infrequently in medical practice. Such individuals may not have the ability to link sex with the risk of pregnancy or may not be able to look after a child.

Minors

The age of majority in Scotland and England is 18. For patients under that age who themselves do not have the mental capacity to consent, consent to treatment can be given by the person holding parental responsibility for that minor. This treatment can include contraception, abortion and, it is thought, even sterilization but *only* where that sterilization is *incidental* to other therapeutic treatment (e.g. hysterectomy because of severe menorrhagia).

Where sterilization is the only purpose of the treatment, however, the House of Lords, in 1987, gave the clearest possible instruction that the decision to sterilize a child under the age of 18 should only be made by a High Court Judge, warning '*A doctor performing a sterilization operation with the consent of the parents might still be liable in criminal, civil or professional proceedings*' (Lord Templeman). Thus any doctor planning to sterilize (with the sole intent of rendering infertile) an adolescent who is under 18 years of age and has a learning difficulty should seek the Court's approval.

Adults

With adults who lack sufficient mental capacity the situation is more complicated. In English and Scots law no one can give consent on behalf of the 'mentally incompetent' adult. If emergency treatment is considered necessary, then to provide it without consent would, however, be considered legal and court approval would not be essential. It would be wise to discuss the case with another medical colleague and if possible record the fact of that discussion.

In the case of abortion it might be argued that an unplanned pregnancy does not constitute an emergency in the sense of a threat to the health of the mother (unless there are serious complications of pregnancy). However, once a decision has been taken that abortion is in the mother's best interests then it is also in her best interests to terminate the pregnancy at the earliest possible gestation.

When treatment is not an emergency, time can be taken over the decision. Following a case in England in 1989 involving the sterilization of a woman of 36 with a mental age of 5, Lord Brandon declared '...a doctor can lawfully operate on, or give other treatment to, adult patients who are incapable, for one reason or another, of consenting to his doing so, provided that the operation or other treatment concerned is in the best interests of the patient'.

In the case cited above, the House of Lords, although emphasizing that they could not require doctors to apply to the Courts before undertaking such a radical measure as sterilization, said that they trusted that doctors would choose to do so.

In 1993, the Official Solicitor set out the procedure for applying to the Courts in England for consent to sterilize a child or mentally incapacitated adult.

In Scotland the appropriate procedure is for the Court of Session to be petitioned to appoint a 'Tutor Dative' to give the necessary consent.

It is probably not necessary to go to court if a reversible method of contraception is being considered.

In reality, every case is different and faced with such decisions it is important that a second medical opinion is obtained and that the hospital or regional legal department is consulted. Doctors who are members of a medical defence organization should seek advice from the organization.

CONFIDENTIALITY

Keeping the patient's secrets is central to medical ethics. It is stated within the Hippocratic Oath and the obligation of confidentiality is, in theory at least, absolute. Breach of confidentiality may be permitted in what are described as 'very exceptional circumstances'. The doctor may be legally compelled to reveal confidential information or he may find it necessary to relax the rule of confidentiality in the interests of public safety. In all, the General Medical Council (GMC) lists eight possible exceptions to the rule (BMA 1993).

Young people

In the context of family planning, perhaps the biggest problem of confidentiality lies with teenagers. Allen (1991) reported that almost 75% of young people under 16 and 50% of 16–19 year olds worry that their GP either must or might involve their parents in contraceptive consultations.

In 1993 a leaflet entitled *Confidentiality and People under 16* (Ch. 1) was circulated by the British Medical Association (BMA) to all GPs which clarified the legal position with respect to provision of contraceptive services to young people. It is advisable that in all such cases the doctor is able to support the fact that his or her decisions were made in the best interests of the patient. It is also important that young people under 16 who are seeking contraceptive advice should be aware that although the doctor is obliged to discuss the value of parental support, he or she is not legally entitled to inform the parents and it would be a serious breach of confidentiality if the doctor did so in the face of a prohibition by the child. It is important that young people are made aware of the profession's code in this respect so that they can be encouraged to seek help without fear.

ABORTION

The history of termination of pregnancy in the UK is interesting, reflecting as it does the social and moral history of this country. In the early years of the twentieth century many unwanted pregnancies occurred because of the lack of contraception. 'Back street' abortions were common, as were their complications which were not infrequently fatal. The moral climate was against therapeutic termination.

In England, the Offences Against the Person Act 1861 and the Infant Life Preservation Action of 1929 made it an offence to procure a miscarriage, the latter referring to the possibility of the child being born alive. This Act does not apply to Scotland.

In 1938 Alec Bourne, a gynaecologist in St Mary's Hospital, London, deliberately carried out a termination of pregnancy on a 14-year-old girl who had been raped. He reported himself to the Director of Public Prosecutions and was duly prosecuted. He was found not guilty thus clarifying that termination could legally be carried out when there was danger to health and life.

In 1967 Parliament passed the Abortion Act which came into effect in 1968 and was amended by Section 37 of the Human Fertilisation and Embryology Act 1990. It is applicable in England, Wales and Scotland but not in Northern Ireland. The grounds on which abortion may be carried out are well known and covered in Chapter 10.

Termination of pregnancy must be carried out in NHS hospitals or in places approved by the Secretary of State. Two forms must be completed, Certificate A stating the grounds for termination and the Notification of Termination Form, which notifies the abortion procedure. This must be done within 7 days. *Failure to meet this requirement can lead to prosecution and a fine.*

Conscientious objection to abortion

Where doctors or nurses object on ethical or moral grounds to abortion those objections are respected. The Abortion Act of 1967 does, however, require them to provide necessary treatment in an emergency. Outwith the emergency situation, doctors who object to abortion do have a duty to refer the patient to another doctor who does not hold moral objections. Such referral must take place without delay and it must not be left to the patient to find such help.

Special circumstances

Termination of the pregnancies of women lacking full mental capacity or of minors are subject to the same conditions. Provided that the operation is carried out in the best interests of the patient it will be regarded as legal. The issues of consent and confidentiality already examined apply.

A husband has no right enforceable at law to stop his wife having, or a registered medical practitioner performing, a legal abortion.

LITIGATION

The increase in medical litigation in the United Kingdom affects obstetrics and gynaecology to a considerable and disturbing degree. Table 11.1 shows the nature of claims notified in 100 consecutive gynaecological cases of litigation (James 1991).

Fertility control

Fertility control, especially sterilization, contributes significantly to gynaecological claims. Specific legal issues and the risk of litigation vary according to the method of contraception. General rules apply, however, to all family planning consultations.

When providing a method of contraception, information must be given about its efficacy, side-effects and risks (including risk of failure) together with proper and appropriate instructions for its

Table 11.1 Legal claims notified in 100 consecutive gynaecological litigation cases

Nature of complaint	No. of claims
Failed sterilization	25
Operative complications	25
Contraception	10
Urinary tract damage	10
Retained swabs/instruments	3
Others	27

Source: James 1991.

use. A balance must be reached between fully informing the patient and putting her off using the method at all. Too much information may be counterproductive but too little may lead to litigation.

It is a dilemma to which there is no clear answer and every doctor must ensure that what he or she discusses is as adequate as they, in all conscience, feel is necessary. In the event of a complication occurring, if due warning has been given and duly noted in the case records then the recourse to litigation may be pre-empted.

Barrier methods

There are no legal restrictions on the provision of barrier methods of contraception which can be purchased over the counter. By virtue of their low risk of side-effects these methods have a very low risk of litigation.

Hormonal contraception

Hormonal contraception is still only available on prescription. Regulations concerning pill prescription are controlled by the Medicines Act 1968 and the Pharmacy and Poisons Act 1933.

1. Only a medical practitioner may prescribe the pill.
2. A nurse may supply and reissue pills to the patient in accordance with the doctor's directions written on the prescription. This permits a useful degree of delegation both within general practice and in clinics. But even with special training, nurses are not yet permitted to prescribe the COC.
3. Prescriptions must be in writing and must be dated.
4. Prescriptions must not be indefinite in terms of quantity, duration and validity.
5. Each container should be labelled with the name of the patient, the product, the place and the date of issue.
6. Clinics which dispense supplies of hormonal contraception including emergency contraception (Chs 3, 4 and 9) from large so-called 'clinic packs' must ensure that these are correctly packaged and labelled with the patient's name and that a copy of the manufacturer's package insert is included.
7. Arrangements should be made for inspection of storage facilities at intervals of not more than 3 months by the pharmacist or person in control of the clinic. A written record of the inspections should be kept, dated and signed, confirming that the storage system is satisfactory.

The risk of litigation associated with the provision of hormonal contraception lies mainly in the incidence of side-effects. Claims have arisen alleging inappropriate prescribing leading to cerebro-vascular accidents and other serious side-effects; failure to advise correctly about possible drug interactions and failure to advise about cessation of the pill prior to surgery.

It is conceivable that cases might arise over failure of the method as a result of inadequate or inappropriate instructions for use and even, in the future, over the very long-term risks of hormonal contra-ception, including breast cancer (Orr 1992).

Some patients will insist on using a method of contraception, particularly the combined pill, against medical advice. The doctor can only do his or her best to ensure that the patient understands the risks that she may be exposing herself to, but it may be difficult to refuse to prescribe the method. In these cases discussion of the risks should be carefully documented and the doctor's advice recorded in the notes.

Particular care should be taken when counselling women about the use of long-acting methods which do have the potential for abuse. In some countries there have been reports of women being given injectable methods of contraception without informed consent or indeed without any consent (WHO 1993). Concerns have been raised in the United States of America over women being required by the courts to use Norplant as a condition of probation or custody of their children (Forrest & Kaeser 1993).

Implants which have to be surgically removed give rise to particular ethical and moral problems. In the USA some women have implants inserted postpartum free of charge under government programs for which they are no longer eligible when they want the implant removed.

In the UK, where contraception is free, there can be a fine line between encouraging a woman to 'keep trying a little longer' in the face of unacceptable side-effects in the hope that they will settle, and putting pressure on someone to continue using a method which becomes very expensive if it is discontinued prematurely.

Emergency contraception

Emergency contraception administered after ovulation has occurred may act by inhibiting implantation. Some people regard this as infringing the Offences Against the Person Act of 1861 where it is an offence for anyone unlawfully to administer a drug or use an instrument to procure an abortion whether the patient is pregnant or not. The argument hinges on the definition of abortion.

Norrie (1991) argues that 'before a pregnancy can be terminated it must have commenced'. In the United Kingdom the law does not define the start of pregnancy but it is widely believed that the courts will accept that it does not start until implantation is complete. Therefore, contraceptives which act before implantation or which prevent it are not abortifacients. Indeed, in 1983, prior to the licensing of the combination oestrogen–progestogen postcoital contraceptive, the Attorney General ruled: 'I have come to the conclusion that this form of postcoital treatment does not constitute a criminal offence...'. He based this conclusion on the fact that preventing implantation is not 'procurement of a miscarriage' (Dando P R (MDU), personal communication).

Pregnancies do occur despite emergency contraception. Most women choose to have a termination, but if pregnancy continues there is always the possibility of congenital malformation. It is not necessary for a woman to sign a consent form prior to being given emergency contraception since consent is implied by her voluntarily taking the tablets. Information about possible failure and its consequences should, however, be given and documented (Ch. 9)

Intrauterine devices

It is important that the doctor inserting a device has been trained in the technique, that proper counselling is given before insertion so that informed consent can be obtained, and that the method used for the insertion is recorded in the notes.

Perforation of the uterus is a not uncommon cause of litigation.

Missing threads should never be interpreted as an expulsion without an ultrasound confirmation of an empty uterus and/or a plain X-ray to exclude perforation.

IUD users should be made aware of the risks of failure of the IUD and of the risk of ectopic pregnancy. Ectopic pregnancy is notoriously difficult to diagnose and may be catastrophic in its consequences. All doctors should maintain a high index of suspicion of ectopic pregnancy in IUD users and should always investigate women with any suggestive features.

Although the risk of pelvic infection associated with IUD insertion is small, it should be covered in the routine counselling. The IUD is a good example of a method where a detailed discussion of the risks and side-effects can put the patient off the method for ever.

Sterilization

Vasectomy and tubal occlusion have become increasingly popular in the last 20 years. Some people, however, have moral objections based largely on religious beliefs which regard the procedure as irreversible interference with the ability to reproduce. The objection of the Catholic Church is more direct in that sterilization is regarded as a mutilation of the body leading to the cessation of a natural function (Mason & McCall-Smith 1991).

Sterilization differs from other surgical procedures in that it is almost always requested by the patient. It is, however, essential that proper counselling is offered to patients. Adequate counselling must include discussion of the nature and irreversibility of the procedure, its failure rate, risks and long-term effects (Ch. 8).

It is a moot point whether a doctor is ever justified in refusing a request for sterilization even in someone who is comparatively young or who is nulliparous and the patient should certainly be referred for a second opinion.

Consent forms for sterilization should incorporate written warnings about the possible failure of the procedure (Ch. 8). These should not replace verbal discussion and should preferably be signed immediately following counselling and witnessed by the advising doctor. Although discussion with both partners as part of the counselling procedure may be thought appropriate, the consent may only be taken from the partner undergoing the procedure.

Unfortunately, legal claims associated with both male and female sterilization are not uncommon. Patients sue for sterilization failures sometimes alleging that they were not told about the possibility of failure. If an adequate consent form has been signed and it has been recorded in the notes that the patient has been told about failure rates it will be difficult for the plaintiff to convince the court that adequate counselling did not take place.

If it can be proved that the procedure has been negligently performed, there can usually be no defence and these claims attract high damages.

Complications arising from surgery also give rise to litigation, particularly following vasectomy, but these may be successfully defended if it has been recorded in the notes that the potential complications were discussed and that the procedure was correctly performed. Negligence cannot be inferred simply from failure of the procedure.

Litigation may also be avoided if complications are recognized promptly and managed appropriately and if a full explanation is given to patients after the event.

Therapeutic abortion

Failure to effect a complete abortion may lead to litigation. Sometimes the continuing pregnancy is not diagnosed until late or, more commonly, there are retained products leading to secondary bleeding or infection or both, requiring further hospitalization and surgery. Again, full counselling beforehand is essential, and if difficulties have been encountered with the procedure detailed documentation must be made and explanation given to the patient as soon as possible. Routine follow-up by the surgeon or the referring doctor should overcome the problem of pregnancies continuing unrecognized after failed abortion.

How to avoid litigation

From these comments the steps that can be taken to avoid litigation should be apparent. The 'golden rules' are:

1. Explain everything clearly to the patient so that consent is properly obtained.
2. Keep adequate notes.
3. Explain to the patient if things have gone wrong and express regret if appropriate. Take great care in offering an apology lest it be taken as an admission of fault.
4. Give written information wherever possible and ensure that the patient reads the consent form.

In other words, talking to the patient and careful recording go a long way to avoiding or minimizing the risk of litigation. Recording should be factual and never include personal or potentially offensive remarks. This holds for all record keeping. Patients now have a statutory right to read any entry in their own notes made since November 1991.

The process of a claim

An early indication of possible litigation is the patient's solicitor requesting production of the patient's notes implying that a possible claim for damages may follow. If, following a study of these records, the patient is advised that he or she has grounds for a claim then certain procedures will be followed. These differ between England and Scotland. In all the complexities of preparation for a legal case, it is imperative that the doctor has the guidance of and follows instructions from his or her defence organization or the Authority's legal advisers. The doctor must prepare a factual account of what happened and should stick very strictly to the contemporary notes and records. It is then that the need for good, comprehensive, and factual record keeping will be particularly appreciated.

Medical defence organizations and NHS indemnity

Until January 1990 doctors were obliged to be members of a defence organization which provided, in a sense, a buffer between the doctor and the law. One of their purposes was, and still is, to help, support and guide a doctor who becomes the target of a claim.

From January 1990 the NHS Indemnity Scheme was introduced. Health Authorities and Trusts take financial responsibility for negligent acts of hospital and community health service doctors and dentists. GPs are still required to provide their own insurance through the defence organizations. Doctors who are wholly employed in a NHS Hospital or Trust need not, theoretically, have other insurance. It is advisable, however, that insurance cover is taken out not only for private practice, where it is necessary, but also for protection in disciplinary cases and for so-called 'Good Samaritan' activities. The defence organizations also continue to provide a valuable advisory service for doctors.

MEDICAL RESEARCH

Without research there would be little progress in clinical medicine. Research into many aspects of contraception and fertility control is essential.

It is interesting that a licence must be obtained in order to experiment on animals (Animals (Scientific Procedures) Act 1986) and on human embryos (Human Fertilisation and Embryology Act 1990) yet there is no legal requirement governing research on adults or children. This may well change as European Union (EU) legislation is developed.

There are, however, many guidelines and safeguards on research. Local research ethics committees, although not required by law, are encouraged by the Department of Health. Their task is to scrutinize research projects from an ethical standpoint before granting approval. They will assess the means of recruitment, the information given to the subjects about the research and the adequacy of the consent forms, the scientific validity of the project and the competence of the researchers.

The Department of Health demands that all research undertaken on NHS premises should have such approval. Funding for a research project is not likely to be forthcoming without such approval and most peer-reviewed journals insist that manuscripts submitted for publication state that ethical committee approval was obtained for the research being described.

The World Medical Association Declaration of Helsinki which was modified in 1989 gives clear principles for experimentation on human subjects. Fundamentally, it highlights the fact that the patient's interests must come first and emphasizes the need for appropriate and adequate information to be given to the subject of any research project.

Written consent must be obtained from all subjects taking part in research. Consent must be based on full information given in as unbiased a way as possible and without pressure on the patient. Written information about the study and what it asks of participants must be available to all participants. Risks must be discussed.

Young people of sufficient maturity and understanding can consent to taking part in research and parental consent is necessary for the participation of minors deemed unable to understand.

Randomized controlled trials have become central to most modern research. Here patients are randomly divided into two or more groups and given different treatments (often including a placebo) the effects/outcomes of which are monitored. In a 'double blind' randomized trial both the doctor giving the treatment and the subject receiving it are unaware of what is being given thus removing any element of personal bias or preference. There are those who argue that these types of scientific trials are the only valid ones but doubts have been raised about the ethics of them. For example, subjects who are receiving a placebo may be denied the best chance of treatment (Brazier 1992).

The outcome of such trials is usually reviewed at regular intervals so that if one treatment proves to be particularly effective, or indeed particularly ineffective, the trial or one arm of it can be stopped.

A useful summary on these and other aspects of research can be found in the BMA's handbook, *Medical Ethics Today – Its Practice and Philosophy* (BMA 1993).

ETHICAL ASPECTS OF ACQUIRED IMMUNODEFICENCY SYNDROME (AIDS) AND HUMAN IMMUNODEFICIENCY VIRUS (HIV)

The appearance of AIDS as a worldwide problem has created new ethical problems many of which are still vigorously debated and as yet unresolved. Many of the ethical concepts already examined are particularly highlighted in the case of HIV positive patients and those with AIDS. Some family planning clinics now offer routine testing for HIV infection on request.

Consent

The social and medical implications for the patient found to be HIV positive or to have AIDS are so profound that as things stand at the present time the consent of the patient must be obtained before testing. Full counselling must be given to the patients before testing and in the event of a positive result counselling must be available.

Random testing, for epidemiological purposes in antenatal clinics for example, has been carried out strictly anonymously. This avoids the problems of named testing. But whether such programmes are lawful or ethical is debatable.

Confidentiality

The serious implications for the HIV positive person, in terms of employment and life insurance for example, are such that it is imperative that the strictest confidentiality is maintained. But this raises profound ethical dilemmas. There are risks to other people including health care workers. It is noteworthy that the General Medical Council requires any professional who suspects that he or she may be HIV positive to undergo testing and if positive to obtain advice on whether to continue practising or not. Disciplinary action will result against those who do not follow this requirement or who deliberately conceal their positive status. But the reverse is not the case – there are no formal rules to require patients to be tested.

In the UK neither AIDS nor HIV are notifiable conditions. Whether the law will change remains to be seen.

Can a doctor disclose that a patient has AIDS or is HIV positive? As we have seen, doctors owe patients a duty of confidentiality but this duty is not absolute where the safety of others is concerned. It has been pointed out that to breach a patient's confidentiality, there has to be a 'clear and significant risk of the patient causing harm to others' (Brazier 1992). The problem is not an easy one and here again a legal opinion may have to be sought in the individual case.

THE INFERTILE COUPLE

Recent developments in treatment for infertile couples which raise particular ethical questions are assisted conception techniques and surrogacy. Fundamental to all this is the basic question – do all couples have a right to procreate? If the answer is yes, then there are almost no limits to which medical treatment should go in the quest for successful conception.

In vitro fertilization (IVF)

In 1982 the Warnock Committee was set up to consider 'recent and potential developments in medicine and science related to human fertilization and embryology; to consider what policies and safeguards should be applied including the social, ethical and legal implications of those developments; and to make recommendations'. Final implementation of the report took place in 1990 through the Human Fertilisation and Embryology Act. The Human Fertilisation and Embryology Authority (HFEA) was established as a result and this is the present controlling body on all treatment and research involving the use of embryos or *frozen* (but not fresh) gametes.

Gamete intrafallopian transfer (GIFT)

The transfer of gametes directly into the fallopian tubes allows fertilization to take place within the tube and GIFT thus raises fewer ethical issues than IVF. Since only fresh gametes are used, the HFEA in the UK has no jurisdiction over GIFT as it has over IVF. This leaves the way open for poorly-organized and badly-monitored units to conduct the procedure, often for considerable financial gain.

Surrogacy

The involvement of a third person in the treatment of infertility raises ethical problems which, for some, are the greatest of all.

Donor insemination (DI) has long been employed in the management of infertility where the male is azoospermic. Matters of public health importance are raised particularly in relation to transmission of infection. Ovum donation can be part of IVF if egg production in the female is absent. In both these procedures, questions of genetic and legal inheritance arise.

Commercial surrogacy was banned in the UK after the Warnock Report. The Surrogacy Arrangements Act 1985 forbids the development of commercial surrogacy agencies in Britain. Otherwise, surrogacy is not illegal. However, profound ethical, moral and social issues remain.

GENDER SELECTION

Apart from doubts as to the *efficiency* of most of the procedures presently available for gender selection, there are many ethical and moral issues. (Aborting a fetus of the 'wrong' sex is an efficient but at present illegal procedure.)

The BMA's Medical Ethics Committee concluded in 1993 that sex selection for social and/or medical reasons was acceptable (BMA 1993). This was not supported by the annual representative meeting which concluded that sex selection was justified for strictly medical reasons only.

Following a consultation document in 1993 (HFEA 1993), the HFEA supports sex selection techniques for medical reasons but to date is against sex selection for social reasons. It also feels that the data on sperm-sorting techniques as a method of sex selection do not support their use.

USE OF FETAL TISSUE FOR RESEARCH AND TREATMENT

Tissue obtained from aborted fetuses may be used for research and (with the exception of fetal ovaries) for the treatment of medical conditions such as Parkinson's disease. Informed consent must be obtained from the mother of the fetus and the use of tissue is subject to strict guidelines (Polkinghorne 1989). In 1994, following a widespread public consultation, the HFEA recommended that eggs from fetal ovaries should not (for the time-being) be used for the treatment of infertility.

The debate on these and other related issues continues.

REFERENCES

Allen I 1991 Family Planning – Pregnancy Counselling Projects for Young People. London Policy Studies Institute
BMA 1993 Medical Ethics Today – Its Practice and Philosophy. BMA, London
Brazier M 1992 Medicine, patients and the law. Penguin, Harmondsworth

Dunstan G R 1989 Doctor's decisions: Ethical conflicts in medical practice. Oxford University Press, Oxford

Forrest J D, Kaeser L 1993 Questions of Balance: Issues Emerging from the Introduction of the Hormonal Implant. Family Planning Perspectives 25: 127–132

HFEA 1993 Sex Selection: Public Consultation Document. HFEA, London

James C 1991 Risk Management in Obstetrics and Gynaecology. Journal of the Medical Defence Union 7 (2) 36–38

Mason J K, McCall-Smith R 1991 Law and medical ethics, 3rd edn. Butterworth, London

Norrie K 1991 Family planning practice and the law. Dartford

Orr C 1992 Contraception. In: Chamberlain G (ed.) How to avoid Medico-legal Problems in Obstetrics and Gynaecology. RCOG, London.

Polkinghorne J 1989 The Polkinghorne Report. Review of the guidance on the research use of fetuses and fetal material. HMSO, London

World Health Organization 1993 Fertility Regulating Vaccines. Report of a meeting between women's health advocates and scientists to review the status of the development of fertility regulating vaccines. 17–18 August 1992. WHO, Geneva

Appendix 11.1

ETHICAL PRINCIPLES FOR PRACTICE AND RESEARCH

Respect for persons: the duty to respect the self-determination and choices of autonomous persons, as well as to protect persons with diminished autonomy (e.g. young children, persons with mental retardation and those with other mental impairments). Respect for persons includes fundamental respect for the other; it should be the basis of any interaction between professional and client.

Beneficence: the obligation to secure the well-being of persons by acting positively on their behalf and, moreover, to maximize the benefits that can be attained.

Nonmaleficence: the obligation to minimize harm to persons and, wherever possible, to remove the causes of harm altogether.

Proportionality: the duty, when taking actions involving risks of harm, to so balance risks and benefits that actions have the greatest chance to result in the least harm and the most benefit to persons directly involved.

Justice: the obligation to distribute benefits and burdens fairly, to treat equals equally, and to give reasons for differential treatment based on widely accepted criteria for just ways to distribute benefits and burdens.

(United States, National Commission for the Protection of Human Subjects, 1979; Beauchamp and Childress 1994).

12. Screening and reproductive health

Patricia Last

Screening

Screening for pelvic disease
Cervical cancer
  Risk factors
  Diagnosis
  Prevention of invasive cervical cancer
  Taking a cervical smear
Cervical intraepithelial neoplasia (CIN),
  carcinoma in situ
  Management of women with
    abnormal smears
  Frequency of cervical smears
Cancer of the ovary
Cancer of the endometrium
Other pelvic conditions
When to examine

Screening for breast cancer
Screening techniques
  Breast self-examination
  Clinical examination

  Mammography
Management of the patient with a
  breast lump

Other screening
Weight
Blood pressure
Urine testing: haemoglobin estimation
Rubella screening
  Recommended schedule

Who should screen?

Health promotion
Smoking
Alcohol
Exercise
Video display terminals
In general

Resources

Appendix

Apart from routine medical examinations at school, most women do not have any physical examination until they attend for family planning advice in their late teens or early twenties. The family planning consultation therefore offers an excellent opportunity for screening and for promoting health. The supervision necessary for women using various contraceptive techniques has been discussed in the relevant chapters. Screening will be considered as a separate entity although in many cases the examinations will overlap.

The screening procedures recommended in this chapter represent a counsel of perfection. No-one should be refused contraception just because she does not wish to avail herself of the screening facilities offered. The approach of the clinic personnel should not be so authoritarian that an overweight smoker feels too guilty to attend. The vaginal examination and smear test sometimes recommended at the first visit can be omitted if the patient feels unable to accept them.

SCREENING

Health screening is the examination of symptom-free persons in an attempt to discover early disease or the predictors of disease. The examination of those with symptoms is disease diagnosis and is quite separate.

The theory of screening is based on the belief that disease caught early in its progress or even before it is clinically manifest will respond more readily to treatment, with lower morbidity and mortality rates than disease left to become clinically well established and symptomatic. Not all diseases will respond favourably to early detection and certain rules are used as guidelines for a screening programme (Wilson & Jungner 1968).

Screenable disease   The disease to be screened for must:

1. Be serious enough to justify the search.
2. Be common enough to give a reasonable pick-up rate.
3. Develop slowly with a fairly long pre-symptomatic phase.
4. Be amenable to treatment which must be available and acceptable to the patient. Furthermore, there must be an advantage in treating the disease at a stage before the patient would otherwise present.

Screening test   The screening test must be:

1. Simple and easily applied.
2. Positive in the majority of persons who have the disease or its predictors. This demands a high sensitivity i.e. a test which produces few false negatives.
3. Negative in the majority of persons without the disease. This demands a test of high specificity i.e. one producing few false positives.
4. Acceptable and not harmful to the patient.
5. Economically possible within the current resources of the health care service in the country concerned.
6. Capable of giving reproducible results independent of observer variation.

Useful definitions   Two particularly useful definitions are:

1. The *prevalence* of a disease is the finding of an abnormality in a well-defined population examined for the first time.
2. The *incidence* of a disease is the finding of new cases in the same screened population when examined at specific intervals.

SCREENING FOR PELVIC DISEASE

Cancer is common. 32% of all women will get cancer at some time in their lives. While 8.6% will get breast cancer, 1.41% will get ovarian cancer, 1.8% will get cancer of the cervix and 1.3% will get cancer of the uterus (CRC 1994a). Some 9% of all cancers in women are gynaecological.

Cancer in women under the age of 45 is uncommon. The exception to this statement is carcinoma in situ of the cervix, which has a peak incidence in the 25–34 age group. The incidence of other genital tract cancer rises dramatically in the age group 45–54.

There is also a geographical variation in these cancers. While there is an increased risk of ovarian and breast cancer in the South of England compared with the North, the risk of cervical and uterine cancer is greater in the North (CRC 1994b).

Cervical cancer

Cervical cancer is the eighth commonest cancer in women; it accounts for 3% of all cancers. In England and Wales it has a 5-year survival of 58% (Table 12.1).

In 1992 there were 1860 deaths from this disease in the UK. While death rates are highest in the over 65s, the highest numbers are diagnosed in 35–39 year olds with a second peak at 65–69 years.

Table 12.1   Ten commonest cancers in UK women 1988

Site	No. registered	(%) All cancers	Rate/ million	5-year relative survival % 1981 (E&W only)
1 Breast	29 870	18	1021	62
2 Skin (non-melanoma)	17 455	11	597	97
3 Lung	13 627	8	466	7
4 Colon	10 639	6	364	37
5 Ovary	5 832	4	199	28
6 Rectum	5 145	3	176	36
7 Stomach	4 975	3	170	10
8 Cervix	4 943	3	169	58
9 Uterus	4 179	3	143	70
10 Bladder	3 716	2	127	–

Source: CRC 1994d Fact Sheet 1.3.

Table 12.2   Cervical and breast cancer in women under 55 in England and Wales

		Under 35	35–39	40–44	45–49	50–54
New registrations	Breast	524	983	1480	1891	2058
(1986)	Cervix	642	487	336	337	278
(Cancer stats 1986 HMSO 1991)						
Rates per 100000	Breast		53.2	94.3	136.8	154.4
Mortality (1990)	Breast	140	232	511	713	954
(Mortality stats:	Cervix	97	130	133	128	121
Cause 1990 HMSO 1991)						
Death rates per 100000	Breast		13.9	27.8	47.6	69.3

Although only 15.5% of cases occur in women under 35 years old, it is the most common cancer in this age group *(but deaths from breast cancer are higher than deaths from cervical cancer in women under 35)* (Table 12.2). Although there has been little change in the overall incidence of cervical cancer, there has been a decrease in the mortality rates over the past 20 years. There is also a striking effect of birth cohort on mortality rates. Women born around 1951 have twice the risk of dying from cervical cancer compared with those born 10 years earlier (CRC 1994c)

Risk factors

The actual cause of cervical cancer is not yet known. It is epidemiologically linked with young age at first intercourse and multiple sex partners (or partners who have had multiple partners). There is a strong possibility that a sexually transmissible infection – possibly human papilloma virus (HPV) – is linked to development of cervical cancer. Prophylactic vaccines and specific therapeutic immunization against the high-risk viral subtypes are under active research.

The disease seems to favour women in the lower socio-economic groups and women in the developing world. Smoking is an added risk factor and it has been suggested that a chemical in inhaled cigarette smoke affects the immune cells in the cervix and inhibits their protective action against the papilloma virus.

Diagnosis

The diagnosis of cervical cancer can usually be made on the appearance of the cervix on speculum examination. It is a rare condition and even a family planning doctor will see less than five cases in the course of a professional lifetime. Taking a cervical smear may be helpful in diagnosis, but in 10–15% of pathologically proven cervical cancers, smears fail to show any neoplastic cells. Any patient with a suspicious looking cervix or with persistent postcoital or irregular intermenstrual bleeding should be referred for further investigation despite a negative smear result.

In 1963, the World Health Organization stated that invasive carcinoma of the cervix is a preventable disease. If preventable, why not prevented?

Prevention of invasive cervical cancer

The majority of invasive cervical cancers are preceded by a neo-plastic non-invasive process – cervical intraepithelial neoplasia (CIN) – which cannot be diagnosed by the naked eye but which may be detected by exfoliative cytology. Since CIN is virtually 100% curable, cervical screening by smear test must rank as one of the most important screening procedures available to women. In countries with extensive screening programmes, the registration rates for cervical cancer are falling.

National screening programme   Screening for cervical cancer has been in place in the UK since 1967, but it was not until the late 1980s that the National Co-ordinating Network (NCN) was created in an attempt to bring together the wide variety of specialists involved in an effective screening programme. This culminated in 1994 in the appointment of a National Co-ordinator who will administer both the breast and cervical screening programmes for the UK.

Over the past four years the NCN has published a wide range of literature related to cervical screening aimed at monitoring, auditing and standardizing all aspects of quality in the programme. *Assuring the Quality and Measuring the Effectiveness of Cervical Screening* is the latest in the series (March 1994). This document attempts to draw together all the elements necessary for a successful screening programme.

Most important too has been the collection of data. In 1992–93 in England, 1 570 893 women were screened. Results were negative in 94.9%, 4.4% were abnormal (borderline, mild or moderate dyskaryosis) and 0.7% were positive (severe dyskaryosis). In all, some 80000 women had an abnormal smear. Over the past 5.5 years 83% of the target population (age 20–64) have had a smear test, and in the same period, 12.5 million women have been tested (Government Statistical Service 1994).

Taking a cervical smear

The competence of the smear taker is a vital element in a successful programme. All staff, doctors or nurses entrusted with taking smears must be properly trained both in the taking of the smear and the correct response to the result sent from the laboratory. *Taking Cervical Smears* (a video and accompanying booklet) produced by Dr Margaret Wolfendale (British Society for Clinical Cytology 1989) is now widely used as a teaching aid by the large numbers of practice and family planning nurses currently training for the screening programme. Doctors also need specific training.

The commonest error in taking a smear is failing to take an adequate sample from the squamo–columnar junction, the area where neoplastic change occurs. In nulliparae, and in women past the menopause, the squamo–columnar junction may be well within the cervical canal and it is not always possible to scrape this area.

Technique   The technique used is as follows:

1. Place the patient in the dorsal or left lateral position.
2. With good illumination insert the speculum, lubricated only with water and expose the cervix.
3. If the presence of an invasive carcinoma is suspected on clinical examination, refer the woman for a gynaecological opinion irrespective of the smear result.
4. Insert a wooden or plastic spatula into the cervical os and rotate through 360° (Fig. 12.1).

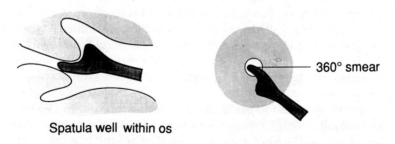

360° smear

Spatula well within os

Fig. 12.1   Taking a cervical smear. Rotate spatula through 360°.

5. Spread the scrapings from the spatula thinly and evenly onto an indelibly-named glass slide (using a pencil not a ball-point pen).
6. Fix immediately with a spray or by immersing the slide for 10–15 minutes in equal parts of absolute alcohol and ether.
7. Proceed to vaginal examination after carrying out the cervical smear.
8. Complete all sections of the request form, which must accompany each smear to the laboratory.

Choice of spatula   Many new spatulas have been introduced over the past few years. They must prove themselves both as being more effective in sampling the squamo–columnar junction, and in the area of cost, before being recommended (Fig. 12.2).

Endocervical brushes are very efficient at sampling the endo-cervical canal. They are not necessarily better than cervical spatulas at sampling the squamo–columnar junction. Therefore, they should not replace the spatula, but should be used in conjunction with it. Most cytopathologists prefer the brush smear and spatula smear mounted separately on two slides. However, this should be checked with the local laboratory.

Indications for use of an endocervical brush sampler:

1. No endocervical cells on a previous smear.
2. Previous cone biopsy.
3. A patient with symptoms whose cervix looks normal.
4. Requested by the cytolaboratory.

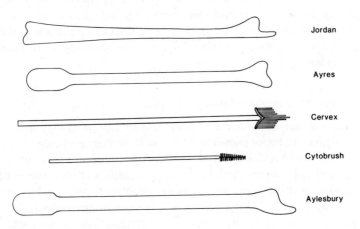

Fig. 12.2   Types of sampling spatula.

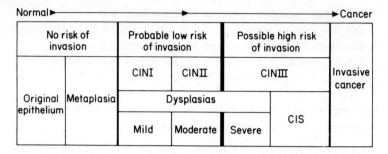

Fig. 12.3 Three stages of cervical intraepithelial neoplasia: CIN cervical intraepithelial neoplasia, CIS carcinoma in situ (Anderson M C, personal communication).

Cervical intraepithelial neoplasia (CIN), carcinoma in situ

Exfoliative cytology identifies cellular abnormality but cannot diagnose the severity of the histological change. Three stages of CIN are recognized (Fig. 12.3).

1. CIN I – equivalent to mild dysplasia.
2. CIN II – equivalent to moderate dysplasia.
3. CIN III – equivalent to severe dysplasia and carcinoma in situ.

Reversion to normal can occur in CIN I, especially in women under 30 years of age. Reversal to normal in cases of CIN II and III is uncommon.

In some 30% of cases there will be discrepancy between the cytological assessment and the eventual histological grade. It is not uncommon to find CIN II or even CIN III in a patient referred to colposcopy despite having had smears showing only mild dyskaryosis.

Management of women with abnormal smears

The prevalence of abnormal cervical smears can be as high as 5%. This figure can be increased to 11% when cytology and colposcopy are used together (Giles et al 1988). An abnormal smear is not diagnostic of cervical cancer; it only identifies the presence of potential for disease and indicates the need for further evaluation. Normally the cytologist's report will contain suggestions for the appropriate management. If there is any doubt about this a personal approach to and discussion with the cytologist is the best plan.

The NCN published *Guidelines for Clinical Practice and Programme Management* edited by Dr Ian Duncan in 1992. Among the recommendations are:

1. CIN II and CIN III should be treated once diagnosed.
2. CIN I may be treated or kept under close surveillance.
3. A woman should be referred for colposcopy the first time that she has a moderately or severely dyskaryotic smear.
4. A smear showing borderline nuclear or mildly dyskaryotic change should be repeated 6 months later and consideration given to colposcopic referral if it is not then normal.
5. There should be a minimum of two consecutive negative smears at least 6 months apart following a borderline or mildly dyskaryotic smear before surveillance is reduced to the frequency of a woman with no previous abnormality, preferably 3-yearly.
6. Cervical cytology screening is not justified in teenagers.
7. To minimize the anxiety for those receiving abnormal smear results, all women undergoing cervical screening should be provided with detailed information (both verbal and printed) at all stages of screening both before and after the smear.

It should be remembered that these are only recommendations and that local policies may differ somewhat. In Lothian, for example, teenagers who have been sexually active for more than one year are offered a cervical smear.

Doctors should be clear about the facilities for investigation and treatment available locally. It is pointless to discuss theoretical possibilities with a patient. Where a colposcopic service exists, cone biopsy will be avoided in the majority of women with abnormal smears. Instead they will be treated by locally destructive techniques such as cryosurgery, laser vaporization or cautery using loop excision. Cone biopsy will still be necessary for the few patients in whom the abnormal epithelium extends up into the cervical canal and where its upper edge cannot be delineated.

Frequency of cervical smears

All programmes will screen women age 20–64 who are, or have been, sexually active and who still have a cervix. Smears are repeated every 3–5 years.

There is evidence now to suggest that women over 50 who have had regular smears which have always been negative can be omitted from routine recall, but this has not yet been accepted as routine clinical practice.

Every effort should be made to ensure that the maximum number of sexually active women are screened at regular intervals. Frequent repeat smears in women without risk factors are unnecessary.

The Intercollegiate Working Party on Cervical Cytology Screening reported in November 1987 (RCOG 1987). Among its recommendations are:

1. All women should be regularly screened from the age of 20.
2. 3-yearly screening for women between the ages of 20 and 64 should be available where resources permit.
3. Women of 65 and over who have had three consecutive negative smears – the last one no more than 3 years previously – may be excluded from further screening.

Instructions on the management of the cervical cancer screening programme, together with the definition of the responsibilities of doctors and nurses, are fully outlined in DHSS circular HC(88) 1:HC(FP)(88)2.

Although abnormal smears are uncommon under the age of 20, they have been reported in girls as young as 16. The above recommendations are, therefore, minimum requirements and, if the service and the laboratory can cope, and if financial constraints permit, the age range for smears should be expanded. Ideally one would like to offer a cervical smear:

1. At the beginning of sexual activity.
2. 1 year later to eliminate a false negative report.
3. Regularly thereafter with a maximum interval of 5 years.
4. More frequently to women at greater risk of cervical cancer – those who start having intercourse at an early age, who have multiple partners (or whose partners have multiple partners), who have a history of sexually transmissible diseases, particularly genital herpes or genital warts, and those who have previously had abnormal smears.

A diagnostic smear is indicated for any women who has symptoms. Any woman who has never had a smear and who was or is sexually active should be offered one even if she is over the age of 65.

A computerized call and recall system is now in place in all regions. However, computers can only work well if they are given accurate information. Unhappily, human beings are not overly cooperative in such a scheme. Women move house not infrequently, and the majority change their name at least once, if not twice, during their lives. Inevitably some women will escape the call/recall net. Opportunistic screening should be offered to women who have never had a smear or have not had a smear within the past 3–5 years.

Remember, pre-clinical cancers are now presenting at an earlier age. Many women dying from cervical cancer are those who have never had a cervical smear.

The Health of the Nation (Department of Health 1992) set the following target: 'to reduce the incidence of invasive cervical cancer by at least 20% by the year 2000 (from 15 per 100 000 in 1986 to no more than 12 per 100 000)'.

The family planning clinic offers the opportunity to carry out smears in women who would not/have not visited their own GP for this. Every effort must be made to integrate with GP services so that there is no duplication.

Every woman must be given a definite result of every cervical smear she has.

Cancer of the ovary

This cancer is uncommon in young women but when it does occur it may be extremely aggressive. Every woman having a cervical smear should have a bimanual pelvic examination to identify any pelvic mass. If any abnormality is found, the woman should be referred for a gynaecological opinion.

Where there is a strong family history of ovarian cancer, women can be referred to a specialist ovarian cancer screening clinic. A blood sample for CA125 antigen and a family tree will serve to check whether there is a genetically determined risk. Some 5–10% of all ovarian cancers may be hereditary and where two first-degree relatives have had ovarian cancer before age 50, a woman may have a lifetime risk as high as 1:3. There are approximately 40–60 new cases of ovarian cancer in the UK in these high-risk women each year.

The Cancer Research Campaign (CRC) is currently funding further research to assess population screening of older asymptomatic women for ovarian cancer.

A decision analysis model was used to answer the question, 'Will a one-time screen improve the average life expectancy in a cohort of 40-year-old women?'. The result showed an average lifetime gain of just 1 day using transvaginal ultrasound and CA125 together (Schapira et al 1993).

Fact sheets on various cancers in both men and women have been produced by the CRC (see useful addresses).

Cancer of the endometrium

This is rare before the menopause. A healthy 50-year-old woman has a lifetime probability of 2.5% of having uterine cancer and a 0.2% risk of dying from it.

No screening or special surveillance is indicated at a family planning clinic. Current hormone replacement regimens incorporate regular monthly progestogen to protect the uterus from possible endometrial hyperplasia which may predispose to cancer.

Other pelvic conditions

Management of non-malignant conditions is dealt with in Chapter 16. If the patient is told about the presence of these abnormalities without adequate explanation, much anxiety can be caused; this should be carefully avoided.

When to examine

Ideally pelvic examination should be carried out on all new patients (it is necessary for those using the diaphragm or IUD), but should not be insisted upon. There is no justification for performing regular yearly pelvic examinations in healthy young women just to identify ovarian tumours.

SCREENING FOR BREAST CANCER

In the UK, 1 in every 12 women will develop a breast cancer at some time in their lives. Each year in the UK some 26 000 women are newly diagnosed and some 16 000 die from it.

Breast cancer screening using mammography is nationally available for women aged 50–64, yet each year in England and Wales, 4800 women under the age of 50 are diagnosed as having breast cancer (1800 in the same age group have cervical cancer).

It is important to be aware of breast abnormalities and their possible significance. While only 1 in 10 breast lumps is due to cancer, cancer is not rare in young women.

In women eligible for breast screening in 1992–93, 1.6 million women were invited and 1.16 million were screened. 6597 new cancers were detected and 1497 of these were 1cm or less in size (NHS 1994).

Screening techniques

Breast self-examination (BSE)

There is evidence that the earlier breast cancer is detected and adequately treated, the longer the life expectancy, and it is to this end that screening is directed.

Although the Forrest Report cast doubt on the cost-effectiveness of BSE, there is evidence that women who are taught and who practise it have smaller tumours at an earlier clinical and pathological stage than those who do not. The likely impact of BSE on breast cancer mortality is difficult to assess, although the potential benefits of the lead time gained must not be ignored when assessing the costs and benefits of BSE.

Every woman should be breast aware. Part of this awareness is self-examination. It seems sensible for every woman to examine her own breasts on a regular basis, preferably just after the menstrual period. This is particularly important in women over the age of 35 and under the age of 50 in whom breast cancer is not rare. Excellent leaflets are available from the Health Education/Promotion Bodies and the Women's Nation-wide Cancer Control Campaign and Breast Cancer Care (see useful addresses). In addition, many breast clinics and departments of surgery produce their own (Appendix 12.1). Such leaflets should be available in family planning clinics and in doctor's surgeries.

It is important to stress to every patient that if she detects an abnormality she should report at once to the clinic or her doctor and not wait until her next routine visit is due.

The fear of disfiguring treatment for breast cancer may explain the reluctance of many women to examine their own breasts or even to report breast lumps once they have been found. Less mutilating surgery is a widely accepted practice now. If women were told about this it might well encourage them to seek help as soon as they discover a lump in the breast.

Clinical examination

Breast examination should be carried out by the doctor or the nurse using the same thorough technique as is taught for breast self-examination, and should be offered annually to those at particular risk of breast cancer. They include women:

1. With a history of benign breast disease and/or biopsy.
2. With a strong family history of breast cancer, especially in a first-degree female relative aged less than 50.
3. Who have no children or had their first child after the age of 35.
4. Who have already had cancer of one breast.

Mammography

Although this is not suitable for screening young women attending for family planning, it may be offered to women with high risk indicators where facilities are available. Breast ultrasound is now widely available for symptomatic young women.

Management of the patient with a breast lump

Patients with multiple discrete lumps or a generalized increase in density in the breasts on clinical examination should be re-examined after the next menstrual period. Symmetrical bilateral lesions and those associated with bilateral tenderness often resolve after the onset of menstruation. A young woman with a breast lump which 'comes and goes' should not be referred *straight away* to a surgeon. *But any* woman with a breast lump which is constant i.e. does not change in size at different times in the menstrual cycle, must be referred to a specialist.

Although only 1 in 10 lumps is malignant, it is important to identify that one case. There are no characteristics of the malignant lesion. Many malignant tumours present as smooth, mobile, well-circumscribed lesions and it is important to recognize this fact. It is, however, most unlikely that a well-circumscribed lesion that has been present for several years will be found to be malignant.

OTHER SCREENING

Weight

Routine weighing is unnecessary. Overweight patients should have their weight checked and be advised about appropriate diet. Weight should be correlated with height and the woman given her ideal weight from national charts. Most women are weight-conscious and need little encouragement to monitor their own weight. Care must be taken not to make a woman so embarrassed by weight that she stops coming for family planning advice. The leaflet *Healthier Eating and Your Heart*, produced by the Coronary Prevention Group, is of interest even to women who are not overweight, and should be available in the clinic or surgery. The Health Education Promotion Bodies have information leaflets and the Department of Health runs a literature line (see useful addresses).

Blood pressure

As a screening base, the blood pressure (BP) should be recorded on *all* new patients, but this ideal is rarely achieved. Even in routine medical examinations at school, BP may not be recorded. Renal disease and coarctation of the aorta are rare but certainly not unknown in completely fit young people. A baseline BP is valuable before a patient becomes pregnant. This simple test, which in women not taking the pill need only be carried out once by the clinic sister, should, therefore, not be beyond the resources of *every* family planning clinic.

All women using hormonal contraception should have their BP recorded regularly (Chs 3, 4).

Urine testing: haemoglobin estimation

These tests are not recommended routinely but should be carried out if indicated by symptoms or examination.

Rubella screening

Maternal rubella infection before 16 weeks gestation can lead to severe fetal abnormality. Safe, effective rubella vaccine is available and great efforts have been made to offer vaccination at school to all girls aged 13. Although this has proved very successful in some areas, the resource is greatly under-used in others. In 1980 and 1981 uptake averaged only 84%. The effectiveness of rubella vaccination is now well established.

In 1988 mumps, measles and rubella vaccinations (MMR) became available to all babies and young children. It is unknown whether immunity will persist into adulthood.

In 1994, a national measles and rubella campaign was launched. The purpose of the campaign is twofold; to prevent the measles epidemic which is predicted to occur in 1995 and to improve immunity against rubella especially in males. Whilst immunization of schoolgirls has reduced the susceptibility to rubella in this group to 1–2%, the figure for comparable males is 20%. Infected males increase the infection rate in susceptible pregnant women by chance social contact. The number of infected pregnant women was just 2 in 1992, but associated with a rubella outbreak in young men, the figure was 22 in 1993.

The family planning consultation offers an ideal opportunity to check the immune status of women before they embark on a pregnancy. A history of past infection or vaccination does not exclude determining the current immune status.

Recommended schedule

1. Nulliparous women should be offered a blood test to evaluate their immune status. If resources for this are not available, women who give a history of rubella vaccination at school or previous rubella infection may be excluded. However, some such women may be rubella-susceptible.
2. Arrange vaccination for rubella-susceptible women either at the clinic, by the GP or at a special community health clinic.
3. Ensure that no woman who is pregnant or suspected of being pregnant is vaccinated.
4. Warn the woman not to conceive within the next month and provide her with efficient contraception to try to ensure that she does not do so. The importance of this has been questioned following evidence that vaccine virus rarely causes fetal abnormality (Hinmann et al 1983). Tookey and colleagues (1991) suggest that the vaccine virus is not teratogenic, and the need to give the above advice to women is now of questionable scientific basis. With litigation in mind it is probably, however, wise. Those who do become pregnant inadvertently can at least be reassured and termination of pregnancy is not mandatory.
5. If screening is carried out in a clinic or hospital, notify the GP of the result.
6. Give the patient the result in writing. Ask her to keep it and take it to the antenatal clinic when and if appropriate.

Leaflets and posters about rubella are available from the Health Education/Promotion Bodies and should be displayed in family planning clinics and GP surgeries. It is particularly important to give these leaflets to women who are shown to be rubella-susceptible.

WHO SHOULD SCREEN?

Having considered the individual woman, the diseases for which she should be screened and the frequency at which screening procedures should be carried out, it is proper to consider who should undertake these examinations. All the tests described, including bimanual pelvic examination, cervical smear taking, instruction in breast self-examination and breast examination itself can be undertaken by specially trained nurses. Training of these nurses can be undertaken by the doctors with whom nurses work, or by the appropriate hospital department. The Board of Education of the Royal College of Nursing has approved course modules for training nurses in screening procedures. Details may be obtained direct from the College.

HEALTH PROMOTION

Health is a very special commodity. It cannot be bought or sold, nor can it be forced upon people. The family planning consultation offers an excellent opportunity to give women simple, sensible advice. This is particularly important for those who are planning a pregnancy.

Smoking

This is one of the better known risks to health and the incidence of carcinoma of the lung increases year by year. Lung cancer will overtake breast cancer as the primary cause of cancer deaths in women in England and Wales if the present rate of increase is maintained. This has already happened in Scotland.

The Health of the Nation target is, 'to reduce the prevalence of cigarette smoking in men and women age 16 and over to no more than 20% by the year 2000'.

Ischaemic heart disease is not an important cause of death or disability in women under the age of 54, but in older women it is one of the main causes of mortality and morbidity. There is a very strong correlation between ischaemic heart disease and smoking.

The risk of cervical neoplasia and ectopic pregnancy has also been shown to be increased among smokers.

Every encouragement should be given to women to give up smoking. After 10 years of non-smoking the risk of smoking-related disease is no greater than in the general population. This fact should be a great encouragement to women to give up the habit.

The family planning or well woman consultation is an appropriate time to offer advice. There are many aids for those who wish to give up smoking, and information about these should be available in clinics and surgeries. The Health Education/Promotion Bodies (see useful addresses) have excellent literature on the subject.

Alcohol

Alcohol is the only freely available mood-changing drug in the UK and its misuse among women is increasing. The damaging effects to health are as great as those arising from smoking and the use of illicit drugs, yet are less well publicized. Advice on 'sensible drinking' can be given without offence when discussing family planning, and is particularly important as part of pre-pregnancy counselling.

Exercise

Moderate exercise is good. Most housewives reckon that they work very hard in the home, but this exercise is insufficient. Exercise should be undertaken on a regular basis at least three times a week for 20 minutes within the limits of tolerance and in a properly planned fashion. Such exercise should raise the pulse rate above 100 beats per minute and sustain it at this level for 5–10 minutes. Clinic personnel should be able to recommend one or two suitable books or exercise tapes to help patients with keep-fit programmes.

Video display terminals

Many young women who use video display terminals are concerned about continuing to do so when they are pregnant. There is no evidence that video display terminals present any hazard to pregnant women. However, the seeds of doubt have been sown and women are often not prepared to take this risk.

In general

Health promotion is a general and gradual affair. It is important that information is reinforced without 'nagging'. The family planning or well woman consultation is an ideal opportunity for showing an interest in all aspects of a woman's health and offering her help and advice on how to stay healthy. Help sheets and leaflets on a wide variety of subjects produced by the Health Education/Promotion Bodies are available to clinics and general practices.

The reassurance which comes from finding no abnormality on screening is important in improving the patient's confidence in her own good health. Women should be made aware of the difference between tests which are medically indicated, e.g. taking the blood pressure of an oral contraceptive user, and screening tests, which are offered as an additional part of the family planning service. If patients do not wish to avail themselves of the latter they can be omitted. However, it is a sad reflection on current health care resources that valuable screening tests are often omitted because of the shortage of staff, time or space.

RESOURCES

Health information is widely available and some sources and telephone helplines are listed in the useful addresses section.

REFERENCES

British Society for Clinical Cytology 1989 Taking Cervical Smears. A video and accompanying booklet. BSCC Secretariat
Cancer Research Campaign 1994a Incidence – UK, Fact Sheet 1.1. CRC, London
Cancer Research Campaign 1994b Atlas of Cancer Incidence in England and Wales, Fact Sheet 19. CRC, London
Cancer Research Campaign 1994c Cancer of the Cervix Uteri, Fact Sheet 12. CRC, London
Cancer Research Campaign 1994d Fact Sheet 1.3. CRC, London
Department of Health 1992 The Health of the Nation. HMSO, London
Government Statistical Service 1994 Cervical Cytology 1992–93. Summary of Information from KC53 England. DH Statistics Division (SD2B)
Giles J A, Hudson E, Crow J, Williams D, Walker P 1988 Colposcopic assessment of the accuracy of cervical cytology screening. British Medical Journal 1: 1099–1102
Hinmann A R, Bart K J, Orenstein W A, Preblud S R 1983 Rational strategy for rubella vaccination. Lancet i: 39–41
National Co-ordinating Network 1994 Assuring the quality and measuring the effectiveness of Cervical Screening. Farmery E, Muir-Gray D (eds) NCN, Oxford
National Co-ordinating Network NHS Cervical Screening Programme 1992 Guidelines for Clinical Practice and Programme Management. Duncan I D (ed.) NCN, Oxford
National Health Service Breast Screening Programme Review 1994. Patnick J (ed.) ISBN.1. 87 1997 968
Royal College of Obstetricians and Gynaecologists 1987 Report of the Intercollegiate Working Party on Cervical Cancer Screening. RCOG, London
Schapira M M, Matchar D B, Young M J, 1993 The Effectiveness of Ovarian Cancer Screening. Annals of Internal Medicine 118: 838–843
Tookey P A, Jones G, Miller B H R, Peckham C S 1991 Rubella Vaccination in Pregnancy. Communicable Disease Report Review No 7 Volume 1
Wilson J M G, Jungner G 1968 Principles and Practice of Screening for Disease. WHO Public Health Papers No. 34. WHO, Geneva

Appendix 12.1

BREAST SELF-EXAMINATION

Instructions for patients

1. Sit in front of a mirror stripped to the waist. Be sure you are sitting up straight. Look at your breasts carefully.
2. Is there any inequality between the size of your breasts? Has one breast recently become lower than the other?
3. Now look at the nipple area. Has one nipple become turned in? Is there any discharge? Always inspect the inside of your 'bra' for signs of a discharge. Do not squeeze the nipple or areola.
4. Now look at the skin of the breasts. Is there any puckering or dimpling? Is there any rash or change in skin texture? You may have to lift the breasts to see the under surface.
5. Raise your hands above your head and concentrate on the upper part of the breast that leads into the armpit. Is there any swelling or skin puckering?
6. Lean forward and examine each breast in turn. Is there any unusual change in outline, any puckering or dimpling of the skin or any retraction of the nipple?
7. Lie down in a relaxed and comfortable position. You may find it convenient to carry out this part of the examination with a soapy hand when having a bath.
8. First examine the left breast with the right hand. Use the front part of the flat of the hand, keeping the fingers together. It is important to learn how hard to press when examining the breasts; too hard will dull the sensation and too soft will not allow you to feel deeply enough. Never pinch the breast; if you do, you may feel lumps even in a normal breast.
9. Slide your hand over the breast, above the nipple, starting at the armpit and moving across to the centre of the body, pressing in to feel for lumps.
10. Repeat this action passing the hand from the outside inwards below the nipple.

11. Finally slide your hand across the nipple, making sure you have felt all parts of the breast.
12. Feel for lumps along the border of the pectoral muscles and in the armpits.
13. Now carry out items 8-12 with the left hand on the right breast.

(Printed by permission of BUPA Medical Centre, London)

13. Sexually transmissible diseases

Alexander McMillan

Prevalence

Genitourinary medicine clinics

Examination of the female patient

Bacterial infections
  Gonorrhoea
    Clinical features
    Diagnosis
    Treatment
  Syphilis
  Non-specific genital tract and chlamydial
  infections
    Clinical features
    Diagnosis
    Treatment
  Bacterial vaginosis
    Clinical features
    Diagnosis
    Treatment

Protozoal infestation
  Trichomoniasis
    Clinical features
    Diagnosis
    Treatment

Fungal infection
  Candidiasis
    Clinical features
    Diagnosis
    Treatment

Viral infections
  Herpes simplex virus
    Natural history
    Clinical features
    Diagnosis
    Treatment
    Genital herpes in pregnancy
  Human papilloma virus
    Clinical features
    Management
  Human immunodeficiency virus (HIV)
    Epidemiology
    Clinical features
    Course of infection
    Diagnosis
    Management
    Follow-up and treatment
  Hepatitis A virus
  Hepatitis B virus
  Hepatitis C virus
  Hepatitis D virus
  Molluscum contagiosum virus
  Epstein Barr virus
  Cytomegalovirus

Arthropod infestations
  Phthiriasis
  Scabies

Appendix

Doctors who provide family planning services deal with a young sexually active population, some of whom may be at risk of sexually transmissible diseases (STDs). Indeed, the doctor may be the first individual in whom a young person confides that he or she has acquired a sexually transmitted infection. Many infections are symptomless but signs may be noted during routine examination. It is therefore important that the practitioner should be aware of the clinical features of the more common sexually transmissible infections in adults.

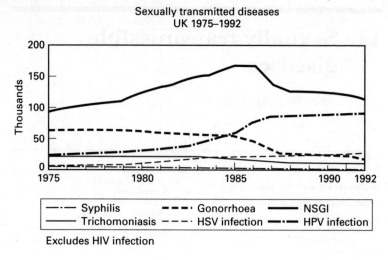

Fig. 13.1   Sexually transmitted diseases UK 1975–1992. Excludes HIV infection.

PREVALENCE

The prevalence of sexually transmissible diseases varies geographically, but Fig. 13.1 illustrates the trends in their prevalence in the United Kingdom (UK) over the past 17 years. The number of patients with gonorrhoea has declined since the early 1970s, and the increasing importance of viral infections, particularly with human papilloma virus (HPV) and of non-specific genital infection, is obvious. Although the incidence of trichomoniasis has fallen over the past 15 years, bacterial vaginosis, a newly described cause of vaginal discharge, is being recognized with increasing frequency.

The human immunodeficiency viruses (HIVs) with their propensity for heterosexual transmission and congenital infection are, of course, of great concern to doctors who may be asked for advice by infected individuals.

GENITOURINARY MEDICINE CLINICS

Ideally, all patients in whom a sexually transmissible disease is suspected should be referred to a genitourinary medicine clinic. In the UK, the Venereal Diseases Regulations (1916) allowed for the establishment of clinics for the diagnosis and treatment *in confidence* of STD. Today, these clinics provide facilities for the collection of the most appropriate anogenital material for microbiological examination. In addition, trained counsellors and contact tracers are immediately available. As most departments are within hospitals there is ease of access to additional diagnostic services, such as ultra-sonography, that may be required in the investigation of a patient with, for example, suspected pelvic inflammatory disease (PID). As referral to a genitourinary medicine clinic is not always possible, the family planning doctor or general practitioner may need to undertake appropriate investigations.

EXAMINATION OF THE FEMALE PATIENT

Appendix 13.1 outlines the examination for suspected STD. This schedule can of course be modified to suit individual requirements. The investigation of women with vaginal discharge is outlined in the algorithm (Fig. 13.2).

It must be stressed that concurrent infections are common and every effort should be made to exclude other infections when one is discovered.

BACTERIAL INFECTIONS

Gonorrhoea

Gonorrhoea is caused by *Neisseria gonorrhoeae*, small kidney-shaped Gram-negative cocci arranged in pairs. In adults it is almost always sexually acquired. Although gonococcal vulvovaginitis may result from accidental contamination, in children the infection may indicate sexual abuse.

Although the prevalence of strains of *N. gonorrhoeae* that are relatively insensitive to antibiotics has been increasing for several decades, it was the discovery in 1976 of β-lactamase-(penicillinase) producing *N. gonorrhoeae* (PPNG) that caused concern amongst physicians. These organisms are endemic in South East Asia and in West Africa but account for only a small proportion of strains in developed countries. In the UK, the prevalence of infection associated with PPNG has declined in the past few years.

Clinical features

In men

1. Most patients with urethral gonorrhoea develop urethral discharge and dysuria 2–10 days after sexual intercourse with an infected partner. There is usually a profuse mucopurulent

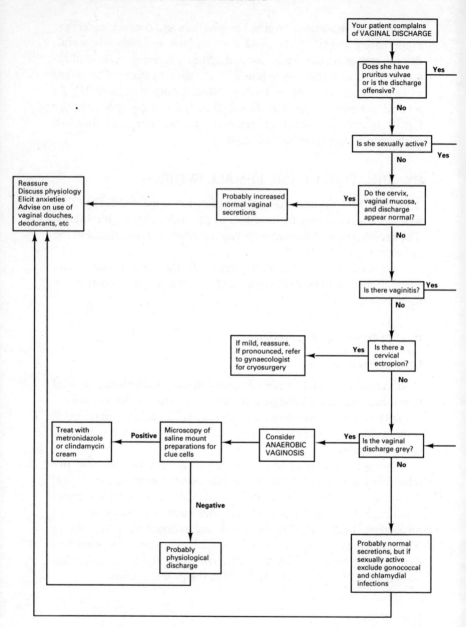

Fig. 13.2 Investigation of vaginal discharge

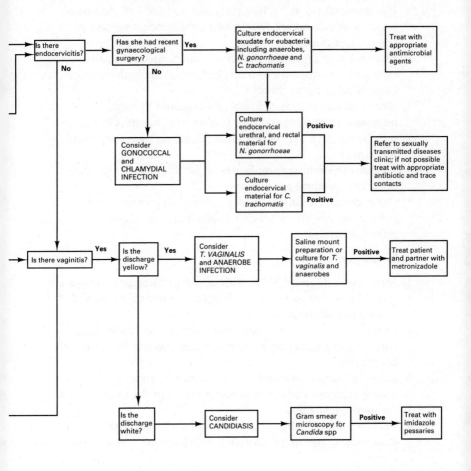

(McMillan A 1986 British Medical Journal 293: 1357–1360).

urethral discharge but less severe urethritis is not uncommon. It is important to note, however, that up to 5% of men with urethral infections are *symptomless* (and hence represent a reservoir of infection).

2. Pharyngeal gonorrhoea, resulting from orogenital sexual contact is mostly symptomless, but occasionally the patient complains of a sore throat.

3. Rectal infection, almost invariably acquired through homosexual anal intercourse, is often symptomless but there may be features of proctitis (anal discharge, pain, bleeding, tenesmus).

4. Epididymo-orchitis complicates about 5% of men who have untreated urethral gonorrhoea.

5. Other complications, such as periurethral, prostatic and seminal vesicle abscesses and disseminated gonococcal infections are rare.

In women

1. Most women (about 80%) with uncomplicated gonorrhoea are *symptomless*. Some, however, complain of increased vaginal discharge and dysuria.

2. In the absence of concurrent infections, the only abnormal clinical finding may be a mucopurulent exudate from the cervical os.

3. Infection of the paraurethral glands may be manifest as mucopurulent exudate on gentle massage of the distal urethra through the vagina.

4. PID complicates about 15% of women with untreated gonorrhoea, and its presentation may be acute, subacute or chronic.

5. Bartholinitis with abscess formation may develop in 10% of infected individuals, and, less commonly, disseminated gonococcal infection (presenting as a febrile illness with polyarthralgia and vasculitic skin lesions, or as a septic arthritis) may result.

6. As in the male, pharyngeal and rectal gonorrhoea are usually symptomless.

In prepubertal girls   The parents usually notice a discharge on the girl's underclothes, and on examination there is redness and swelling of the vulva and a purulent vaginal discharge. Other causes of vulvovaginitis include foreign bodies in the vagina (also thread-worms), faulty hygiene or urinary infection.

Table 13.1 Sites infected with *Neisseria gonorrhoeae* in a woman with uncomplicated gonorrhoea

Site	Percentage of infected women from whom *N. gonorrhoeae* is isolated from that site
Endocervix	85–90
Urethra	65–75
Anorectum	25–50
Pharynx	10–15

Diagnosis

In men For men with suspected urethral gonorrhoea, a smear of exudate is prepared on a microscope slide, using a plastic, disposable inoculating loop (Nunc Products, Denmark), fixed by passing gently over a spirit lamp flame and sent to the laboratory. Material, collected on an applicator stick tipped with cotton wool, should also be sent in the appropriate transport medium for culture (Appendix. 13.1). For the diagnosis of rectal and pharyngeal gonorrhoea, culture of the appropriate material is essential.

In women Material for culture from women should be obtained from all possibly infected sites (Table 13.1). As a single set of cultures may fail to identify about 7% of infected women, they should be repeated once, about 1 week later.

Note: As culture of material from a high vaginal swab yields negative results in about a third of infected women, this examination is unreliable for the diagnosis of gonorrhoea. When facilities are limited, however, an endocervical swab at least should be taken. As gonococci may not survive in the transport medium, it is sometimes helpful to send appropriately fixed smears to the laboratory. Serological tests for gonococcal antibodies are useless for routine diagnosis.

In young girls For young girs with suspected gonorrhoea, Gram-stained smears of vaginal exudate should be examined, and culture of vaginal, urethral, anorectal and pharyngeal material should be undertaken.

Treatment

Although the choice of antimicrobial agent should depend on the sensitivity pattern of the gonococcal isolate, treatment often has to be commenced before this is known. With a knowledge of the drug sensitivities of the strains prevailing in the community, a suitable drug can usually be selected easily.

In geographical areas where PPNG strains are uncommon, the penicillins remain the drugs of first choice , but other antimicrobial agents may be used (Table 13.2). Where PPNG strains are more prevalent, β-lactamase stable antimicrobial agents must be used as first line treatments. In the UK, such drugs are also used in the treatment of individuals who have acquired their infection in areas where PPNG are common. As there may be difficulty in patient compliance, single-dose treatment should be given whenever

Table 13.2   Some schedules for the treatment of uncomplicated gonorrhoea in adults

Antimicrobial agent	Dosage	Comments
Penicillins		
Ampicillin	2 g stat orally*	
Ampicillin	3.5 g stat orally*	
Amoxycillin	3 g stat orally*	
Amoxycillin with clavulanic acid (potassium salt) (Augmentin)†	3 g/250 mg stat orally*	
Cephalosporins		
Cefuroxime†	1.5 g im stat*	Hypersensitivity
Cefuroxime axetil†	1.5 g orally stat*	in penicillin
Ceftriaxone†	250 mg im stat	hypersensitive patients
Tetracyclines		
Doxycycline	300 mg stat orally	Nausea as side-effect Avoid in pregnancy
Minocycline	300 mg stat orally	Vertigo as side-effect Avoid in pregnancy
Spectinomycin†	2 g im stat	
Acrosoxacin†	300 mg stat orally	Safety in pregnancy not established
Ciprofloxacin†	250 mg stat orally	

* Given with probenecid in an oral dosage of 1 g.
† Useful ... infection with β-lactamase producing strains of *Neisseria gonorrhoeae*.

possible. Single-dose treatment of pharyngeal gonorrhoea in both sexes and rectal infection in men, however, is usually ineffective; infections at such sites must be treated with a course of anti-microbial agents e.g. ampicillin 250g by mouth every 6 hours or ciprofloxacin 250mg twice daily by mouth for 5 days.

As some 40% of patients with gonorrhoea have a concurrent chlamydial infection, some clinicians give simultaneous treatment for this (see below).

In women and in men with pharyngeal and rectal gonorrhoea, cultures should be repeated *twice* after treatment.

In all cases, contact tracing must be undertaken.

The possibility of sexual abuse must be considered in prepubertal children with gonorrhoea and the appropriate action taken to ensure the safety and future well-being of the child.

Syphilis

Syphilis, caused by *Treponema pallidum* ssp. *pallidum*, is uncommon in the UK (Fig. 13.1). It is most frequently acquired by sexual intercourse with an infected partner, but congenital infection also occurs. Serological screening for treponemal antibodies of all pregnant women has reduced the prevalence of congenital syphilis in developed countries. For a detailed description of the clinical features and diagnosis of syphilis, the reader is referred to one of the standard textbooks of sexually transmissible diseases.

Non-specific genital tract infection and chlamydial infection

The prevalence of non-specific (NSU) or non-gonococcal (NGU) urethritis has increased over the past 15 years. Although chlamydiae can be detected in the urethras of about 50% of these men, the aetiology in other cases is uncertain. However, anaerobes and mycoplasmas, including *Mycoplasma genitalium* and *Ureaplasma urealyticum*, may play some role.

Amongst adults, the oculogenital serovars of *Chlamydia trachomatis* are sexually transmitted; for example, the organism can be detected in the cervices of about 80% of the sexual partners of men with chlamydial urethritis. Adult chlamydial ophthalmia is usually the result of autoinoculation of infected material from the genital tract.

Clinical features

In men

1. After an incubation period of about 3 weeks, men with chlamydial urethritis complain of a mucoid or mucopurulent urethral discharge and dysuria of variable severity. About 25% of infected men, however, are *symptomless*.
2. Proctitis may result from chlamydiae acquired through anal intercourse.
3. Epididymitis is the most common complication of untreated chlamydial infection.
4. Chlamydiae probably play a part in the aetiology of reactive arthritis (including Reiter's disease).

In women

1. Most women with a chlamydial cervical infection are *symptomless* but some complain of increased vaginal discharge, and dysuria is an occasional feature.
2. There may be no specific signs. The cervix may appear normal or there may be an endocervicitis with mucopus exuding from the os.
3. PID may complicate up to 15% of women with an untreated chlamydial infection of the cervix with subsequent infertility and an increased risk of ectopic pregnancy. In general, the clinical features are less pronounced than those of gonococcal infection. The pelvic pain tends to be of lower intensity and fever is less frequent. Mild adnexal tenderness is usual.
4. Occasionally, perihepatitis is a complication: there is an acute onset of pain in the right hypochondrium, the pain being exacerbated by deep inspiration, nausea, anorexia and low grade pyrexia. There is tenderness over the liver and a friction rub may be heard.
5. Reactive arthritis may complicate chlamydial infection in women.

Diagnosis

Until recently, the diagnosis of chlamydial infection depended on the isolation of the organism in tissue culture. As this can be difficult, time-consuming and expensive, and as transport problems were common, facilities for chlamydial detection were not available in many areas. With the development of immunological methods for the detection of antigen, most practitioners should now have access to a chlamydial diagnostic service. The laboratory will advise on the system to be used. Most published data show that the results of culture and antigen detection correlate well.

1. Endocervical material should be obtained by inserting a cotton wool applicator stick into the cervical canal and rotating gently.
2. As the diagnostic yield is lower than when an endocervical swab is taken, there is little advantage in collecting material from the urethras of women even when they complain of dysuria.
3. A cotton-tipped wire swab (Medical Wire Co. Ear Nose and Throat swab) is used for the collection of urethral material from men.

Kits for the rapid detection of chlamydial antigen are now available and some are suitable for use in the clinic, results being available in about an hour.

Treatment

Tetracyclines and the macrolides are equally effective in the treatment of adult chlamydial infections.

1. Oxytetracycline 250 mg by mouth 4 times per day for 7 to 14 days is useful in the treatment of *men* with NGU, including that caused by chlamydiae. Recurrence of urethritis, however, occurs in about 30% of individuals.
2. Erythromycin stearate 500 mg twice daily by mouth for 7 days is preferred in the treatment of *women* with chlamydial infection of the cervix as an early pregnancy may be undiagnosed (tetracyclines being contraindicated in pregnancy).
3. A similar regimen is used in the treatment of women who are the known sexual partners of men with NGU. There is epidemiological evidence that the recurrence rate of non-chlamydial NGU is higher after resumption of sexual intercourse with a partner who has not been treated with antimicrobials.
4. A single oral dose of 1 g of azithromycin, a long-acting macrolide, is also highly effective in the treatment of uncomplicated chlamydial infection in non-pregnant individuals.
5. In the treatment of chlamydial PID, erythromycin or doxycycline can be given and, as there may be a concurrent anaerobe infection, metronidazole should also be prescribed.

6. Two tests of cure should be undertaken, about 2–4 weeks after completion of treatment, and only if those are negative should sexual intercourse be resumed.

Contact tracing is *essential* in all cases.

Bacterial vaginosis

This condition is being recognized with increasing frequency as a cause of increased vaginal discharge. It is associated with infection with a variety of anaerobes including *Bacteroides* spp. and *Peptostreptococcus* spp. and with *Gardnerella vaginalis*; lactobacilli are absent. In contrast to trichomoniasis and candidiasis, the vagina is not inflamed. The pathogenesis of bacterial vaginosis is uncertain, but animal model systems suggest that hormonal influences may be important. There is no clear evidence that this is a sexually transmissible disease.

Clinical features

1. Increased vaginal discharge, greyish white in colour with a fishy odour, particularly after intercourse.
2. Pruritus vulvae is *not* a feature unless there is concurrent infection, e.g. with *Candida* spp.
3. A greyish discharge may be noted at the introitus, and on speculum examination the walls of the vagina may be coated with a discharge that is sometimes frothy.
4. Vaginitis is not a feature.

Diagnosis

Diagnosis is clinical, supplemented by a few simple microbiological tests.

1. The pH of the vaginal discharge is measured using narrow-range (pH 4–6) pH paper (Whatman) held in a pair of forceps, and avoiding the alkaline cervical secretions. The pH of vaginal secretions is normally less than 4.5 but in bacterial vaginosis it is greater than 5. Note, however, that the pH of vaginal fluid can be greater than 5 in women who do not have the condition.
2. A loopful of discharge is suspended in a drop of isotonic saline (8.6 g NaCl/l) on a microscope slide, covered, and examined microscopically using a ×40 objective. Polymorphonuclear

leucocytes are few but 'clue cells' – epithelial cells that appear granular because of adherent bacteria – are usually obvious. The exceedingly mobile curved rods of *Mobiluncus* spp. may also be noted.

3. Although the 'sniff test' (performed by mixing some vaginal secretions with a drop of potassium hydroxide, 25% w/v, on a slide and immediately sniffing to detect the characteristic ammoniacal odour of volatile amines) is said to be a sensitive and specific test for bacterial vaginosis, it is subjective and requires some degree of practice.

4. Culture of vaginal discharge for *G. vaginalis* and anaerobes is not helpful diagnostically.

Treatment

Metronidazole 400 mg by mouth twice daily for 5 days, or clindamycin cream are both effective, but recurrence is common. There is no clear evidence that treatment of the sexual partner is indicated.

PROTOZOAL INFESTATION

Trichomoniasis

Trichomoniasis is caused by the protozoan flagellate *Trichomonas vaginalis* that colonizes but only rarely invades the mucosa of the lower urogenital tract. The organism is sexually transmitted. In recent years, the incidence of the disease has declined, perhaps because of the widespread use of metronidazole in a variety of conditions.

Clinical features

In women

1. A thin, yellow, offensive vaginal discharge, vulval soreness, dysuria and dyspareunia are the classic symptoms.

2. The vaginal wall is reddened and a frothy, yellow discharge pools in the posterior fornix; punctate red spots on the ectocervix ('strawberry cervix') may be noted. These features, however, are not always present and are not pathognomonic of trichomoniasis.

3. Up to one quarter of infected women are *symptomless*.

In men

1. Most men who are infected with *T. vaginalis* are *symptomless*, but a few present with a non-gonococcal urethritis.
2. Trichomoniasis can occasionally be identified in urethral material or urine from men who are known sexual contacts of women with trichomoniasis.

Diagnosis

1. In women, saline mount preparation of material from the posterior fornix is examined microscopically at a magnification of ×400. Urethral smears or a centrifuged deposit of urine from men can be examined similarly. The protozoa are recognized by their size (10–30 μm in length), oval shape, rapidly-moving anterior flagella, undulating membrane and their jerky movement.
2. Material in Stuart's or Amies' medium can be sent to the laboratory for culture, a method considered more sensitive than microscopy.
3. The rapid detection in secretions of trichomonal antigen by latex agglutination is also a possible diagnostic test.
4. Sometimes, trichomonads may be found in Papanicolaou-stained smears, but this method is not recommended for routine diagnosis.

Treatment

1. Metronidazole 200 mg by mouth every 8 hours for 7 days is usually curative.
2. The regular sexual partners of women with trichomoniasis should be treated similarly, even when the protozoan cannot be detected in genital secretions.
3. Patients taking metronidazole should be advised to avoid alcohol (because of unpleasant side-effects from their interaction) until treatment has been completed.

FUNGAL INFECTION

Candidiasis

Vulvovaginal candidiasis is caused by yeasts of the genus *Candida*, particularly *Candida albicans*. This yeast is saprophytic in humans, but certain conditions favour its transition to a pathogen, and these

Table 13.3   Conditions that favour transition of *Candida albicans* from saprophyte to pathogen in the genitalia

Pregnancy
Diabetes mellitus
Other endocrine disorders (e.g. hypothyroidism, hypoparathyroidism)
Oral antimicrobial agents
Debilitating conditions
Local trauma
Immunosuppressive drugs, including corticosteroids
Human immunodeficiency virus infection

should be considered when a woman presents with candidal vulvovaginitis (Table 13.3). Candidal balanoposthitis may be the presenting feature of diabetes mellitus in men.

Clinical features

In women

1. Pruritus vulvae and burning of variable severity are the principal features; there may be associated superficial dyspareunia.
2. Erythema of the vulva that sometimes extends to the perineum, perianal region, genitocrural folds and the medial aspects of the thighs.
3. Oedema of the labia minora is common.
4. Vaginitis is less frequently found but there may be a curdy white vaginal discharge with white adherent plaques.
5. Primary cutaneous candidiasis affects the genitocrural folds and outer aspects of the labia majora. The lesions are initially papular with small satellite vesicles or pustules, but progress to superficial ulcers.

In men

1. Pain or itching of the penis and often a subpreputial discharge.
2. The prepuce may be oedematous and fissured, resulting in phimosis. Usually the glans is reddened with multiple maculopapules that may progress to superficial ulceration.

Diagnosis

Material from the posterior fornix of the vagina or from plaques can be examined microscopically for pseudohyphae after mounting in a drop of saline. Yeasts may also be seen in Gram-stained smears. *Candida* spp. can be cultured, but the presence of yeasts does not imply that they are the cause of vulvovaginitis.

Treatment

1. Nystatin vaginal tablets, each containing 100 000 units nightly for 14 nights; in addition, nystatin cream (100 units/g) can be applied to the vulval area.
2. As nystatin is yellow and can stain underwear, it is often preferable to use one of the imidazoles such as clotrimazole (Canesten) given as a single 500 mg pessary. Clotrimazole cream (1%) can be applied topically twice daily.
3. A single oral dose of 150 mg fluconazole is efficacious in non-pregnant women with candidiasis.
4. Relapses after treatment are common. In such cases it may be helpful to examine the male partner and treat him with an antifungal cream if he has symptoms.
5. Wearing nylon pants or tight trousers should be avoided to reduce the production of a hot humid environment in the anogenital region, a factor that promotes fungal growth.
6. In women with frequent recurrences of vaginal candidiasis, suppressive therapy should be considered. A single clotrimazole 500 mg pessary can be used about a week before the expected onset of menstruation, or, depending on when symptoms usually occur, immediately post-menstrually. If this regimen fails, a single 100 mg clotrimazole pessary can be used twice weekly, initially for 3 weeks and then weekly for 3 months.
7. Asymptomatic candida found, for example, on a routine cervical smear does not require treatment.

VIRAL INFECTIONS

Table 13.4 indicates the viral infections that are sexually trans-missible. The more common are discussed below.

Herpes simplex virus

The prevalence of herpes simplex virus (HSV) infection of the genitalia has been increasing over the past 20 years. In most areas of the UK, HSV 2 has been considered to be the principal type that affects the genitalia. However, HSV 1 is the infecting type in about

Table 13.4   Viruses transmissible by sexual contact

Herpes simplex virus (HSV 1 and 2)
Human papilloma virus (HPV)
Hepatitis B virus (HBV)
Hepatitis A virus (HAV)
Hepatitis C virus (HCV)
Human immunodeficiency viruses (HIV 1 and 2)
Molluscum contagiosum virus
Epstein Barr virus (EBV)
Cytomegalovirus (CMV)
Marburg virus

40% of women and in about 25% of men with primary genital herpes. In most cases, this type of virus has been acquired from orogenital contact. In developed countries, the prevalence of antibodies against HSV 1 in adolescents has been declining, and it has been suggested that the increasing incidence of genital herpes may reflect lack of protection against HSV 2 by prior exposure to type 1 virus.

Symptomless infections are common. More than 80% of those whose sera contain antibodies against HSV 2 have had no clinical features of infection. Transmission can occur when a symptomless individual is excreting the virus in genital secretions.

After replicating in the skin or mucous membranes the virus is transported via the axon to the neurones in the sacral ganglia. Further replication occurs and the virus then spreads via the sensory nerves to the skin or mucous surface, where clinical signs of infection may develop. After resolution of the primary disease, the virus becomes latent or hidden in the ganglia. Reactivation by mechanisms that are uncertain is followed by transport of viral genomes to the skin surface where replication can occur. This occurrence may or may not be associated with the development of clinical signs.

Natural history

The long-term natural history of genital herpes is uncertain.

1. Within 1 year about 55% of individuals who have had symptomatic primary herpes associated with HSV 1 and 90% who have had primary HSV 2 infection will develop a recurrence (Corey 1986).

2. In general, there is a longer interval between the primary
   episode and recurrence in patients who have had HSV 1
   infection compared with those who have had HSV 2.
3. Recurrent episodes seem to be less frequent with HSV 1
   infection.
4. It is as yet unknown whether the recurrence rate decreases
   with time.

Clinical features

Primary genital herpes develops after a variable latent period.

1. Systemic symptoms are common, particularly in women and
   include fever, headache, malaise and myalgia.
2. Pain in the vulva or penis, dysuria and increased vaginal
   discharge.
3. Tender enlargement of the inguinal lymph nodes usually
   develops more than 1 week after the onset of the illness.
4. Lesions are initially papular but quickly become vesicular and
   ulcerate. They persist for up to 2 weeks until crusting.
5. *In women,* extensive ulceration of the labia majora, labia
   minora, adjacent skin, introitus, perineum, perianal region,
   vagina and cervix is found.
6. *In men,* ulceration of the coronal sulcus, glans penis, prepuce,
   shaft of the penis and perianal region may be noted; in the
   uncircumcised, phimosis with secondary bacterial infection
   may develop.
7. *In both sexes,* herpetic proctitis may be a feature.
8. New lesion formation is noted during the first 10 days.
   Sacral radiculitis, presenting as constipation, urinary
   retention and paraesthesiae in the distribution of the sacral
   nerve is an uncommon complication of primary HSV 2
   infection.
9. Systemic features usually resolve within 7–10 days and genital
   lesions usually heal within about 21 days.
10. Clinical features in women tend to be more severe than those
    in men.
11. Clinical features of first-episode genital herpes in individuals
    who have been exposed previously to HSV are believed to be
    less severe than those suffering truly primary genital infection.

Recurrent genital herpes   Clinical features in general tend to
be less severe than those of primary disease.

1. Systemic symptoms are not a feature, but prodromal symptoms occur commonly and consist of a tingling sensation in the affected area or shooting pains in the distribution of the sciatic nerve.
2. Lesions are similar to those of the primary disease but are usually much less extensive and heal more quickly.

Diagnosis

It is good to make a definitive diagnosis by virological methods so that proper counselling can be undertaken.

1. Material obtained by gently scraping the base of an ulcer using an applicator stick tipped with cotton wool should be sent in the appropriate transport medium (e.g. Hank's) for viral isolation in tissue culture.
2. The detection of HSV antigens by immunofluorescence or enzyme-linked immunoabsorbent assay (ELISA) may become a practical alternative to tissue culture in the non-pregnant woman.
3. Blood should be taken at the first clinical attendance, and again 10–14 days later, for serological studies, particularly using complement fixation test (CFT). Individuals with primary infection will develop antibodies in this interval. The CFT, however, cannot detect initial infection with HSV 2 in the presence of HSV 1 antibodies.

Treatment

Primary or initial infections

1. Acyclovir (Zovirax) 200 mg orally 5 times per day for 5 days is the treatment of choice. Compared with placebo, the lesions heal more rapidly, pain is relieved more quickly, new lesion formation ceases, and systemic features resolve more speedily. Recurrences, however, are not abolished or reduced in frequency.
2. Patients should be warned about the possible risk of auto-inoculation of other parts of the body, particularly the cornea, and about the need for detailed attention to hygiene.
3. Resumption of sexual intercourse should be delayed until the lesions have healed.

Recurrent disease   The use of acyclovir is less certain. Although the clinical course of the disease is shortened somewhat, in general this is of marginal benefit to the patient. When given early, for example during the prodromal stage, acyclovir may reduce significantly the duration of the recurrence.

Suppressive treatment   Acyclovir 200mg orally 4 times per day, or 400mg twice daily reduces the frequency of recurrences and may be useful in the occasional patient with very frequent or disabling recurrences. The subsequent recurrence rate may be reduced.

Acyclovir has few side-effects but its safety in pregnancy has not yet been established.

Counselling plays an important part in the management of patients with genital herpes and adequate time should be allotted for this.

Genital herpes in pregnancy

Primary infection in the third trimester of pregnancy may be associated with prematurity, abortion, intrauterine growth retardation and neonatal herpes infection. Over one-half of infants born to mothers with primary HSV infection at term are likely to become infected and develop overt disease with its high mortality rate. In these women, caesarean section reduces the risk of neonatal infection. The risk to babies born vaginally to women who have recurrent HSV at term is low, but caesarean section should be undertaken if genital lesions are present at term. As 60% of women who deliver babies with HSV infection do not have any clinical features of the infection or a history of genital herpes, routine screening during pregnancy is not considered appropriate.

Human papilloma virus

Warts are caused by the human papilloma virus (HPV) of which there are over 60 types, as determined by DNA–DNA hybridization studies. Most genital warts are associated with types 6 and 11 but types 16, 18 and 31 are sometimes detected in tissues. The importance of the latter types is that DNA sequences that hybridize with HPV types 16 and 18 are identified frequently in biopsies from women with premalignant and malignant disease of the genital tract. Whether the association is causal or casual remains uncertain. Certainly, HPV DNA sequences homologous to those of HPV types 16 and 18 can be found in healthy tissues. The role of co-factors, such as cigarette smoking, in carcinogenesis is also unclear. Vulval intraepithelial neoplasia (VIN) has also been associated with HPV infection (Campion & Singer 1987), but progression to malignant disease appears to be uncommon in young women. Similarly, the significance of penile intraepithelial neoplasia found in male contacts of women with HPV infection and cervical intraepithelial neoplasia (CIN) is uncertain.

The virus is highly contagious through sexual contact, but the latent period is variable, being on average 3 months from exposure. Genital warts in prepubertal children should raise the possibility of sexual abuse.

Clinical features

1. The most common manifestation of genital HPV infection is the fleshy hyperplastic wart (condyloma acuminatum).
   In women these lesions are located at the introitus or at the labia majora and minora, perineum, perianal region, vagina, urethra and cervix.
   In men they are found most frequently in the coronal sulcus and frenum, but also on the prepuce, skin of the shaft of the penis, within the distal urethra, in the perianal region and on the scrotum.
   Although condylomatous lesions of the cervix are noted in only about 6% of women with genital warts, cytological or colposcopic evidence of HPV infection is found in at least 25% of cases. There are often associated dysplastic-like changes of variable severity. Although spontaneous regression of the milder dysplastic changes has been described, the natural history of these lesions is unknown.
2. At least 50% of women with vulval intraepithelial neoplasia complain of pruritus vulvae, burning and pain. The lesions are single or multiple, macules or papules on the skin that may be white and lichenified; mucosal lesions are usually erythematous macules. Blanching is noted after the application of 5% acetic acid. Some lesions are pigmented. Biopsy is essential for diagnosis (Campion & Singer 1987).
3. Subclinical infection with HPV of the skin of the penis is now well-documented.

Management

1. Every effort should be made to exclude a concurrent sexually transmissible disease (about one-third of patients are likely to

Table 13.5   Treatments available for condylomata acuminata

Treatment	Method of use	Comments
Antimitotic/antimetabolite		
Podophyllin resin	Suspension 20–25% w/v in liquid paraffin or ethanol, applied topically once weekly. Protect surrounding surfaces with petroleum jelly. Wash off after six hours.	Batch variation in potency. Avoid use on cervix, vagina or anal canal. Avoid in pregnancy (can be absorbed systemically, resulting in peripheral neuropathy in mother and stillbirth/abortion).
Podophyllotoxin	0.5% solution applied twice daily for 3 days; further treatments at 7-day intervals.	Possibly more satisfactory than podophyllin. Avoid in pregnancy and on above sites.
5-fluorouracil	Cream applied topically.	Burns frequent. Avoid in pregnancy.
Destructive methods		
Trichloracetic acid	50% solution applied carefully to surface of wart.	Burns frequent.
Cryotherapy Electrocautery Laser ablation Scissor excision		If extensive, may require general anaesthesia.
Immunomodulatory		
Inosine pranobex	Orally, used in conjunction with podophyllin.	Efficacy not proven.
Alpha interferon	Intralesional or subcutaneously.	Initially, side effects common (fever, malaise). Efficacy uncertain. Expensive.

have concurrent infection). Treatment of, say, trichomonal vaginitis or anaerobic balanoposthitis often facilitates the treatment of genital warts. In the absence of specific antiviral chemotherapy, treatment is largely symptomatic. Although the condylomata acuminata eventually undergo spontaneous regression, perhaps as a result of cell-mediated immunity, persistence for many months is common. As the lesions are psychologically disturbing and as they may become secondarily infected and bleed, some form of therapy is usually indicated.

2. At the first consultation, counselling about the infection and its protracted course should be undertaken. The sexual partner should be encouraged to attend for examination, counselling and treatment, if necessary.

3. The use of condoms to prevent the spread of infection should be encouraged.

4. Table 13.5 indicates some treatments that are available for condylomata acuminata. With every treatment, however, recurrence is common.

Cervical screening policy   Although the natural history of the dysplastic-like changes associated with HPV infection is unknown, it seems reasonable, given the association between certain types of HPV and cervical cancer, to offer regular cervical screening to women who have had genital warts or who are known sexual contacts of men with warts. Local policies will usually dictate whether screening can be more frequent than the standard 3-yearly examination.

Human immunodeficiency virus (HIV)

The human immunodeficiency viruses (HIV 1 and 2) selectively infect and destroy cells that bear the CD4 antigen – T4 (helper/inducer) lymphocytes and cells of the macrophage/monocyte system. After entry into the cell, the viral genomic RNA is transcribed into DNA by reverse transcriptase and some becomes circularized and integrated into the host cell genome. Throughout the course of HIV infection, there is constant replication of the virus, with progressive impairment of the immune system, as manifest by the decrease in CD4 cells in the peripheral blood. In addition, brain cells – microglia, astrocytes and possibly neurones – can be infected by HIV and, even in the absence of secondary infection, neuropsychiatric features may develop.

Epidemiology

HIV can be detected in blood, semen, cervicovaginal secretions, breast milk and saliva. There is little evidence, however, that the latter fluid is important in the transmission of infection. In developed countries, men who have had unprotected *anal intercourse* with an infected man constitute the group at greatest risk of HIV infection, but recent data show clearly the propensity for *heterosexual spread*. Indeed, in central Africa, the majority of infected individuals, both men and women, have acquired the virus heterosexually. There is evidence that the presence of a concurrent sexually transmitted disease, particularly an ulcerative condition, such as genital herpes, facilitates infection with HIV.

As the duration of HIV increases, so does infectivity through sexual intercourse, whether homo- or heterosexual. Infection from *artificial insemination* with infected semen is rare.

Intravenous drug users who share contaminated syringes and needles are also at risk of HIV infection. Since the introduction of self-exclusion policies and screening of donated blood for anti-HIV, the risk of acquisition of the virus through blood transfusion in developed countries is now very low. Heat treatment of blood products such as Factors VIII and IX has reduced significantly the risk of infection to haemophiliacs.

Although there have been reports on the probable infection of *neonates* by breast feeding, most infants have acquired HIV from an infected mother before or during parturition. There is good evidence that infection can occur very early in pregnancy, but by no means every infected mother transmits the infection to the fetus. The risk of neonatal infection varies from 22% to 51% and it is likely that there is a direct relationship between duration of maternal infection and risk to the child. In women with symptomatic infection, pregnancy may influence adversely the outcome. Recent studies have suggested that treatment of the mother with zidovudine during pregnancy may reduce the risk of transmission to the fetus.

Clinical features

1. Many HIV-infected individuals are *symptomless,* the infection only being detected by serological testing.
2. Within a few weeks of infection, and before antibodies become detectable, some patients develop a mononucleosis-like illness with pyrexia, malaise, skin rash, sore throat, lymphadenopathy, diarrhoea, arthralgia and, sometimes, neurological features.

These symptoms usually resolve within 3 weeks, but the lymphadenopathy may persist.

3. Persistent generalized lymphadenopathy is a common clinical finding, even in symptomless infected individuals. The lymph nodes are enlarged (>1 cm in diameter) but discrete and usually not tender. The spleen may also be enlarged.

4. Although there may not be other clinical features, dermatological abnormalities are common (and may occur in the absence of lymphadenopathy) and include seborrhoeic dermatitis of the face and scalp, facial warts, extensive tinea pedis and cruris, pityriasis versicolor, multiple molluscum contagiosum, extensive folliculitis and purpura (resulting from thrombocytopenia).

5. Oral manifestations include candidiasis, hypertrophic gingivitis and oral hairy leukoplakia.

6. The development of herpes zoster, persistent weight loss and diarrhoea are associated with a deteriorating immune system.

7. The secondary neoplasms and infectious diseases that constitute the acquired immune deficiency syndrome (AIDS) are tabulated (Table 13.6).

Table 13.6 Neoplasms and secondary infectious diseases in HIV infection

NEOPLASMS
Kaposi's sarcoma
B-cell lymphoma

INFECTIONS Protozoa	Fungi	Bacteria	Viruses
Pneumocystis carinii	*Candida* spp.	*Mycobacterium tuberculosis*	Cytomegalovirus
Toxoplasma gondii	*Histoplasma capsulatum*	Atypical mycobacteria	Herpes simplex virus
Cryptosporidium spp.	*Cryptococcus neoformans*		J C virus
Isospora belli		*Salmonella* spp.	
Microsporidium spp.		*Campylobacter* spp.	
		Streptococcus pneumoniae	
		Nocardia spp.	

8. HIV infection may present as a dementing illness without evidence of other secondary infections.
9. Features of AIDS in children include failure to thrive, lymphadenopathy, disseminated candidiasis, *Pneumocystis carinii* pneumonia, disseminated mycobacterial infection, lymphocytic interstitial pneumonia and parotitis.

Course of infection

The natural history of HIV infection is still uncertain. Up to 50% of individuals who have been infected for 10 years have not developed serious infectious diseases or neoplasms. There is no doubt that the incidence of AIDS increases as the duration of HIV infection increases, but the prognosis in an individual is not entirely predictable. Serial estimations of the number of CD4 cells in the peripheral blood, and HIV p24 antigen testing may be useful, however, in assessing prognosis.

Diagnosis

In a family planning setting it is generally the 'worried well' individual who seeks help and advice and, hopefully, reassurance. Careful, sympathetic, knowledgeable counselling, even before embarking on blood testing to establish the diagnosis, is essential. Pre-test counselling is time-consuming, and should be carried out with great sensitivity and should take into account:

1. The anxiety felt by individuals about themselves, particularly the possibility of having to face not only the stark reality of the diagnosis and ultimate prognosis but also the effect on their partner and their families.
2. Fear and embarrassment that secret hidden parts of their lives will be revealed.
3. Concern that their general practitioners will not keep them on their lists nor dentists be prepared to treat them.
4. Implications for future applications for mortgages, life insurance and even jobs.
5. Provision of up-to-date information about the disease, current tests and the relevance of false-negative results. Myths must be dispelled.
6. Advice on contraception, safer sex techniques and alteration of lifestyle as appropriate.

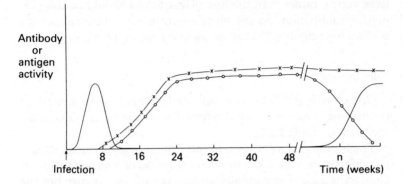

Fig. 13.3 Time course of detection of human immunodeficiency virus antibodies or antigens in the serum of an infected individual.

——— = antigen
—o— = antibody against the core antigen p42
—x— = antibody against the enveloped antigen p41.

In most cases the infection is detected by testing serum for antibodies against core antigens (e.g. by ELISA). There is, however, an incubation period before serum antibodies become detectable (Fig. 13.3) which may vary from a few weeks to 3 months, or, rarely, longer. In general, if blood obtained 3 and 6 months from exposure has yielded negative results, testing can be discontinued.

Although core antigen may be found in the serum before antibodies become detectable, this is not always so, and antigen detection is not recommended for routine testing. Detection of p24 antigen in the later stages of infection, however, often precedes the development of AIDS.

A different type of virus (HIV 2) has been recognized in West Africa, but there is little evidence of its widespread distribution elsewhere.

As sera showing positive results in one test will always be checked by another system a 'false-positive' report is most unlikely. Technical errors (e.g. a wrongly labelled blood tube) can and do occur, however, and it is good practice to obtain a second blood sample from a patient who has no clinical features of HIV infection before telling him or her the result.

Note: Blood is a source of contamination in a person who is HIV positive. Gloves should be worn for venepuncture, and the thicker latex variety rather than the fine plastic gloves should be used for pelvic examination. As the virus is sensitive to chemical agents, sodium hypochlorite 2% can be used to decontaminate surfaces.

Management

Counselling When an infected individual is identified counselling is essential. Some issues that should be considered are indicated in Table 13.7.

The means of transmission of the virus should be explained and the appropriate steps taken to avoid the spread of infection to others. Contact tracing is not usually undertaken in this country but the individual is encouraged to inform his/her sexual partner of the infection and to persuade him/her to attend a specialist clinic for counselling and, if requested, serological testing.

Within a relationship, considerable anxiety is often encountered when one partner is seropositive for HIV and the other is apparently uninfected. Anal intercourse should be avoided, but if this is to occur, a more robust sheath, lubricated with a water-soluble lubricant, should be used.

In addition to the risk to the fetus, there has been some suggestion that pregnancy can affect adversely the course of the infection in women with late stage disease. When pregnancy occurs in a sero-positive individual, the risk should be explained to the patient in a

Table 13.7 Points to be considered in counselling a symptomless HIV-infected individual*

---

1. *Means of transmission* of the virus and the avoidance of spread of infection to others.
2. *Lack of risk* to others through social contact.
3. *Natural history* of infection *uncertain* – Note research in antiviral chemotherapy and prospects for the future.
4. Medical and dental. The individual should *inform* practitioners of his/her infection. Otherwise *only* trusted individuals should be informed. Attendance at self help groups may be useful.
5. Regular attendance at a specialist clinic (genitourinary medicine or an infectious diseases unit) for counselling, clinical examination and investigation should be encouraged. Clinical deterioration and progressive impairment of cellular immunity may be indication for antiviral therapy.

---

* Counselling is time-consuming and should be undertaken only by those familiar with HIV infection. Particularly in the months following diagnosis, frequent counselling sessions are often required. At each visit, the patient should be encouraged to discuss his/her feelings.

sympathetic manner. Although termination should be discussed, taking into account the known predictors, it is the individual's and the partner's decision whether to continue with the pregnancy or not. If she decides against termination, the woman must receive the optimal antenatal care. Although in developed countries breast feeding by seropositive women is not recommended, this advice may be different in developing countries where breast milk may be the only safe source of infant nutrition.

Contraception The knowledge that HIV is transmissible sexually has created the need for policies on contraceptive provision for affected individuals which not only prevent unwanted pregnancy but also protect the partners from infection. It must be remembered, however, that the most effective contraceptive is the one that they are prepared to use (see Ch. 2).

1. *Condoms* meeting BSI requirements should be recommended, either alone or in addition to other contraceptives, as protection against transmission of HIV and other STD (pp. 169–172).
2. *Female barriers*. There is no good evidence that diaphragms alone are protective against HIV transmission but some benefit may accrue when they are used with spermicides containing nonoxynol-9. The female condom offers more protection.
3. *Spermicides*. Creams, jellies, pessaries, foams, films or sponges containing nonoxynol-9 may provide an additional barrier to HIV infection, but the irritant effect of this agent in some individuals may be disadvantageous (pp. 172–179).
4. *Hormonal contraception*. The combined pill (COC) is known to depress the immune system but there is no evidence that it affects the progression of HIV disease. Because of its effectiveness it is particularly suitable, but women in high-risk groups should be encouraged to ask their partners to use a condom in addition.
   The progestogen-only pill (POP) can be an effective method in conjunction with condoms.
   Injectables have less effect on immunity and on liver function than COCs. Since no motivation is required they are a very appropriate method of contraception for HIV-positive women. Hormonal contraception is dependent on there being no concomitant liver disease – liver function should be checked in all drug users and ex-drug users before it is prescribed.
5. *Intrauterine devices* are not recommended for HIV-positive women or for those at risk of infection. If such women already have an IUD in situ they would be best advised to change to

another effective method. The presence of an IUD increases the risk of PID in the HIV-positive woman who is already immunocompromised, and recurrent acute episodes might lead to more rapid disease progression. Insertion may cause transient inflammatory reaction with trauma to the endometrium, which may facilitate virus entry. IUDs increase the discharge of monocytes and lymphocytes into the vagina and are often associated with heavier, longer and irregular menstrual bleeding, all of which could increase the risk of transmission of the virus.

6. *Sterilization.* There is no evidence that this is contraindicated for either partner.
7. *Postcoital contraception.* There is no contraindication to hormonal PCC, but an IUD should not be used (see above).

Follow-up and treatment

Table 13.8 outlines the management of a newly diagnosed HIV-infected individual. Although there is much variation from clinic to clinic in the details of management, it is the author's policy to assess symptomless individuals at 3-monthly intervals. At these consultations it is important to discuss issues regarding lifestyle, general health, worries and fears, and to offer referral for appropriate counselling and psychological and social support.

A physical examination is undertaken and note made of any new findings such as the development of extensive oral hairy leukoplakia that may indicate progressive disease.

Blood is taken for:

1. Haematological tests – haemoglobin, white cell count, platelet count.
2. Immunological tests – CD4 cell count, β_2-microglobulin concentration
3. p24 antigen estimation.

When the CD4 cell count in the peripheral blood falls below $200/mm^3$, there is increased risk of the development of opportunistic infections, and prophylaxis against *Pneumocystis carinii* pneumonia should be offered to individuals who have had counts of less than $200/mm^3$ on at least two occasions over a 1 month period.

In addition, consideration should be given to the provision of prophylaxis against *Toxoplasma gondii* reactivation in patients in whose sera specific IgG antibody has been detected. Co-trimoxazole

Table 13.8 Assessment of a newly diagnosed symptomless HIV-seropositive individual

	Comments
1. Repeat anti-HIV test	Need to exclude technical error.
2. History	Note sexual history, past history of sexual diseases, drug use, occupational risk, blood or blood product transfusion, residence abroad, menstrual cycle, obstetric history, social circumstances.
3. Physical examination	Note particularly, skin and mucosal abnormalities, lymphadenopathy, hepatic or splenic enlargement. Genital examination for warts, candidiasis.
4. Haematological examination	May be anaemia, leucopenia or thrombocytopenia.
5. Plasma enzyme tests of liver function	Often minor elevation of alanine aminotransferase.
6. Immunological tests:	
(a) Peripheral blood CD4 count	Normally > 500/mm^3. Repeat in 1 month to establish baseline.
(b) Serum immunoglobulins	Often elevated.
(c) β_2-microglobulin	Elevated in later stages of disease.
7. Serum HIV p24 antigen estimation	Detected in very early and again in late disease.
8. Serological tests for:	
(a) *Toxoplasma gondii*	Possible reactivation in late stage disease; consider prophylaxis.
(b) Cytomegalovirus	Possible reactivation in late stage disease. Avoid transfusion of CMV antibody positive blood if recipient anti-CMV negative.
(c) Syphilis	Past infection. Aggressive course if untreated.
(d) Hepatitis B virus	Possible reactivation in late disease.
(e) Hepatitis C virus	May produce chronic hepatitis/cirrhosis.
9. Cervical cytology/coloscopy	Increased risk of HPV infection; annual screen.
10. Chest X-ray	Baseline film.
11. Pyschological assessment	

(Septrin forte) tablets, given daily or 3 times per week, offer useful protection against both infections, and is still the agent of first choice. Reactions to this drug, however, are common (e.g. skin rash), and may be severe. Pentamidine esithionate, given by nebulizer, at monthly intervals is an alternative approach, but the drug given in this form does not protect against disseminated *P. carinii* infection (rare) or against the development of toxoplasmosis. Dapsone may also have a role in prophylaxis against both infections. It is important to note that drug reactions are very common in HIV-infected individuals and it is frequently necessary to modify treatment or prophylactic regimens in these patients.

Zidovudine is a reverse transcriptase inhibitor that has proved useful in improving the duration and quality of life in late-stage HIV disease. It is, however, toxic, the principal effect being on the bone marrow, with the development of anaemia and leucopenia. In vitro studies have shown that the virus becomes less sensitive to the effects of zidovudine when it has been used in treatment for several months; the clinical significance of this finding is still uncertain. Didanosine and zalcitabine are other nucleoside analogues that may be helpful in the treatment of symptomatic patients who are intolerant of zidovudine, or who show disease progression whilst receiving the latter drug. Combination treatment with nucleoside analogues is currently under investigation.

Hepatitis A virus

The sexual transmission of hepatitis A virus (HAV), particularly amongst homosexual men, is well documented, the virus being acquired by the faecal–oral route. Hepatitis A vaccine should be offered to those who have oral–anal sexual contact with different partners, and whose serum gives negative results for anti-HAV IgG.

Hepatitis B virus

Although hepatitis B virus (HBV) infection is endemic in certain geographical areas (e.g. South East Asia), in temperate climates most infections are acquired by the inoculation of infected blood (e.g. by sharing contaminated syringes and needles) or sexually, mostly through homosexual contact. Heterosexual transmission is also now considered important.

As the detection of e antigen in serum is associated with active viral replication, infected individuals who are e-antigenaemic are the most infectious and should be counselled about their infectivity to sexual contacts and, during parturition, to a child.

Hepatitis B vaccine is available and, at least in the short term, provides a high degree of protection against infection. The vaccine should be offered to men who have sex with other men and to female sex industry workers.

Hepatitis C virus

Hepatitis C virus is usually acquired parenterally e.g. by sharing contaminated syringes and needles. Although the virus can be transmitted sexually, the degree of risk is still uncertain; condom use during sex with an infected partner should be encouraged. Chronic liver disease is a common sequela of infection.

Hepatitis D virus

Hepatitis D virus is a defective RNA virus that is almost always found in association with hepatitis B virus (which it requires for its replication). Although most individuals who have been infected have acquired the virus by the parenteral route, sexual transmission is possible, and condoms should be used during sexual intercourse with an infected partner.

Molluscum contagiosum virus

Molluscum contagiosum, caused by a pox virus, presents as hemispherical, umbilicated, pearly, flesh-coloured skin nodules 2–5 mm in diameter. When acquired through sexual contact, they are found on the penis, vulva and inner aspects of the thighs. The diagnosis is clinical but can be confirmed by electron microscopy of the core of a lesion that has been removed using a needle and fine forceps. Treatment is by curettage, electrocautery or piercing with a sharpened orange stick, the tip of which has been dipped in iodine solution.

Epstein Barr virus

Epstein Barr virus (EBV) is a transforming herpes virus that causes infectious mononucleosis and possibly an enervating illness, and has been implicated in the aetiology of Burkitt's lymphoma, and the B cell lymphomas that develop in HIV infection. The virus is shed from the oropharynx and, until recently, kissing was considered the principal means of transmission. However, infection of epithelial cells of the uterine cervix has been shown, suggesting that EBV can be transmitted sexually.

Cytomegalovirus

Cytomegalovirus (CMV) is another herpes virus that can be acquired by sexual contact and congenitally. CMV can be isolated from semen and cervicovaginal secretions, and there is direct evidence of sexual transmission. Young children, however, may also be the source of maternal infection. Of pregnant women with primary CMV infections, 30–40% transmit the virus to the fetus. In 10% of cases, congenital infection may result in neonatal death or later complications, particularly a sensori–neural deafness.

There is, however, little information on whether termination should be offered to women who have had primary CMV infection in pregnancy. Permanent damage is more likely if infection occurs in the first half of pregnancy. Information to pregnant women on how long conception should be delayed after primary infection is not available. Viral shedding from the cervix certainly can continue for many months after clinical features resolve.

ARTHROPOD INFESTATIONS

Phthiriasis

Phthirus pubis (the crab louse) is 1.2–2 mm in length and infests the strong hairs of the pubic and perianal areas, abdomen, thighs, axillae and, rarely, the eyebrows, eyelashes and beard. The louse is transferred by sexual contact but can be acquired from clothing. Itch is the principal symptom.

Treatment Treat with malathion or carbaryl lotion (1%w/v)

Scabies

Scabies is caused by the mite *Sarcoptes scabiei* var. *hominis*. Most infestations are acquired by non-sexual contact.

1. The principal symptom is itch which is particularly noticeable at night and develops up to 6 weeks after a first infection, but earlier in second or subsequent attacks.

2. Burrows may be found on the hands and wrists, extensor surfaces of the elbows, feet and ankles, penis and scrotum, buttocks, axillae and, less frequently, elsewhere. When hygiene is good, burrows may not be apparent.
3. An erythematous rash with urticarial papules not associated directly with the presence of the mite, is also noted in infested patients; penile and scrotal lesions are common.
4. Indurated nodules are sometimes found on the genitals and elsewhere.

Treatment   Treat with γ-benzene hexachloride, but this agent should be avoided during the first trimester of pregnancy. Benzyl benzoate application is also useful, but causes stinging in children and should not be used on them.

REFERENCES

Campion M J, Singer A 1987 Vulval intraepithelial neoplasia: clinical review. Genitourinary Medicine 63(3): 147–152
Corey L 1986 Genital herpes simplex virus infections: natural history and therapy. In: Oriel J D , Harris J R W (eds) Recent advances in sexually transmitted diseases, 3rd edn. Churchill Livingstone, Edinburgh, p. 71–108
McMillan A 1986 Vaginal discharge. British Medical Journal 293: 1357–1360

FURTHER READING

Adler M W 1993 ABC of AIDS, 3rd edn. British Medical Association, London
Holmes K K et al 1990 Sexually transmitted diseases, 2nd edn. McGraw–Hill, New York
McMillan and Scott G R ,1990 Colour aids in sexually transmitted diseases. Churchill Livingstone, Edinburgh

Appendix 13.1

SUGGESTED ROUTINE FOR EXAMINATION OF WOMEN FOR SEXUALLY TRANSMISSIBLE INFECTIONS

1. Examine woman in semilithotomy position in a warm, well-lit room.
2. Inspect mouth and, if indicated, take material from tonsils or tonsillar fossae for culture for *Neisseria gonorrhoeae.*
3. Inspect skin (note particularly, lesions suggestive of scabies or secondary syphilis, icterus, needle marks, ectoparasites).
4. Collect blood for serological tests for syphilis and, if indicated, for hepatitis B virus and human immunodeficiency virus infection (in latter, only after counselling).
5. Inspect pubic area for *Phthirus pubis* infestation, warts or molluscum contagiosum.
6. Palpate inguinal lymph nodes (if enlarged, note whether uni- or bilaterally enlarged and whether tender or not).
7. Inspect labia majora, labia minora, urethral orifice, introitus, perineum and perianal region. Note swelling of Bartholin's gland.
8. With the right forefinger in the vagina, gently massage urethra and look for expression of mucopus. Using an applicator stick tipped with cotton wool, collect secretions and prepare slide for microscopy. Collect more secretions and send for culture for *N. gonorrhoeae.*
9. Palpate Bartholin's glands and inspect expressed secretions. If mucopus exudes, collect for microscopy and culture for *N. gonorrhoeae*
10. Pass speculum and inspect vaginal walls. Note character of secretions.
11. Using applicator sticks tipped with cotton wool, collect material from posterior fornix for microbiological examination for *Trichomonas vaginalis* (saline mount), *Candida* spp. (Gram-stained smear) and bacterial vaginosis (saline mount and Gram-stained smear).
12. When indicated, a cervical smear must be taken *before* other tests are performed.
13. Gently wipe cervix with cotton wool held in sponge-holding forceps and note characteristics of cervical secretions (perfectly adequate

specimens for microbiological examination can be obtained during menstruation).

14. Using an applicator stick tipped with cotton wool, collect material from the endocervical canal and smear on a slide for later microscopic examination. Send another swab in transport medium for culture for *N. gonorrhoeae*.
15. Collect material from the endocervical canal for microbiological examination for *Chlamydia trachomatis* (see text).
16. Pass an applicator stick tipped with cotton wool about 3cm into the anal canal and send in transport medium for culture for *N. gonorrhoeae*.
17. Undertake bimanual vaginal examination, unless contraindicated.

Transport medium for *Neisseria gonorrhoeae*

Using charcoal-impregnated swabs for the collection of material, Stuart's medium has proved valuable. In Amies' modification, the charcoal is incorporated into the medium, thereby allowing the use of untreated swabs. The clinician must be guided by the local laboratory on which transport system to use.

14. Sexuality and family planning

John Bancroft

The functions of sex
Fertility
Pleasure
Pair-bonding and fostering intimacy
Asserting masculinity or femininity
Bolstering self-esteem
Achieving power or dominance in
  relationships
Expressing hostility
Reducing anxiety or tension
Risk taking
Material gain

**The unfolding of sexuality and the
evolving of sexual relationships**
Adolescence
The couple and early marriage
Early parenthood
Middle age

Common forms of sexual difficulty
Female problems
  Loss of enjoyment

  Loss of sexual interest
  Sexual aversion
  Orgasmic dysfunction
  Vaginismus
  Dyspareunia
Male problems
  Premature ejaculation
  Erectile dysfunction
  Ejaculatory failure
  Loss of sexual desire
Problems that involve both partners

Sexual effects of contraceptive methods
Hormonal contraception
Intrauterine devices (IUDs)
Diaphragms
Condoms
Withdrawal (coitus interruptus)
Natural methods of fertility regulation
New methods of male contraception
Sterilization

Helping with sexual difficulties

Family planning is only necessary because people engage in sexual behaviour. The implications of this statement are often overlooked or ignored, as is shown by the neglect in contraceptive research, the lack of appropriate training for staff working in family planning clinics and primary care, and the shortage of provision of appropriate help when issues or problems relating to sexuality arise.

During a family planning consultation, issues of sexuality are or should be open for discussion. By seeking advice on contraception, an individual or couple is implicitly stating their involvement, current or intended, in a sexual relationship, and one in which, at least for the time being, they do not wish to bear children. This is important for two principal reasons. First, the impact of a particular contraceptive method on the individual or the sexual relationship needs to be considered; this reflects on the direct consequences as well as the psychological effects of the method. Secondly, the obvious sexual implications make talking to the family planning doctor or nurse an opportunity to express concerns or seek advice about broader aspects of sexual life. Increasingly, individuals or couples contact family planning clinics simply to seek such help, often reluctant to approach their general practitioner (GP), either for reasons of confidentiality or uncertainty about how the enquiry will be received.

Doctors and nurses working in family planning therefore need to be informed about the impact of contraceptive methods on sexual life and to feel comfortable enough to discuss broader issues of sexuality to allow patients to express their concerns.

In many cases, listening and empathizing will be helpful. In others, simple advice, requiring some general understanding of sexuality rather than special expertise, may be all that is required. Occasionally, referral to those with special training in the management of sexual problems will be appropriate.

In any case, the health professional should be able to respond in ways which make it easier, rather than more difficult, for patients to express their concerns. There are many in the medical profession who believe that it is intrusive to enquire about their patients' sexual lives. In some circumstances that is the case. But when discussing contraception it *is relevant*, and the important aim is that one's approach should allow patients to respond in the way that suits them best; to say little or nothing if that is their choice, or to respond feeling secure that one's comments will be listened to appropriately. There is little doubt that a key factor in determining whether a patient discusses sexual concerns with a doctor or nurse, is the patient's expectation of whether or not the response would be sensitive and unembarassed.

THE FUNCTIONS OF SEX

Although reproduction is the fundamental purpose of sex, the human species is one in which sexual behaviour has come to serve a variety of other functions. In understanding patients' sexual concerns, it is often helpful to have a clear idea of the range of these functions. Not infrequently, problems arise in a sexual relationship because the two participants are, at the time, using sex for different and conflicting purposes. Fertility remains an important and influential factor even for those seeking contraceptive advice.

Fertility

In general, in our society, the majority of men and women expect and want to have children at some stage in their lives, although many are happy to delay this stage until they have established themselves in a relationship and a career, and feel economically secure enough to start a family. Other pressures may play a part and reflect individual characteristics, cultural or religious influences.

In some cultures, a young woman may feel a powerful need to demonstrate her fertility even when she does not want a child at that point in her life. These are societies where traditionally a woman is only regarded as worthy of marriage when she has proved herself to be fertile. The relevance of such influences in European societies is complex but of considerable interest. Up to the end of the nineteenth century there was a striking contrast in this respect between the north of Europe (e.g. Scandinavian countries, northern Germany) and the south or Mediterranean regions. In the north, the importance of proving fertility before marriage was evident; in the south, the emphasis was on proving virginity.

There are signs that these contrasting patterns still apply with greater acceptance of single motherhood in the north, more evidence of 'double standards' of sexual morality and the 'virginity ethic' in the south. But whatever the social context, some young women may approach contraception with an ambivalent attitude because of this underlying, quite possibly unconscious, need to prove their fertility. To embark on many years of contraception, *not knowing whether you will be fertile at the end of it*, can cause concern for some.

Religion can also be a powerful influence. In the Catholic Church, women are encouraged to believe that sexual pleasure is acceptable only if it is associated with the possibility of conception. The majority of women in the Catholic Church, and other religions with similar teaching, escape from this restraint on their sexual expression and come to terms with their need for effective contraception – but not all.

Pleasure

Perhaps the primary, or most basic reinforcer of sexual behaviour is the pleasure that can be experienced, a combination of sensual pleasure and the uniquely sexual pleasure associated with orgasm. In some individuals this becomes a powerful motivation for their behaviour; for others it is of secondary importance. In either case it will reflect that individual's capacity for sexual responsiveness and orgasm, and this capacity can be affected by psychological factors – relationship problems, illness, including depression, drugs and sometimes contraception.

Pair-bonding and fostering intimacy

This becomes the most rewarding factor for many people, particularly after the excitement of a new relationship has subsided. In an exclusive sexual relationship, the couple do things together which they would not do with others. This is the essence of sexual intimacy. The effectiveness of sex in fostering such intimacy stems from the inherent psychological risks that are involved; in particular the risks of being rejected, laughed at, found unattractive, or losing control in ways which one's partner finds off-putting. To express ourselves fully in a sexual relationship we therefore need to lower our defences. To do so and to feel safe in the process provides a particularly powerful form of bonding between two people. Experiencing and giving pleasure no doubt contributes to this process, but may be less crucial to bonding than the experience of emotional security that is engendered. It is for this reason that the bonding effect of sexuality within a relationship is so readily threatened by sexual involvement outside the relationship.

Asserting masculinity or femininity

'Gender identity' is how we feel about ourselves as male or female. Too much importance is possibly attached to this aspect of our personal identity and it is much more important to concern ourselves with the 'type of person' we are, rather than how masculine or feminine we are. Nevertheless, gender remains a powerfully reinforced characteristic in our society.

During childhood, sexuality is relatively unimportant to gender identity; at that stage, a sense of gender is established in terms of non-sexual interests, activities, and peer-group relationships. Following puberty, when secondary sexual characteristics develop and hormonal and social milieu change, sexuality becomes important. How attractive or effective we feel in sexual terms becomes an important reinforcer of how masculine or feminine we feel, amongst other things. Much of early adolescent sexuality can be understood in this way. Throughout our lives, particularly at times when gender identity is threatened in other ways (e.g. when facing redundancy or the effects of ageing), we may use our sexuality for this purpose.

Bolstering self-esteem

Feeling sexually attractive to others, or succeeding in one's sexual endeavours, may generally improve self-esteem (and conversely, in the face of sexual failure, lower it).

For both these functions, reinforcing gender identity and bolstering self-esteem, there are differences as well as similarities in the ways in which men and women use sexuality. For example, a man's capacity to 'perform' sexually may become central to his sense of manhood, particularly his ability to develop an erection. This is of considerable importance in understanding problems of erectile dysfunction.

Achieving power or dominance in relationships

The 'power' of sexuality tends to be regarded as an aspect of masculinity, with the male, for both social and physical reasons, typically being in a position of dominance. However, sex can be used to control relationships by both men and women and, as such, is often an important aspect of the dynamics of a relationship. Power may be exerted by controlling access to sexual interaction, determining the form that a sexual encounter takes, and whether the process has a positive or negative effect on the partner's self-esteem. While this can continue to be a factor within an established relationship, it is also an important and interesting aspect of early 'courtship' behaviour.

Whereas women have legitimate reasons for fearing the abuse of power by men in sexual interaction, the extent to which women control normal sexual exchanges is perhaps under-estimated. Typically, during 'courtship', the man makes obvious approaches; the woman decides whether or not they should be allowed to progress to the next stage. This pattern, while tending to become obscured once sexual relationships are established, can nevertheless be influential in determining the response to 'rejection'; men get used to the idea that their requests for sex may be turned down, women may feel particularly vulnerable if they invite sexual activity, and the invitation is rejected or ignored.

Expressing hostility

An important aspect of the 'dominance' issue of male–female sexual interaction, is the use of sexuality to express hostility. This is of most relevance to the problem of rape and sexual assault. Many instances of sexual assault or coercive sex can be seen as an extension of dominance or power, usually by the male over the female. There are also instances when the sexual assault can be understood as an expression of anger, either against the individual woman, or against the woman as a representative of other women, or against the man whose property the assaulted woman is seen to be. There is much controversy about the extent to which rape should be understood as either an act of aggression or a sexual act. To understand many cases of rape and sexual assault it is necessary to understand how aggression and sexual arousal can interact.

For many people, anger and sexual arousal seem incompatible; for them sex becomes difficult if not impossible until anger subsides. For others, anger can enhance sexual arousal, and aggressive sex can become a means of expressing the anger. This is the basis of much of the sexual assault that occurs within established relationships although, mainly because of the physical dominance that is required, it is largely an expression of anger that men use towards women. A woman has other ways of expressing her anger through the sexual relationship; she may deny her partner sexual access; she may deny him the satisfaction of knowing that she enjoyed his love-making, and she may in a variety of subtle ways, make him feel sexually inadequate.

Reducing anxiety or tension

The reduction in arousal that typically follows orgasm may be used as a device to reduce anxiety or tension. While this is an occasional function for most people, it is most likely to become established as an habitual pattern when solitary masturbation is the main sexual outlet. In such circumstances, masturbation may increase in frequency when anxiety or tension is high. Sometimes, when an individual who has developed an habitual pattern of this kind gets involved in a sexual relationship, he or she may find difficulty in using sex in ways that serve the relationship.

Risk taking

Sexual interaction provides a variety of risks, ranging from the relatively benign, such as being found out, to the serious, such as pregnancy or sexually transmissible diseases. Such risk taking has taken on a special and more disturbing significance in relation to the HIV and AIDS epidemic. For some individuals, taking sexual risks is a form of excitement which they seek.

Material gain

Offering oneself as a sexual partner for payment or other material benefits is a well established aspect of human sexuality. Prostitution, the institutionalized form of such sexual transaction, has long been established in most human societies. The social function of prostitution, i.e. the extent to which it serves the needs of a society, has been an issue of considerable debate at various times. A cynical view of marriage sees it as a barter between sex, provided by the woman, and material security, provided by the man. In some marriages, the woman may take this view, making it more difficult for her to realize her own sexual identity. If she feels that her partner is not keeping his side of the bargain, she may tend to withhold hers, denying herself as well her partner the potential benefits of a good sexual relationship.

THE UNFOLDING OF SEXUALITY AND THE EVOLVING OF SEXUAL RELATIONSHIPS

Following the sexual development of the individual and his or her subsequent sexual relationships, a temporal pattern evolves in which particular functions are more important at some stages of the lifespan than at others. Contraception and the choice of method have varying implications through these life stages.

Adolescence

In early adolescence, much of sexuality is to do with re-establishing gender identity and self-esteem. Most of us reach the end of childhood reasonably confident in our identities as children, whether boys or girls, and up till then sex has been largely irrelevant, unless we have been unfortunate enough to have been abused or exploited sexually as a child. With the onset of puberty, bodily changes occur in an unpredictable fashion and hormonal changes have an impact on our emotional reactivity.

Capacity for sexual arousal is heightened, probably reaching its peak for males during the adolescent years, and society informs us in a variety of ways that we should now be evaluating ourselves as sexual beings. Much of early adolescent sexual behaviour, whether it be 'innocent' dating (i.e. with no expectations of sexual interaction), or more obviously sexual exploration, is principally motivated by the need to establish what sort of sexual person we are, whether or not we are successfully masculine or feminine in our sexuality and whether we are sexually attractive to others. Somewhat lower on the agenda is concern about sexual competence – do we know what to do, and can we effectively do it? While struggling with these new and complex issues, the young 'dating' couple will be starting to explore their ability to establish and cope with intimacy. The sense of vulnerability, of emotional risk, will be particularly acute for both boy and girl at this stage, and their earlier experiences at negotiating close relationships will prove important in determining their success.

Not surprisingly, considering the complexity of this new situation, there is much scope for 'dysfunction' of sexual response. The adolescent or young adult male, who is at the peak of his sexual responsiveness, may find it difficult to control his arousal, and rapid ejaculation may be a problem, further lowering his self-confidence. The young woman, until she has developed a sense of security and comfort with her emerging sexuality, may find it difficult to experience orgasm, at least in the presence of her partner.

In most such cases one can justifiably take an optimistic approach and anticipate that with time these difficulties will be resolved. Those whose earlier experiences have made them particularly vulnerable (as a consequence of earlier emotional traumas or sexual abuse) may now start to establish more overt sexual difficulties.

At this stage, the implications of contraception are probably more complex as well as more important than at any other time. Clearly, the teenage girl needs to avoid an unwanted pregnancy which can have disastrous consequences. But her approach to avoiding conception will be inextricably caught up in how she sees herself as a sexual person. While 'going on the pill' may be a sensible way to deal with the issue, it might have other meanings to her. By taking the pill, is she declaring herself 'sexually available' and by doing so, will her suitability as a sexual partner be devalued? Would her self-esteem be better served by avoiding any such forward planning so that sexual activity when it does occur is in the 'heat of the moment'?

A study of young female university students found that women using oral contraceptives were not only more sexually active than their fellow students using other methods of contraception, but were also more sexually interested and more comfortable with their sexual relationships (Bancroft et al 1991a). Their choice of this method of contraception may not simply have improved their sex lives, it may, in the first place, have reflected their greater comfort with their own sexuality.

In the last few years, the emphasis on safer sex and the importance of condoms has added a further complexity to the decision-making of adolescents and young adults. At the time in their lives when they are first exploring issues of intimacy and trust in their sexual relationships, they are advised to act on the assumption that no sexual partner should be trusted. In other words, they should use condoms as a protection against sexually transmissible infection, regardless of what their partner tells them about his or her previous experience. The difficulties of such a situation for an adolescent should not be underestimated, and it is noteworthy how little attention has been paid to helping adolescents learn how to cope with these sensitive negotiations in their early relationships.

The couple and early marriage

Once the relationship is established, particularly after marriage or cohabiting begins, the challenge is to develop the security of the established sexual relationship, which is also starting to lose the powerful impact of 'novelty'. It is at this stage that establishing good communication becomes crucially important to the continuing development of the sexual relationship. If the couple does not establish ways of letting each other know what they enjoy and what they find unpleasant, then problems which otherwise would be sorted out and resolved, will become established.

A common type of problem for the young couple stems from an interesting difference between males and females. As already mentioned, the younger male has a tendency to ejaculate quickly when he is sexually aroused. His developmental task is to learn to control his sexual responses so that he can ejaculate when he wants to. The young female often has to overcome established, socially conditioned patterns of inhibition which tend to delay or prevent her experiencing orgasm; she has to learn to 'let her self go' sexually. Unfortunately, once anxiety enters the situation, as it may do when the couple feel they are facing a problem of adjusting sexually, the effect of the anxiety is to aggravate the man's rapid ejaculation and to further delay or inhibit the woman's response. In such circumstances, the young woman, after a few years in which she is frequently aroused but seldom satisfied sexually, finds that she is losing interest, preferring not to get involved so that she avoids further disappointment and frustration. Her male partner, aware of his poorly controlled ejaculation, fails to establish confidence in his sexual performance, making him vulnerable, sooner or later, to other problems such as erectile failure.

Approximately half of the young to middle-aged men who present at sexual problem clinics with erectile problems report life-long lack of control over their ejaculation.

Occasionally, in couples who have delayed sexual intercourse until after marriage or until they start cohabiting, the woman may be unable to tolerate vaginal intercourse; spasm of her perivaginal muscles makes penile insertion difficult or impossible. This condition is known as vaginismus. Usually it results from a tendency for a woman's pelvic floor muscles to go into spasm as soon as insertion of anything into the vagina is attempted (they may find it difficult or impossible to use tampons). Such women may be responsive and able to enjoy love-making until vaginal entry is attempted. In other cases, the vaginismus is part of a more general aversion towards sexuality. This is a problem typically of the young woman and seldom develops as a secondary problem after a woman has experienced satisfactory sexual intercourse.

In the young couple, failure to fulfil the broader expectations of the relationship can also lead to withdrawal from the sexual relationship by one or other partner. Thus, for the young man or woman who finds their partner failing to give them the emotional and practical support they expected while continuing with their individual-oriented interests, it may become increasingly difficult to engage in sexual activity which will be sexually pleasurable for both.

Contraception at this stage is primarily concerned with avoiding unwanted pregnancy. But the choice of method can have various implications which we will consider in more detail below.

Early parenthood

Pregnancy, and the few months following childbirth, pose further needs for sexual adjustment. The woman is likely to experience a diminution of her sexual desire and capacity for sexual enjoyment towards the end of the pregnancy largely because of the major physical and mechanical changes. It may be as long as a year after childbirth before she regains her previous level of sexual interest and enjoyment.

Postnatally, a number of factors conspire to delay her return to sexual enjoyment. She is likely to be tired, and if she is feeding her infant through the night this will be a major factor. Sexual intercourse may be painful for several weeks following a delivery, particularly if she had an episiotomy or perineal tear. Depressive mood changes are common, and these will serve to dampen her sexual interest. The dynamics of her relationship with her partner undergo major change with the arrival of a child and many couples find this disrupts their closeness and in particular their sense of sexual intimacy, at least temporarily.

Resentments may arise in either partner which may have sexual repercussions. How the couple negotiate the return to love-making can certainly test the man's sensitivity to his partner's needs. Breastfeeding, particularly when this is the only form of feeding, delays the return of ovarian cyclicity; the hormonal state of the fully breastfeeding woman is comparable to that after the menopause, with oestrogen deficiency which can impair normal vaginal response and cause discomfort during intercourse (Alder & Bancroft 1988).

The postnatal period, for these various reasons, is one of the commonest times for sexual difficulties to arise, which, if the couple have not developed the appropriate methods of resolving them, can become established long-term difficulties. The commonest of such long-term problems is the woman's loss of sexual desire.

Middle age

The sexuality of the long established relationship typically encounters some different obstacles. By this stage, the novelty of the sexual relationship has long gone. For many that is not a problem; they have established a comfortable form of sexual intimacy which remains an integral part of their relationship. But for others, a routine quality to the sexual relationship takes its toll. In such circumstances it is all too easy for stresses, at work for example, to distract causing tiredness and to dampen any spontaneous enthusiasm for sexual activity that might occur. Love-making becomes infrequent, and tensions may develop in the relationship as a consequence.

What does this infrequency mean? Does my partner no longer love me, or find me attractive? Is he or she sexually interested or involved with someone else? Not infrequently, such couples can be reassured to find that, when they escape from their normal day-to-day pressures, such as on holiday, they recapture some of their earlier sexual enthusiasm. All too often, the lessons of such a discovery are not learnt, and they return from holiday to their previous routines and pressures, and somewhat barren sexual existence.

Other factors impinging on sexual function become increasingly important with the ageing process. A gradual reduction in the speed and intensity of our sexual responses occurs and physical disease becomes increasingly common. Cardiovascular and neurological diseases are particularly important in men, impairing erectile function. Women experience gynaecological problems which can generally impair their well-being and hence their capacity for sexual interest and pleasure.

As women enter their 40s, menstruation frequently becomes more heavy, prolonged or frequent and directly interferes with their sexual lives. It is common for women passing through the transitional period of the perimenopause to experience a decline in their sexual interest and responsiveness. To some extent, this is a direct result of hormonal changes; oestrogen deficiency will, in some menopausal women, result in impaired vaginal lubrication which makes sexual intercourse uncomfortable or even painful. However, the loss of sexual interest that commonly occurs can only be partially explained in such terms, and we remain uncertain of the causes of such mid-life sexual decline in many women. It may be relevant that the evidence of such decline is most apparent in women from lower socio-economic groups, amongst whom satisfaction with the premenopausal sexual relationship tends to be less (Garde & Lunde 1980).

By the time women are considering the relevance of the menopause, they are often encountering a variety of other new challenges. It is a time when many women are moving on from major commitments of motherhood to consider new alternative roles, when men are contending with the consequences of their age in their career (e.g. threat of redundancy, being overtaken by younger colleagues), as well as the impact of faltering physical health.

Choice of contraception for this age group becomes confounded by other health issues and is considered elsewhere in the book (Ch. 16).

With yet older age groups, the sexual problems we see are mainly erectile problems in men and loss of sexual interest in women. The effects of ageing do have an impact on sexuality but not all negative by any means. These couples are less likely to seek help within a family planning or reproductive health context.

COMMON FORMS OF SEXUAL DIFFICULTY

There are interesting sex differences in the way that sexual problems are presented. Men tend to formulate their sexual problems mainly in terms of sexual function. In general, they are more comfortable with a physical rather than a psychological explanation, and consequently tend to seek more physical types of help. Women are more likely to see their difficulties in terms of the 'quality of the sexual experience' and its relevance to the relationship. They are more likely to feel comfortable with a psychological explanation as well as psychological types of help. In general, physical factors are more commonly implicated in male than in female sexual dysfunction, though the study of physical aetiology in women has been somewhat neglected. In both sexes, we remain very uncertain how psychological problems become translated into the physiological failure of sexual dysfunction, but we can recognize a variety of psychological problems which are commonly associated. (For a more detailed account see Bancroft 1989.)

Female problems

Loss of enjoyment

This is probably the commonest sexual complaint of women. A woman may participate in love-making, but fail to experience the pleasure and excitement which she has been used to. If she does not become aroused, then normal vaginal lubrication and vulval tumescence may fail to occur and vaginal intercourse may become uncomfortable or even painful, further blocking her capacity for enjoyment.

Loss of sexual interest

Frequently this occurs together with the loss of enjoyment; such women have no desire to make love and do not enjoy it when it occurs. But in many cases the capacity for enjoyment, once love-making is underway, may remain; the woman simply does not experience any spontaneous sexual desire. As with men, factors leading to loss of sexual desire are varied and often difficult to identify. Mood change is particularly important in women, not only as chronic depressive illness but also as the variations in depressive mood around menstruation that some women experience. Many women are aware of feeling more sexually interested and arousable at certain stages of the menstrual cycle, though the timing of this varies from woman to woman. But those women who typically feel low premenstrually usually lose sexual interest at that time, and find the postmenstrual phase the best time for them sexually.

In some women with marked perimenstrual mood changes, their capacity for sexual desire becomes restricted to a few days post-menstrually, and not infrequently this is eventually lost as well. Unresolved conflicts or resentments in the relationship can underlie both loss of enjoyment and interest. In recent years, it has become much more common for women with such problems to reveal earlier sexual traumas or abuse.

Women contending with life-threatening forms of cancer, such as breast or gynaecological cancer, may react psychologically to both the stress of the illness and the impact of treatment (e.g. mastectomy). Physical factors may also play a more direct role. Loss of desire is to be expected in states of ill-health and may specifically be caused by abnormal hormonal states. Testosterone appears to be important for sexual desire in many, if not all women, as it is in men. Substantial reduction in testosterone, as occurs following ovariectomy or other forms of ovarian failure or suppression, may result in loss of desire.

Sexual aversion

In some cases the thought of sexual activity causes so much fear or anxiety that a pattern of avoidance of sexual contact becomes established. Often in such cases the cause can be identified from earlier traumatic experiences, but sometimes the origins of the problem remain obscure.

Orgasmic dysfunction

Some women present specifically with difficulty in experiencing orgasm, either in the presence of their partner or in any situation. This may be part of a more generalized loss of sexual enjoyment, or be relatively specific, with sexual arousal and enjoyment still occurring but failing to culminate in orgasm. Although occasionally drugs may block orgasm in women, in most cases psychological factors are likely to be responsible.

Vaginismus

This tendency to spasm of the pelvic floor and perivaginal muscles whenever vaginal entry is attempted may result from some earlier traumatic experience of vaginal insertion (e.g. rape or a particularly clumsy pelvic examination by a doctor). More often there is no obvious antecedent cause and it appears to be a particular tendency for reflexive spasm of these muscles when challenged to relax. If the problem is simply one of vaginismus, there is a good likelihood that the condition can be treated relatively simply, with appropriate training in vaginal relaxation and use of vaginal dilators. If the vaginismus is associated with more deep-seated psychological problems, often presenting as a reluctance to accept the maturity of a full sexual relationship, the prognosis is much less certain, and such cases may be resistant to treatment.

Vaginismus is usually a primary sexual difficulty affecting women at the start of their sexual lives, often resulting in 'non-consummation' of the sexual relationship. It is unusual for it to arise later in a woman's life after a phase of normal sexual intercourse, particularly if she has experienced childbirth. When it does, it is important to look for local causes of pain or discomfort that might lead to the muscular spasm.

Dyspareunia

Pain when intercourse is attempted is a common and often treatable problem. If it is a recurring problem then anticipation of pain can easily lead to inhibition of normal sexual response thus aggravating the problem by impairing normal vaginal lubrication. The pain or discomfort may occur at the vaginal introitus, resulting from spasm of the perivaginal muscles (as in vaginismus) or inflammation or soreness of the introitus that can follow episiotomy or perineal tear. A Bartholin's cyst or abscess may cause pain simply as a result of sexual arousal, because of the tendency of the Bartholin's gland to secrete in response to sexual stimulation.

Soreness of the vaginal wall is commonly associated with vaginal infections, with persistence of the soreness for some hours after intercourse is attempted, being a common description.

Pain experienced when the partner thrusts deeply, or when certain positions are adopted during love-making suggests some pelvic problem, such as endometriosis, a low-placed ovary or pelvic inflammatory disease.

Sometimes, pain or discomfort results from the vasocongestion that arises in the pelvic tissues supporting the uterus during sexual arousal, particularly if previous surgery or infection has resulted in adhesions.

Although dyspareunia can be the symptom of a psychological problem (e.g. a conversion symptom) this is relatively unusual, and a local explanation for the pain should be carefully sought. This should include a systematic and careful pelvic examination in which an attempt is made to elicit the pain that normally occurs. Often the cause is treatable.

Male problems

Premature ejaculation

Difficulty in controlling ejaculation so that love-making can continue is typically a problem of younger men. It is seldom, if ever, the result of physical disease, though in some older men physical impairment of erection may need prolonged stimulation before an erection develops, by which time ejaculation is difficult to control. Premature ejaculation is made worse by anxiety. Sexual counselling can often help; the first task is to enable the couple to establish tension-free love-making, so that the anxiety which aggravates the ejaculatory problem is reduced. Then the man, with the co-operation of his partner, learns how to delay ejaculation, using such techniques as the 'stop-start' or 'squeeze'.

Occasionally the use of drugs, such as the new serotonin re-uptake inhibitors (e.g. fluoxetine), is justified to pharmacologically delay ejaculation. However, improvement seldom continues once the drug is stopped.

Erectile dysfunction

This is the commonest sexual complaint of men, affecting about 50% of the men who attend our sexual problem clinics, and being increasingly common in older age groups. The aetiology of this problem is varied and still not well understood. Ageing itself plays an important part, for reasons which are also not clear. It is possible, for example, that there may be an age-related loss of responsiveness to crucial neurotransmitters in the central nervous system (CNS) which normally lead to sexual arousal. But there are a variety of physical diseases, many of them associated with age, which impair erectile response, cardiovascular and neurological disease being the most important.

Psychological factors are undoubtedly important and often combine with physical causes to make the problem substantially worse. In younger men with erectile dysfunction, psychological causes are more likely to predominate and a variety of psychological factors can often be identified in such cases. However, we still know very little about the mechanisms which link such psychological problems to erectile failure. In many cases, some form of direct neurophysiological inhibition of erectile response is involved, but research into such mechanisms is at a very early stage.

Many men, having experienced erectile difficulty, lose confidence in their capacity for sexual response, which in some way serves to maintain the problem. Fortunately, in many such cases confidence, and with it sexual function, returns or can be regained with help, either professional or from a sympathetic and supportive partner.

Ejaculatory failure

Taking a long time to ejaculate or being unable to do so at all in the presence of the partner, or intravaginally, does arise, but less commonly than the above two problems. About 6% of men attending Edinburgh sexual problem clinics have this complaint. In many cases, it results from psychological problems, presumably involving inhibition. In some cases, this inhibitory tendency can be seen as part of a more general pattern of emotional inhibition. In other cases, it appears to be more specifically sexual. In a few cases physical factors, such as testosterone deficiency, can be responsible.

A number of drugs can effectively block ejaculation, though usually, in such cases, orgasm is not blocked, resulting in a so-called 'dry run' orgasm. Neurological damage, as can occur in diabetes, and structural damage after transurethral resection of the prostate, may result in retrograde ejaculation into the bladder.

Loss of sexual desire

Spontaneous desire for sexual activity, or sexual appetite, is a difficult concept. For both men and women it involves the capacity to become aroused by sexual thoughts or situations, leading to a state which motivates them to pursue further sexual stimulation, and ultimately orgasm. Some men seek help because they are aware that their sexual desire has markedly declined. In some cases, this is an understandable reaction to other types of sexual dysfunction and it is important to establish whether the loss of desire preceded or followed the onset of the dysfunction (e.g. erectile failure).

A variety of psychological factors appear to be associated with loss of sexual desire, including depression, unresolved tension or resentment in the relationship. Sexual desire is also likely to be blunted if general health is poor, or if the man is chronically tired or stressed. A specific physical cause is a deficiency of testosterone, the principal androgen, which can result from various forms of hypogonadism. Prolactin-secreting tumours of the pituitary may present as loss of sexual desire, the raised prolactin producing effects very similar to those of androgen deficiency.

Problems that involve both partners

It is often said by sex therapists that there is no such thing as an uninvolved partner. While that might be a slight exaggeration, it is certainly true that there are many ways in which one partner can contribute to the difficulties that are mainly presented or experienced by the other. For example, the way in which premature ejaculation can eventually result in loss of interest on the part of the woman. Erectile problems can be aggravated by problems in the woman, such as dyspareunia. Not infrequently, vaginismus can obscure the fact that the man also has an erectile problem. There are also many ways in which problems in communication or subtle ways of causing anxiety or insecurity in one's partner may contribute to or serve to maintain a sexual difficulty.

SEXUAL EFFECTS OF CONTRACEPTIVE METHODS

Having considered the ways in which attitudes to contraception and its significance to the user vary at different stages during the reproductive span, it is appropriate to consider the effects of different contraceptive methods on sexuality.

Hormonal contraception

The contraceptive efficacy of such methods, together with their lack of intrusion into love-making, have probably enhanced the sexual lives of many women. Several large-scale studies have shown that frequency of coitus is higher in oral contraceptive users than in users of other contraceptive methods. However, a recent review of the literature (Bancroft & Sartorius 1990), concluded that a proportion of women react adversely to combined oral contraceptives (COCs), with depressive mood changes, or loss of sexual desire, or both, and that many such women probably discontinue COC use for that reason, not therefore featuring in large cross-sectional studies of regular COC users. However, the size of this proportion experiencing such adverse effects could not be estimated because relevant studies had not been carried out. The sexual effects of progestogen-only pills (POPs) have, until recently, received no attention at all, which is surprising considering that progestogens are used to inhibit sexual desire in male sexual offenders.

The impact of oral contraceptives on sexuality will be compounded by the implications to the couple of using that type of method. Does the male partner simply leave contraceptive management to the woman, giving evidence of his reluctance to take a fair share of the responsibilities of the relationship? Does this cause any resentment in the woman and consequently affect the relationship? Some women dislike the idea of altering their 'body chemistry' by taking a form of medication every day. Others may dislike the direct contact with their partners' ejaculate, which previously had been contained in condoms. It is difficult to disentangle the psychological implications of hormonal contraception from any direct effects on sexuality or well being.

One unique study (Graham et al 1995) has assessed the direct effects of the COC and POP independently from the psychological implications associated with their use as a method of contraception. Volunteers from Edinburgh and Manila (Philippines) who had been sterilized or whose partners had undergone vasectomy took either the COC or POP or a placebo for four months. Careful evaluation before starting on the treatment phase, showed many differences between the two centres. In particular, the Edinburgh women reported more interest in sex, more enjoyment, arousal, closeness to their partners during love-making, and more preparedness to initiate. The Manila women reported a somewhat higher frequency of sexual activity. COC significantly reduced sexual interest in 50% of the Edinburgh women, whilst producing little change sexually in the Manila women. POP, on the other hand, had no apparent adverse effects on sexuality in either centre and some positive effects on mood. Its only negative effect was the expected disruption of the bleeding pattern.

The mechanism for this negative hormonal effect of the COC is not yet understood. It could be an effect of the progestogen. The COC and POP in this study contained the same progestogen, but it was in substantially larger amounts in the COC. Alternatively, it could result from a reduction in free testosterone. Further research is required to answer these questions. Whatever the explanation, this negative effect on sexual interest could result in some women discontinuing a COC early in its use, and in others could produce subtle negative effects on their sexuality which are not really noticed until the COC is stopped, and an improvement in sexuality occurs. The hormonal effects of COCs on sexual interest are probably subtle and easily obscured if there are other problems or negative influences in the woman's sexual relationship (Bancroft et al 1980; 1991b).

Such adverse effects are only relevant for a proportion of women, and for many the advantages may result in net gains in the quality of their sexual lives. The possibility of a negative effect on sexuality, particularly sexual interest, and to some extent on mood, should be considered when helping women to decide on the method which suits them best. The rather positive message about the POP from Graham's study should also be borne in mind when weighing up the alternatives. Newer methods of hormonal contraception, such as Norplant, await assessment in this respect.

Intrauterine devices (IUDs)

There has been little research into the effects of IUDs on sexuality. Any adverse effects that do occur are secondary to the effects of the IUD on menstruation. An important aspect of this method is that the fitting of the IUD is the responsibility of a doctor. For some women this has psychological implications which make the method more acceptable.

Diaphragms

This method, while reasonably effective when used conscientiously, is unacceptable to many women. It interferes with the spontaneity of love-making; either the woman has to disrupt the love-making to go and fit her diaphragm, or she has to anticipate when love-making is likely to occur, which can be particularly problematic for young couples. It also requires handling of the genitalia for fitting and removal, with which some women are uncomfortable. Some women find that a diaphragm interferes with their sexual enjoyment with loss of cervical and some vaginal sensation. Occasionally the male partner is aware of its presence during intercourse.

Condoms

This barrier method has been extensively promoted as offering protection against transmission of the HIV virus. It is disliked, however, by many men who find not only that putting on a condom disrupts the spontaneity of love-making, but also that their erotic sensitivity is noticeably reduced. If premature ejaculation is a problem, this effect can be an advantage. On the other hand, if a man is unsure of his ability to maintain his erection, the process of fitting a condom can pose quite a threat, as he is likely to fear loss of the erection in the process. Many of the disadvantages of condoms could probably be avoided, or at least reduced, if couples learned to use condoms properly.

Withdrawal (coitus interruptus)

Withdrawal of the penis from the vagina before ejaculation occurs has a very long history. For many couples, the level of awareness and focused attention necessary to use this method distracts from the enjoyment and 'abandonment' of the love-making. As the male produces urethral secretions before ejaculation which can contain sperm, this method is particularly unreliable. For some couples, however, this method works quite well, particularly when the woman dislikes intravaginal ejaculation.

Natural methods of fertility regulation

The various methods for identifying the fertile period of the woman's cycle and avoiding sexual intercourse around that time are the only methods of fertility control acceptable to the Roman Catholic Church. They have a high failure rate, and require not only conscientious monitoring of the cycle by the woman but also the preparedness to abstain at the stage of the cycle when some women feel particularly interested sexually. An interesting aspect of the Church's approach to this method is the importance that is attached to the abstinence that is prescribed, the implication being that the self-control required is beneficial to the relationship. In fact, the method can be used with avoidance of vaginal intercourse without avoidance of love-making and mutual orgasm. It may well be true, however, that for some couples the pacing of their sexual activity and the periods of abstinence which result may enhance the enjoyment of their love-making when it does occur.

New methods of male contraception

Apart from the condom, the traditional male method, considerable effort is being made to develop alternative forms of reversible male contraception. The method most likely to succeed, which is currently being evaluated by the WHO, is the suppression of testicular function (and hence spermatogenesis). This can be achieved in various ways, but unless testosterone levels are maintained, a predictable loss of sexual interest will result. High doses of exogenous testosterone serve the double purpose of suppressing spermatogenesis by means of negative feedback on the pituitary, whilst maintaining circulating testosterone levels.

As yet such methods appear to work without adversely affecting the man's sexuality, although possible effects on his mood or aggression have not yet been satisfactorily excluded (Anderson et al 1992). It is an interesting fact that concern about possible effects of a male method on the man's sexuality has been in the forefront of researchers' minds, whereas female methods have been in use for decades with negligible concern about possible adverse sexual effects on the woman.

Sterilization

A number of studies have now followed up men and women who have been sterilized and the general impression is of either no effect or an enhancement of the couple's sexual life thereafter (Bancroft 1989). The selection of the method is an opportunity for the couple to demonstrate their sharing of responsibilities and their joint problem solving. The sexual relationships of couples where the woman had been sterilized were found to be less positive than those where the man had undergone vasectomy (Alder et al 1981).

Clearly, the reasons for the decision to choose sterilization are relevant to the consequences; sterilization carried out for medical reasons, often soon after childbirth, is more likely to be followed by an adverse reaction and feelings of regret. It is also important that the person being sterilized is not doing so because of pressure from the partner. Apart from these aspects, however, and providing there are no postoperative complications, there are no reasons why either method should adversely affect sexual response or enjoyment.

HELPING WITH SEXUAL DIFFICULTIES

The ability not only to facilitate the patient's expression of concern about his or her sexual difficulties, but also to listen empathetically, can be of considerable help. Not infrequently, this will be the first time the patient has actually talked about the problem, and being able to do so may make it much easier to get the problems and likely causes into perspective. In many cases there will be a lack of relevant information about normal sexual response and what to expect. This can be readily rectified. Common examples are the assumption that couples should experience orgasm simultaneously to be normal, or that women should experience orgasm simply as a result of vaginal intercourse.

By talking with the couple, it is often possible to help them gain a better understanding of each other and what the sexual experience means to each of them. Enabling the couple to talk more openly and comfortably about their sexual feelings is often half the battle. This can pave the way for the couple to sort things out for themselves.

An important responsibility in the family planning setting is to identify cases of dyspareunia and establish whether any treatable condition, such as a vaginal infection, is present. The impact of other physical problems, such as cardiovascular or neurological disease, on sexual function may require more specialized diagnostic assessment. It certainly should not be assumed, for example, that because a man has diabetes, his erectile problems are simply the result of the diabetes.

Simple advice can be helpful; not only suggesting particular things to do (e.g. involving masturbatory techniques or vibrators, using the 'stop-start' technique for rapid ejaculation), but also 'giving permission' to the couple to try something that they might previously have felt was 'not normal' or not acceptable. Encouraging them to see that 'normal sex' does not have to involve vaginal intercourse, and consequently the inevitable erection, can reduce the pressure on the couple and allow them to relax and enjoy their love-making in new ways.

Such simple counselling is unlikely to do any harm, and hence it is entirely reasonable for the non-expert to provide this type of help. What is required is a modest amount of knowledge, as covered in this chapter, and the ability to talk about it comfortably and without embarrassment. If such a simple approach fails to help, then referral to the specialist should be considered. Vaginismus probably warrants early referral, as do cases of ejaculatory failure, sexual aversion and loss of sexual desire, which are often difficult to assess as well as treat. However, it is important to establish clearly with the patient or couple whether such referral is really what they want at that time.

REFERENCES

Alder E, Bancroft J 1988 The relationship between breastfeeding persistence, sexuality and mood in the post-partum woman. Psychological Medicine 18: 389–396

Alder E, Cook A, Gray J, Tyrer G, Warner P, Bancroft J 1981 The effects of sterilization: a comparison of sterilized women with wives of vasectomized men. Contraception 23: 45–54

Anderson R A, Bancroft J, Wu F C W 1992 The effects of exogenous testosterone on sexuality and mood of normal men. Journal of Clinical Endocrinology and Metabolism 75:1503–1507

Bancroft J 1989 Human sexuality and its problems. 2nd edn. Churchill Livingstone, Edinburgh

Bancroft J, Sartorius N 1990 The effects of oral contraceptives on well-being and sexuality. Oxford Reviews of Reproductive Biology. 12: 57–92

Bancroft J, Davidson D W, Warner P, Tyrer G 1980 Androgens and sexual behaviour in women using oral contraceptives. Clinical Endocrinology 12: 327–340

Bancroft J, Sherwin B B, Alexander G M, Davidson D W, Walker A 1991a Oral contraceptives, androgens, and the sexuality of young women: I. A comparison of sexual experience, sexual attitudes, and gender role in oral contraceptive users and nonusers. Archives Sexual Behavior 20: 105–120

Bancroft J, Sherwin B B, Alexander G M, Davidson D W, Walker A 1991b Oral contraceptives, androgens, and the sexuality of young women: II. The role of androgens. Archives Sexual Behavior 20: 121–135

Garde K, Lunde I 1980 Social background and social status; influence on female sexual behaviour. A random sample of 40-year old Danish women. Maturitas 2: 241–246

Graham C A, Ramos R, Bancroft J, Maglaya C, Farley T M M 1995 The effects of steroidal contraceptives on the well-being and sexuality of women: a double-blind, placebo-controlled, two centre study of combined and progestogen-only methods. Submitted for publication

15. Gynaecological problems in the family planning consultation

Anna Glasier

Vulval, vaginal and cervical conditions
Bartholin's cyst and abscess
Lichen sclerosis
Atrophic vaginitis
Vaginal wall cysts
Congenital malformations
Cervical ectropion ('erosion')
Cervical polyp

Pelvic masses

Menstrual dysfunction
Menorrhagia
Menstrual irregularity
Intermenstrual and postcoital bleeding
Management
Treatment

Postmenopausal bleeding
Management
History
Examination

Oligomenorrhoea and amenorrhoea
Causes
Management
Investigation

Hirsutism
Management

Dysmenorrhoea
Management
Investigation
Treatment

Menstrual migraine

Premenstrual syndrome (PMS)
Management
Investigation
Treatment

Pelvic pain
Management

Dyspareunia

Vaginal discharge

Urinary problems
Urgency and frequency
Stress incontinence
Management
Treatment
Dysuria
Management

Prepregnancy counselling

Bleeding in early pregnancy
Management
History
Examination
Pregnancy test
Referral

Recurrent miscarriage

Infertility
Management
Take a history
Give advice about the fertile time of the cycle
Commercial kits for identifying the LH surge
Initial investigations which may be useful
Referral to a specialist

A wide range of minor gynaecological problems may become apparent in the course of the family planning or well woman consultation. Not all are related to contraception and many can be dealt with without referral to a gynaecologist. In large clinics it may be helpful to have access to a standard gynaecological textbook (Shaw et al 1992).

VULVAL, VAGINAL AND CERVICAL CONDITIONS

Bartholin's cyst and abscess

A Bartholin's cyst arises as the result of an obstruction to the duct of the Bartholin's gland. It presents as a cystic swelling in the labium majorum. Cysts are not usually larger than 5–6 cm in diameter and are painless. Infection of a Bartholin's cyst can result in abscess formation presenting as a hot, red and very painful swelling. Recurrent infections may occur if the abscess bursts and drains spontaneously. Both cysts and abscesses are dealt with surgically and should be referred to a gynaecologist – the latter as an emergency.

Lichen sclerosis

Lichen sclerosis is a condition of older women (50–70 years) and may be noted in the course of a well woman examination. The vulval skin looks thin and atrophic and white patches may be present. The patient often complains of itching. The condition may be associated with malignancy and the patient should be referred to a specialist for consideration of a vulval biopsy.

Atrophic vaginitis

Oestrogen deficiency in postmenopausal women results in thinning of the vaginal epithelium. In atrophic vaginitis, the walls of the vagina look reddened with occasional punctate bleeding points. Atrophic vaginitis is a common cause of postmenopausal bleeding. It responds rapidly to local oestrogen cream or pessaries given for 2 weeks. Most vaginal oestrogen preparations are absorbed systemically. Prolonged treatment may therefore have the same effect on the endometrium as oral unopposed oestrogen and should not usually be given for more than 3 months without additional cyclical progestogens. The new very low dose (25 μg oestradiol) preparations are probably safe to give for much longer without added progestogens.

Vaginal wall cysts

Thin-walled vaginal cysts can arise anywhere in the vagina but are most common in the upper portion. They are remnants of the lower Wolffian duct. They are regular in outline and rather translucent in appearance. These cysts can usually be ignored although if they appear to be enlarging over the course of time the patient should be referred to a gynaecologist. Vaginal wall cysts should not be confused with vaginal adenosis, a rare condition in which multiple glandular cysts occur, often accompanied by profuse mucus secretion. Vaginal adenosis may be premalignant and can occur in young women exposed to diethylstilboestrol (DES) in utero. Women with a history of DES exposure should have regular colposcopic examinations of the vagina and cervix.

Congenital malformations

Rarely, congenital malformations such as vaginal agenesis or vaginal septum may be found on routine pelvic examination or present in patients with sexual difficulties. Referral to a gynaecologist is indicated.

Cervical ectropion ('erosion')

The vaginal surface of the cervix is covered with squamous epithelium and the skin is pale pink and smooth. The cervical canal is lined with columnar epithelium and has a red, glandular appearance. Eversion of the edges of the external cervical os (ectropion) thus exposes the columnar epithelium. The vaginal surface of the cervix may be covered by quite an extensive area of columnar epithelium which appears rough and red ('eroded').

This is usually a chance finding on routine vaginal examination and needs no treatment. Occasionally the exposed columnar epithelium may bleed if touched and can be a cause of postcoital bleeding. An extensive 'erosion' may be associated with a profuse vaginal discharge.

Cervical erosion causing symptoms may be cauterized provided a normal cervical smear has been obtained. Squamous epithelium grows back over the cauterized area restoring a healthy looking cervix. Cautery does result in a very profuse watery discharge and patients should be warned of this. It is better to avoid cauterizing the cervix if the patient is just about to go away on holiday!

Cervical polyp

Single or multiple small, red, so-called 'mucus' polyps may sometimes be found at the external cervical os on routine vaginal examination. They are usually asymptomatic but occasionally may cause intermenstrual or postcoital bleeding. Polyps arise from within the cervical canal and if small (less than 1 cm in diameter) they can simply be twisted off with a pair of polypectomy or sponge-holding forceps. The polyp should routinely be sent for histological examination. Larger polyps, particularly those with a thick stalk, may bleed profusely and should be left for the gynaecologist to remove.

PELVIC MASSES

A pelvic mass may sometimes be diagnosed on routine vaginal examination and if large may also be felt abdominally. Pregnancy should always be excluded. The likely cause is either uterine fibroids or an ovarian cyst and these may often be distinguished on the basis of the history or the examination. Small 'functional' ovarian cysts are not uncommon and usually disappear with menstruation. If a symptomless cyst is found on vaginal examination in a young woman – particularly if she is using oral progestogen-only contraception – it can be left and the examination repeated after the next menstrual period. It is not always possible to distinguish between a uterine mass and an ovarian swelling, even with an ultrasound scan. Women with symptomatic cysts, or cysts which persist after the next menstrual period, should always be referred to a specialist, as should all older women who are found to have a pelvic mass.

MENSTRUAL DYSFUNCTION

Disturbance of menstruation is a problem commonly raised during family planning/well woman consultations. A particular method of contraception may be the cause of the problem: menorrhagia due to an IUD; intermenstrual bleeding associated with low-dose combined oral contraception; irregular menses, resulting from use of the POP; these problems and their management are covered in the relevant chapters. In the absence of a disorder associated with contraception, disturbances of menstruation are often short-lived and bleeding patterns which are normal for that individual may resume within a few cycles. Many women do not require sophisti-cated investigation or treatment but simply reassurance that a particular pattern of menstruation is not sinister. The commonest cause of persistent disturbance is dysfunctional uterine bleeding, defined as excessive bleeding (heavy, prolonged or frequent) of uterine origin that is not due to organic pelvic disease or to a generalized medical condition. It is obviously a diagnosis of exclusion (for review, see Crosignani & Rubin 1990).

A pelvic examination is essential in every case to exclude pathology.

Menorrhagia

Heavy periods are a common complaint particularly in perimenopausal women. Fibroids may be diagnosed on pelvic examination but usually the findings are negative.

Menstrual irregularity

This occurs commonly in adolescents and in the perimenopause and is usually associated with anovulation. It may sometimes be associated with an ovarian cyst.

Intermenstrual and postcoital bleeding

Bleeding between periods (IMB) or after intercourse (PCB) may be due to a local cervical problem (see above) including malignancy or more rarely an intrauterine polyp. Some women bleed around midcycle in response to the fall in oestrogen following the luteinizing hormone (LH) surge.

Management

1. Take a careful history.
2. Pelvic examination to exclude any obvious cause.
3. Cervical smear if due or if abnormality is suspected.
4. *Women under 40 years* complaining of menorrhagia or irregular menses without pelvic pathology do not need dilatation and curettage (D & C) or endometrial biopsy since the chance of finding any abnormality is negligible. Exceptions to this general rule (RCOG 1994) include:
   a. Failure of uterine bleeding to respond to medical treatment.
   b. Persistent intermenstrual bleeding.
5. Endometrial biopsy may be considered in women over 40 and can be done in the clinic/surgery using a disposable sampler.
6. In the absence of any obvious pathology on pelvic examination, an endometrial biopsy may be indicated in women presenting with IMB or PCB.

Treatment

1. Menstrual dysfunction often resolves spontaneously. Reassurance is sometimes all the patient is seeking particularly if she is adolescent or approaching the menopause.
2. In most cases, and in the absence of contraindications, the combined oral contraceptive pill will often restore acceptable cycles – a pill containing 20 µg of oestrogen is usually adequate.
3. Menorrhagia seems to be associated with a local overproduction of prostaglandins which cause increased blood loss and myometrial contractions. It is often improved by the oral administration of prostaglandin synthetase inhibitors such as mefenamic acid or even simply aspirin during menses. Patients appreciate an explanation of the rationale for prescribing these simple analgesics and should be encouraged to take them regularly (e.g. 6-hourly) during heavy bleeding days. If this approach is effective treatment can be prolonged indefinitely.
4. Irregular dysfunctional uterine bleeding responds to cyclical progestogens (norethisterone 10–15 mg/day in divided doses from the 12th day of each month or day 12 of the cycle for 14 days). Progestogens given in this way replace the progesterone which is missing because of the absence of ovulation and stimulate the development of a secretory endometrium which breaks down when the progestogen is withdrawn, thus restoring regular bleeding patterns. It is worth stopping treatment after 6 months or so as the problem may have resolved. Treatment can always be restarted if menorrhagia resumes.
5. If menstrual dysfunction persists despite the above approaches, or if any pathology is found on pelvic examination, the patient should be referred for a gynaecological opinion.

POSTMENOPAUSAL BLEEDING

Irregular and infrequent bleeding episodes are of course common during the menopause but need not be investigated *unless* preceded by one or more years of amenorrhoea.

Vaginal bleeding which occurs in a postmenopausal woman more than 1 year after the last menstrual period should always be investigated.

Management

History

A careful history should be taken paying attention to the following:

1. Date of LMP.
2. Associated pain or discomfort – postmenopausal bleeding (PMB) may simply be the result of a small amount of oestrogen secretion from a surviving ovarian follicle (the ovary having a 'last fling') in which case the bleeding often resembles a normal period and may be accompanied by premenstrual type symptoms and dysmenorrhoea.
3. PMB which occurs after intercourse may be due to atrophic vaginitis.
4. A history of associated discharge may suggest a vaginal infection.
5. A history of weight loss, malaise or apparent weight gain associated with a growing pelvic mass may suggest ovarian or uterine malignancy.
6. It is worth taking a full medical history including a drug history – some patients forget to tell the doctor that they are taking hormone replacement therapy. The history should take account of homeopathic remedies such as ginseng which has some oestrogenic properties.

Examination

1. Pelvic examination may reveal a local vulval, vaginal or cervical cause or a pelvic mass. Local vulval lesions may easily be missed. Atrophic vaginitis (see above) is common in postmenopausal women and, although it may be the cause of the PMB, its presence should not preclude other causes which may coexist.
2. A cervical smear should be taken if there is any suspicion of abnormality or if one is due.
3. Vaginal ultrasound, if it is available in the clinic, may reveal an endometrial thickening if there is a carcinoma but a negative scan does not exclude pathology.
4. Endometrial biopsy using a disposable sampler is thought to be as good as a formal dilatation and curettage for excluding endometrial cancer but may not be possible in elderly women with a narrow cervical os.
5. Even if a benign cause such as atrophic vaginitis is suspected, it is probably advisable to refer women with PMB for specialist opinion.
6. Rarely, a forgotten IUD may be found.

OLIGOMENORRHOEA AND AMENORRHOEA

Infrequent or absent menstruation occurs commonly. Pregnancy should always be excluded. The problem is often short-lived and simple reassurance may be adequate. Depending on the woman's age, need for contraception or desire to start a family, investigation may be delayed for 4–6 months.

Causes

Both may be a result of hypothalamic, pituitary or ovarian dysfunction. Intercurrent illness, particularly endocrinopathy e.g. diabetes or thyroid disease, or diseases which affect nutritional status e.g. Crohn's disease, may be present. Amenorrhoea may be primary or secondary.

Management

Investigation

1. Take a careful history including a history of menstrual patterns since menarche. Problems which appear to have arisen after stopping the pill in fact often pre-date its use and have simply been masked by the pill-induced regular withdrawal bleeds. A history of weight loss, excess exercise, diet (vegetarians seem to be prone to amenorrhoea) or stress should be specifically sought. Recent use of Depo-Provera should be excluded.
2. Examination – in addition to pelvic examination a general physical examination should pay attention to ponderal index, signs of thyroid disease, hirsutism and the presence or absence of galactorrhoea.
3. The measurement of serum gonadotrophin and prolactin concentrations is standard practice. Testosterone estimation is helpful in women with oligomenorrhoea and clinical signs of either polycystic ovarian syndrome (PCOS) such as obesity, acne and hirsutism, or virilization such as clitoromegaly. Thyroid function tests – measurement of thyroxine and thyroid stimulating hormone (TSH) – may be useful. Skull X-ray for examination of the pituitary fossa may be requested particularly if there is hyperprolactinaemia.
4. If biochemical investigations are abnormal, if the problem persists or a pregnancy is desired, refer to someone with a special interest in reproductive endocrinology.

5. If investigations are negative, normal cycles may resume spontaneously within a few months. Review in 6 months.

6. If investigations and clinical signs (and ultrasound scan if available) suggest PCOS and fertility is not required, COC will give regular cycles. Dianette which contains cyproterone acetate (an antitestosterone) instead of a progestogen is particularly useful in someone with acne or hirsutism and provides contraception at the same time.

7. Although women with amenorrhoea or oligomenorrhoea are less likely to conceive than women with regular cycles, ovulation may occur and they should be encouraged to use contraception if they wish to avoid pregnancy. Once the nature of the underlying hormonal disturbance has been established, hormonal contraception may be considered. It is perfectly appropriate to prescribe COC for women with hypogonadotrophic or normogonadotrophic amenorrhoea and indeed it will protect them from osteoporosis accompanying oestrogen lack. Pill use has no effect on their future fertility although the withdrawal bleeding will, of course, continue to mask the underlying disorder. Women with PCOS are at risk of endometrial cancer in later life as a result of long periods of unopposed oestrogen stimulation of the endometrium; for these women, the pill will restore regular cycles and protect them from endometrial cancer. Although COC is not absolutely contraindicated for women with hyperprolactinaemia, the oestrogen component does stimulate prolactin secretion and is better avoided or discussed with a specialist.

HIRSUTISM

This may be a feature of PCOS (p. 370) which can be diagnosed on the basis of an elevated concentration of LH in the presence of a normal circulating follicle stimulating hormone (FSH) and an elevated testosterone concentration, together with an ultrasound scan confirming the typical appearance of the ovaries. In the absence of PCOS, hirsutism may be familial and is common in women whose mothers are of Mediterranean or Asian origin.

Management

1. History and examination to exclude PCOS and/or virilism.
2. Reassurance.

3. Cosmetic advice – bleaching, electrolysis, depilatory creams, shaving.
4. Dianette (p. 371).

Women with signs of virilism (e.g. clitoromegaly) or a markedly elevated serum testosterone concentration or those wishing to conceive should be referred for a specialist opinion.

DYSMENORRHOEA

Dysmenorrhoea (period pain) can be primary or secondary. Primary dysmenorrhoea is often present from menarche, and is probably due to an imbalance of prostaglandins. Secondary dysmenorrhoea occurs in a woman who has not had painful periods previously and may be associated with endometriosis or an intracavity uterine fibroid or polyp.

Management

Investigation

1. Take a careful history including the precise timing of pain. Classical primary dysmenorrhoea is often accompanied by vomiting and diarrhoea.
2. Pelvic examination to exclude underlying pathology. A normal pelvic examination does not exclude endometriosis which may often only be diagnosed on laparoscopy.

Treatment

1. An explanation of the cause of dysmenorrhoea and simple reassurance is often enough. It is true that most young women grow out of it.
2. Simple analgesics – aspirin is a potent prostaglandin synthetase inhibitor. Other non-steroidal anti-inflammatory drugs (NSAID) such as mefenamic acid may be helpful. As is the case with menorrhagia, patients should be advised that they will get more relief by taking the medication at regular intervals and not just in response to pain.
3. Dysmenorrhoea is often improved by the combined pill. If it persists, two or three packets can be taken without a break in order to reduce the frequency of the problem (p. 67).

4. If there is no response to these simple measures, referral to a specialist (preferably one with an interest in dysmenorrhoea) may be indicated.

MENSTRUAL MIGRAINE

Some women complain of severe headaches at the onset of menses. These may result from the relatively abrupt fall in circulating oestrogens at the end of the cycle and seem to be more common among pill users than among women having spontaneous cycles.

Taking two or three packets of the combined pill continuously before having a break may help and, if nothing else, reduces the frequency of the headaches. The application of an oestrogen patch on the last day of pill taking has been reported to be of value but there are few data on this approach.

PREMENSTRUAL SYNDROME (PMS)

PMS is a common complaint and seems to occur more frequently as women approach the perimenopause. The cause is unknown but it is almost certainly related in some way to the balance of steroid hormones. Women may be troubled by physical (bloating, mastalgia, nausea) or mental (irritability, depression, anxiety) symptoms.

Management

Investigation

1. Take a history – true PMS should resolve soon after the onset of menses. If it does not, consider depression, or in older women menopausal symptoms, which may be confused with PMS. A symptom diary for 2–3 months may be helpful.
2. General physical and pelvic examination – women are often reassured to know that there is no underlying pathology.

Treatment

Counselling   An explanation of the nature of PMS and the fact that it is so common often helps. Self-help and support groups are extremely valuable. Some women find dietary advice helpful and a number of publications are available giving this sort of advice.

Drug therapy   This helps some but not others, and the improvement may not last. Women should understand that drugs do not cure the problem but only alleviate it and that finding the right 'treatment' may take some time. Hormonal therapies all have side-effects which may ultimately be worse than the PMS. All have a pronounced placebo effect.

1. Vitamin B6 (pyridoxine) 50 mg/day in the second half of the cycle or for the entire cycle may help.
2. Gamolenic acid (oil of evening primrose) may help, particularly for mastalgia, but it is expensive.
3. The combined pill often relieves symptoms and can be taken bicyclically or even tricyclically (p. 67).
4. Diuretics may relieve symptoms of bloating but should be used with caution.
5. NSAIDs such as mefenamic acid for dysmenorrhoea.
6. Progesterone suppositories or progestogens such as Duphaston during the second half of the cycle may help.
7. Psychotropic drugs e.g. antidepressants/anxiolytics can relieve psychological symptoms and should be used with caution. Serotonin uptake inhibitors (e.g. fluoxetine hydrochloride) show some early promise in the treatment of PMS but should be discussed with a specialist.

PELVIC PAIN

Chronic pelvic pain is a common problem in young women and is often attributed to a gynaecological cause. More often than not, no pelvic pathology such as endometriosis or chronic infection is found.

Management

1. Take a history – include careful exploration of urinary and gastrointestinal tract symptoms. Irritable bowel syndrome is a common cause of lower abdominal pain in young women who may not be constipated but will often admit to a bowel motion 'like rabbit pellets'.
2. Abdominal and pelvic examination.
3. Pelvic ultrasound – for some women a normal pelvis on ultrasound is 'proof' that there is nothing seriously wrong.
4. Exploration of social and psychological factors – a demanding job (especially mother/wifehood), tension at home or low

self-esteem can turn a mild and occasional 'tummy ache' into chronic pelvic pain.

5. There is a school of thought that pelvic pain is due to 'pelvic congestion' and some researchers have demonstrated varices in pelvic veins. Short-wave diathermy may be helpful.

6. Referral for diagnostic laparoscopy – although it often seems pretty certain that no pathology will be found, some women remain concerned until someone has actually 'had a look'.

DYSPAREUNIA

Many women assume that pain on intercourse is the result of an organic problem and the issue is not uncommonly raised during a family planning or well woman consultation. Dyspareunia is described as superficial if it is felt at the vaginal introitus and deep if the pain is felt within the pelvis. It may be primary (i.e. present since the first attempt at intercourse), or secondary. Very rarely is dyspareunia due to an organic lesion such as a pelvic mass but a pelvic examination should be undertaken in order to be able to reassure the patient. Management thereafter is described Chapter 14 on sexual problems.

VAGINAL DISCHARGE

See Chapter 13.

URINARY PROBLEMS

Urinary problems are common in women of reproductive age as well as among postmenopausal women. It is estimated that at least 20% of women suffer from urinary frequency (the passage of urine more than seven times during waking hours and twice or more during the night) and 15% report urgency (a sudden strong desire to micturate, which if unrelieved, may lead to incontinence). Stress incontinence (involuntary leakage of urine on coughing, sneezing etc.) is also common particularly in multiparous women who may not admit to the problem because of the embarrassment it causes. Dysuria may also present quite commonly in the course of the family planning consultation.

Urgency and frequency

These may arise from:

1. Pregnancy or disease outside the urinary tract, including pelvic mass, diabetes, neuromuscular disorders, psychiatric disorders, or diuretic therapy.
2. Renal disease.
3. Disease of the bladder including tuberculosis, interstitial cystitis, functionally small bladder, detrusor instablility.
4. Urethral conditions including urethral syndrome and diverticulum.
5. Surgery (hysterectomy) and radiation.
6. Oestrogen deficiency (menopause).

Stress incontinence

This may be associated with:

1. Congenital weakness of the bladder neck.
2. Childbirth.
3. Trauma e.g. pelvic fracture.
4. Fibrosis following surgery.

Management

1. Take a careful and detailed history. It is important to define the problem exactly since stress incontinence is much more amenable to surgery than urge incontinence or frequency.
2. Pelvic and abdominal examination to exclude mass, prolapse, cystocele.
3. Mid-stream specimen of urine to exclude urinary tract infection (UTI); dipstick to exclude glycosuria.
4. Fluid intake and output chart and urinary diary (which the patient can take to the specialist if referral is required) if frequency or urgency appears to be the problem.

Treatment

1. Any obvious predisposing factors such as UTI should be treated.
2. Menopausal women may benefit from local or systemic oestrogen therapy.

3. Women with stress incontinence who are undecided about surgery or who intend further childbearing may benefit from pelvic floor exercises, if they are properly taught (usually by a physiotherapist) and continued for long enough.
4. Urgency and frequency may be helped by bladder training. The patient reduces her fluid intake, if it is excessive, and uses timed voiding to overcome urgency, slowly increasing the interval between voids.
5. When there is evidence of organic disease or if conservative measures fail, referral to a specialist is indicated.

Dysuria

This may result from:

1. Urinary tract infection.
2. Vaginal infection.
3. Frequency dysuria syndrome (FDS) – sometimes called urethral syndrome – describes a condition of frequency and/or urgency, dysuria, strangury and nocturia without an obvious cause.
4. Oestrogen deficiency.
5. Urethral prolapse or caruncle – the urethral mucosa may occasionally prolapse in elderly women. The everted portion becomes red and inflamed and is sometimes called a caruncle. Often symptomless, it can cause dyspareunia and dysuria.

Management

1. Take a careful history.
2. Examination is indicated if anything other than a simple UTI is suspected.
3. Urinalysis and bacteriological investigation of a mid-stream specimen of urine (MSSU). Chlamydia should be excluded if FDS is suspected. Appropriate antibiotic therapy should be given.
4. Dysuria due to postmenopausal oestrogen deficiency responds well to local oestrogens.
5. Referral to a gynaecologist/urologist for cautery or excision of a urethral prolapse.
6. Recurrent UTI or FDS can sometimes be prevented by simple education. Personal hygiene is important and patients should be instructed to wipe the perineum from front to back to avoid contamination of the urethra. Vaginal deodorants (of dubious

value for anyone) and irritant bath additives should be avoided. Fluid intake should be encouraged particularly when symptoms occur. Alkalinizing agents (e.g. potassium citrate) may be of some help. Regular and complete bladder emptying is essential. Postcoital UTI may be associated with use of a barrier method and a change of method may help.

PREPREGNANCY COUNSELLING

Many women attending a family planning consultation intend to embark upon a pregnancy at some time in the future. If that time is imminent, the nurse or doctor has an opportunity to give some prepregnancy advice or counselling. For many women general advice is sufficient; a few may need specialist help.

Stopping contraception It is a myth that women should stop using the combined pill and change to a barrier method some months before embarking on a pregnancy. Recent use of the pill has no effect on the fetus and, as ultrasound scans are now widely available, conceptions which occur immediately after stopping the pill do not present problems with dating.

Diet There are plenty of leaflets available. Pregnant women should be advised to have a healthy diet and to avoid foods such as unpasteurized cheese or substances which are known to carry organisms such as listeria or salmonella.

Folate supplements Neural tube defects have been linked with folate deficiency. Women planning a pregnancy are advised to take folate supplements in addition to having a balanced diet; 400 µg/day should be taken orally until 12 weeks gestation.

Alcohol and smoking Smoking has been associated with an increased risk of miscarriage, prematurity and intrauterine growth retardation. Pregnancy may offer a good incentive to stop. Alcohol, in small amounts, is not contraindicated but a regular moderate or heavy intake should be discouraged.

Antenatal screening/genetic counselling Women over the age of 35 or those with a family history of genetically transmitted disease may need specialist counselling. The doctor involved in a family planning consultation should be aware of how and to whom in the area couples may be referred.

Rubella status This should be checked, particularly in nulliparous women in their late thirties who were not vaccinated at school (Ch. 12).

BLEEDING IN EARLY PREGNANCY

Women sometimes present to the family planning clinic with bleeding in early pregnancy. They may already know or suspect that they are pregnant or pregnancy may be diagnosed in the course of the consultation. Bleeding may be due to local causes such as cervical 'erosion' or polyp (p. 365) or may be a sign of miscarriage or ectopic pregnancy.

Management

History

Take a careful history including detailed menstrual history and history of accompanying abdominal pain. Unilateral iliac fossa pain rather than period-type pain should raise the suspicion of ectopic pregnancy. Other suspicious symptoms include feelings of faintness and shoulder tip pain. A history of pelvic infection, subfertility or IUD use should be sought specifically.

Examination

The patient's general condition should be assessed. Spontaneous abortion and ectopic pregnancy can both cause heavy bleeding and shock. If the patient is in shock, she should be transferred immediately to hospital preferably with an intravenous line in place. Products of conception distending the cervical os can cause shock in incomplete abortion. If the products are removed digitally from the os, the patient usually recovers immediately. In the absence of shock, abdominal and pelvic examination may distinguish between threatened, incomplete and missed abortion, and ectopic pregnancy. Speculum examination may reveal a local cervical cause of the bleeding and the degree of dilatation of the cervical os can be determined. Products of conception may be seen. Pain on cervical excitation, unilateral forniceal pain and a mass may suggest ectopic pregnancy.

Pregnancy test

This may be helpful but a negative result does not exclude ectopic pregnancy, missed or complete abortion.

Referral

The patient should be referred to hospital as an emergency if ectopic pregnancy is suspected. Threatened abortion can be managed at home by the GP but a scan confirming an ongoing pregnancy is reassuring to the mother. Ultrasound scan is used to distinguish missed and complete abortion and where either is suspected or, if the abortion is incomplete, the patient should be seen by a specialist.

RECURRENT MISCARRIAGE

Some 20–25% of pregnancies end in spontaneous abortion. Some women who miscarry recurrently may ask for advice during a family planning consultation. Most gynaecologists do not investigate couples until three or more pregnancies have miscarried. Women should be reassured that one and even two miscarriages are not uncommon and that their chance of carrying a pregnancy to term next time is high. The only practical advice that can be given is that smoking appears to be associated with miscarriage. Women with recurrent miscarriage should be referred for investigation by a specialist. Useful investigations prior to referral include:

1. Karyotyping of both partners.
2. Full blood count of the mother.
3. Lupus anticoagulant level from the mother.

INFERTILITY

Between 1 in 8 and 1 in 10 couples experience difficulty in conceiving. Some initial advice may be given and, if appropriate, investigations started in the family planning clinic. Depending on the woman's age, investigations should not usually be started until a couple has been trying to conceive for a year, as 90% will succeed within that time.

Management

Take a history

The common causes of infertility are:

1. Failure of ovulation.
2. Tubal disease.
3. Male infertility.

The history should explore these three areas. Women with regular cycles are almost certainly ovulating. Previous abdominal or gynaecological surgery or a history of pelvic inflammatory disease might suggest tubal disease. In the male, a history of undescended testes; hernia repair; mumps; intercurrent disease such as ulcerative colitis treated with drugs that are potentially toxic to sperm; heavy drinking; or smoking, might suggest male infertility.

Give advice about the fertile time of the cycle

With regular cycles, intercourse every other night during the fertile period is adequate. Basal body temperature (BBT) measurement only defines the end of the fertile period. Patients who are keen to do so may be instructed in fertility awareness techniques and use them to achieve a pregnancy.

Commercial kits for identifying the LH surge

These are available to help define the fertile period. They are expensive and many couples find the strain of timing intercourse with such precision somewhat inhibiting.

Initial investigations which may be useful

While a couple waits for an appointment for the infertility clinic, useful investigations include:

1. Serum progesterone in the mid-luteal phase of the cycle
   (e.g. day 21 in a 28-day cycle; day 28 in a 35-day cycle).
   This confirms that ovulation is occurring.
2. In a woman with oligomenorrhoea or amenorrhoea it is worth measuring serum gonadotrophins, prolactin and testosterone concentrations (p. 370).
3. Semen analysis.

Referral to a specialist

If a woman is over 35 years of age, it is probably better to refer after 6 months rather than waiting 1 year. Remember that there may be 2–3 months' wait for an appointment. If you identify a possible cause in the history or examination it may be sensible to refer earlier.

REFERENCES

Crosignani P G, Rubin B 1990 Dysfunctional Uterine Bleeding.
  Human Reproduction 5: 637–638
RCOG 1994 In-Patient Treatment – D & C in women age 40 or less.
  RCOG Guidelines No. 3. RCOG London
Shaw R W, Soutter W P, Stanton S L (eds) 1992. Gynaecology.
  Churchill Livingstone, Edinburgh

16. The menopause

Ailsa Gebbie

Endocrine changes at the menopause
Changes in the perimenopause

Diagnosis of the menopause

Consequences of ovarian failure
Short-term symptoms
Vasomotor symptoms
Psychological symptoms
Intermediate symptoms
Urogenital atrophy
Skin changes
Long-term symptoms
Osteoporosis
Cardiovascular disease

Treatment
Non-hormonal treatment
Oestrogen therapy
Oral oestrogens
Transdermal oestrogens
Subcutaneous oestrogen implants
Vaginal oestrogen delivery systems
Other routes of oestrogen administration
Combined oestrogen–progestogen therapy
HRT without bleeding
Continuous combined HRT
Contraindications to HRT
Absolute

Relative
Complications of HRT
Side-effects of oestrogen
Side-effects of progestogen

Special considerations
Breast cancer
Compliance

Clinical management
Assessment of a woman prior to HRT
History
Examination
Investigations
Monitoring
History
Examination
Duration of use

Contraception in the perimenopause
Pregnancy in older women
Contraceptive methods
Combined oral contraception
Progestogen-only contraception
Intrauterine devices
Barrier methods
Natural family planning

Provision of services

The menopause is a physiological event occurring on average at the age of 50.8 years. Historical texts (Aristotle third century BC) reveal that this average age has remained unchanged for centuries. Most women in the United Kingdom (UK) can anticipate spending at least a third of their lives in the postmenopausal state as this century has seen a striking increase in the average life expectancy of women to just under 80 years.

The menopause is, by definition, the last menstrual period. By convention, this is a diagnosis made in retrospect following amenorrhoea for 12 months. Any subsequent vaginal bleeding should be deemed postmenopausal bleeding and investigated accordingly (Ch. 15).

The transitional phase of fluctuating ovarian function around the time of a woman's last menstrual bleed is known as the 'perimenopause' or 'climacteric'. For most women, this phase of menstrual irregularity lasts around 2–3 years although some women date the onset of symptoms attributable to the menopause as long as 10 years before the actual menopause occurs. The distressing vasomotor and psychological symptoms that cause many women to seek advice from health care professionals are often at their most severe prior to the last period. Women universally refer to the climacteric phase as 'going through the menopause'.

The last decade has seen considerable scientific interest and research in the field of the menopause. Widespread media coverage has made hormone replacement therapy (HRT) a household name and, increasingly, doctors are offering HRT to women both for relief of acute menopausal symptoms and for prophylaxis of long-term sequelae of oestrogen deficiency. Indeed, many women are now demanding the opportunity to take HRT. However, HRT is not a panacea for all the ailments of middle-aged women and, in our present state of ignorance regarding the long-term risks, cannot be universally recommended for all women. Although there is criticism of the medical profession by some who believe that the menopause is being over-medicalized, most women benefit from an individual assessment of their menopausal problems and how the risks and benefits of HRT relate to them.

ENDOCRINE CHANGES AT THE MENOPAUSE

The menopause signals the end of a woman's reproductive years with the onset of irreversible ovarian failure. The exhaustion of the ovaries' store of oocytes leads to the cessation of follicular development and ovulation. This results in:

1. A gradual fall in circulating oestradiol.
2. A rise in circulating gonadotrophins, follicle stimulating hormone (FSH) and luteinizing hormone (LH), as a result of the removal of the negative feedback effects of oestrogen.
3. Amenorrhoea resulting from the absence of endometrial stimulation by ovarian steroid hormones.
4. Very low levels of circulating oestrogen once ovarian activity has ceased. The predominant oestrogen after the menopause is oestrone which originates from the peripheral conversion of adrenal androgens – the postmenopausal ovaries contribute very little to the total oestrogen concentration.

Changes in the perimenopause

The menstrual pattern shows great individual variation, and shortening of the cycle may be the earliest feature. Months of amenorrhoea are often interspersed with spells of regular menstruation although there is generally a lengthening of the cycles as the last period approaches. Long cycles often indicate lack of ovulation and the following menstrual bleed may be particularly heavy due to prolonged stimulation by unopposed oestrogen.

Endocrine changes   At this time endocrine changes include:

1. The ovary becoming progressively unresponsive to gonadotrophin stimulation with a rise in FSH concentration detectable in the follicular phase of cycles.
2. Declining levels of the glycoprotein inhibin produced by ovarian follicles, which in turn cause FSH concentrations to rise.

DIAGNOSIS OF THE MENOPAUSE

Measurement of FSH concentration can be used for diagnostic purposes (>30IU/l indicating menopausal levels). A detectable rise of FSH may be found in the first 7 days of cycles early in the perimenopause. In practice, the diagnosis of the menopause is made clinically and it is only occasionally necessary to resort to biochemical investigation.

FSH measurement may be helpful if:

1. A premature menopause is suspected i.e. in a woman under 45 years.
2. A woman has had a hysterectomy.
3. An older woman is taking the progestogen-only pill (POP) and is amenorrhoeic.

Measurement of oestrogen concentrations, despite being frequently recommended by women's magazines, is not a valid assessment of menopausal status as postmenopausal levels can be similar to those found in the early follicular phase of premenopausal women.

CONSEQUENCES OF OVARIAN FAILURE

Oestrogen deficiency is responsible for the symptoms experienced by women around the time of their last period. Acute, short-term symptoms, although unpleasant, are generally self-limiting and are not a cause of mortality. The two long-term consequences of ovarian failure, osteoporosis and cardiovascular disease, have extremely important implications for future health and represent a huge burden on health resources in the UK.

Short-term symptoms

These symptoms are common, distressing, and cause many previously healthy women to seek medical advice. They are often insidious in onset and frequently misdiagnosed. Quality of life may be severely compromised in some women with menopausal symptoms and should not be ignored in any discussion of the risks and benefits of HRT.

Vasomotor symptoms

1. Hot flushes.
2. Palpitations.
3. Dizziness.
4. Weakness and faintness.

Hot flushes are the commonest menopausal symptoms affecting around 80% of women. They tend to begin before the cessation of menstruation, persist on average for 2–5 years and are universally perceived as unpleasant and embarrassing.

The flush is felt as a sensation of heat affecting the upper chest, neck and face, lasting only a few seconds or persisting for several minutes.

Reddening of the face may occur and intense flushes will often be followed by sweating although some women sweat without an initial flush.

Night sweats with disruption of the normal sleep pattern are often particularly troublesome causing chronic sleep deprivation to both the woman and her partner. Subsequent lethargy and irritability are common.

Flushes can be triggered by stress, hot weather, alcohol and spicy food although most occur without an obvious precipitating factor.

The aetiology and exact physiological mechanism remain unclear. As a result of declining oestradiol concentrations, changes in the thermoregulatory mechanism within the hypothalamus trigger a mistaken perception that the body is warmer than it should be. In response, cutaneous vasodilatation and sweating in the form of a flush occur with a rise in skin temperature of around 5°C.

Psychological symptoms

Many women report psychological symptoms as a problem in the climacteric years but there is little evidence to support an association between the menopause and frank psychiatric disease. Minor psychological disturbances are common and often correlate with the phase of fluctuating hormone profiles prior to the actual menopause. They are listed in Table 16.1. For climacteric women with stressful jobs or in positions of responsibility, many of the symptoms are potentially very disabling. Chronic sleep disturbance from hot flushes and night sweats exacerbates many of these symptoms.

Social stresses can also affect the well being of a woman around the time of her menopause with commonly encountered events such as:

1. Death or illness of an elderly parent.
2. Marital separation or disharmony.
3. Poor job satisfaction.
4. Difficult teenage children. The 'empty nest syndrome' is frequently quoted in this context but grown-up children who remain in the family home are often more of a problem than those who have 'flown the nest'.

Personality, cultural factors and attitudes to the menopause undoubtedly affect the incidence of psychological symptoms in the climacteric. In a society obsessed with youth and sexual attractiveness, feelings of low self-esteem and poor body image as women approach the end of their reproductive life are hardly surprising.

Table 16.1 Psychological symptoms of the menopause

Anxiety
Depression
Feeling unable to cope
Irritability and mood swings
Poor memory
Poor concentration
Difficulty making decisions
Feeling of worthlessness
Emotional lability

Intermediate symptoms

Urogenital atrophy

The tissues of the lower urogenital tract are highly oestrogen-dependent and undergo atrophy as a result of oestrogen deficiency.

1. Dryness of the vagina causes dyspareunia which in turn may result in loss of libido.
2. The vaginal pH increases and the vagina becomes prone to infection with bacterial organisms, as there is loss of the normal colonization with lactobacilli.
3. Dysuria, frequency, urgency and urge incontinence all increase in incidence with advancing age and arise from atrophic change and loss of collagen support around the bladder neck.

Skin changes

1. There is a generalized loss of collagen from the dermal layer of skin postmenopausally.
2. Women frequently complain of thin, dry skin accompanied by hair loss and brittle nails.
3. The common symptoms of widespread joint and muscle aches may also be explained by collagen loss.

Long-term symptoms

Osteoporosis

Osteoporosis is a disorder of bone metabolism characterized by a loss of bone density. Net bone loss occurs because of an imbalance between the amount of bone removed and that formed as bone undergoes the process of remodelling. It is a silent condition until increased bone fragility results in fracture which may occur even in the absence of trauma. Bone density peaks in women in their mid-30s and, thereafter, bone mass declines slowly until women begin to lose bone rapidly at the time of the menopause. Whether or not a woman develops osteoporosis, is determined by her peak bone mass and her rate of bone loss. Osteoporosis is not due to calcium deficiency as the bone present is normally calcified. There is simply not enough bone present.

The risk factors for osteoporosis (Table 16.2) are only, at best, a crude guide to a woman's risk of sustaining osteoporotic fractures. The two major risk factors are being female and postmenopausal!

Table 16.2 Risk factors for osteoporosis

Family history
Premature menopause
Small, slim build
Steroid therapy
Inactive lifestyle
Cigarette smoking
Excess alcohol or caffeine intake

Women are naturally endowed with a much less dense skeleton than men.

Postmenopausal osteoporosis classically affects three main sites:

1. Neck of femur.
2. Distal radius – the Colles' fracture.
3. Vertebral spine – wedge fractures cause the typical 'dowager's hump'.

Fractures are the clinical consequence of osteoporosis and are responsible for much pain and suffering in elderly women. Prevention of postmenopausal osteoporosis represents a major public health challenge. The estimated risks of osteoporotic fractures faced by a 50-year-old woman in her lifetime are:

1. 16% risk of fractured hip.
2. 1–3% risk of dying of complications of hip fracture.
3. 15% risk of fractured wrist.
4. 32% risk of fractured vertebra.
5. An overall 50% risk of sustaining some fracture
(Cummings et al 1989).

Role of oestrogen The role of oestrogen in the prevention of osteoporosis:

1. Oestrogen deficiency at any age causes osteoporosis.
2. Oestrogen will prevent bone loss and, more importantly, reduce the incidence of fractures. Oestrogen therapy for 5 years postmenopausally has been shown to reduce risk of hip fracture by around 50% (Compston 1992).
3. To prevent osteoporotic fractures occurring in women beyond the age of 70, treatment with oestrogen would have to continue for around 10–15 years.
4. As soon as oestrogen therapy is stopped, preservation of bone ceases and bone density will decline at its pretreatment rate.

Alternative therapies   Alternative therapies in the prevention of osteoporosis:

1. Regular weight-bearing exercise, an adequate diet and stopping smoking.
2. Studies on the value of calcium supplements show conflicting results. Dietary deficiency of calcium is rare but there is some evidence that a poor calcium intake in childhood can affect the peak bone density attained. Calcium supplements may decrease the rate of bone loss in very elderly women.
3. Calcitonin, sodium fluoride and various other agents have been claimed to prevent postmenopausal bone loss but oestrogen treatment is more effective.
4. Bisphosphonates such as etidronate are being used in the treatment of established osteoporosis but, as yet, there are no data to support their use in the prevention of osteoporosis.

Bone density screening   Facilities are available in some parts of the UK to perform assessment of bone density by highly accurate machines e.g. dual X-ray absorptiometry. This provides a one-off bone density measurement but unfortunately does not give information on the rate of bone loss, unless serial measurements are undertaken. Bone density measurement is very popular with menopausal women but remains an expensive investigation with, as yet, unproven screening value.

Cardiovascular disease

Cardiovascular disease is the single most important cause of death in both men and women in the western world. Prior to the menopause, deaths in women from cardiovascular disease are uncommon, particularly when compared to men of similar age. Following the menopause, the mortality rate in women from cardiovascular disease catches up with that in men. Women who have sustained a premature menopause have an increased risk of cardiovascular disease.

There is convincing evidence that women using oestrogen postmenopausally have a substantially lower risk of morbidity or death from cardiovascular disease. This reduction in risk is estimated to be about 40% (Stampfer & Colditz 1991). Among women with proven coronary heart disease, oestrogen used postmenopausally in one study reduced the risk of death from myocardial infarction by about 80% (Sullivan et al 1990).

Table 16.3   Effect of oestrogen replacement on lipid and
lipoprotein profiles

Total cholesterol	Decreased
LDL-cholesterol	Decreased
HDL-cholesterol	Increased
Triglycerides	Decreased by transdermal oestrogens but increased by oral oestrogens

Oestrogen is thought to exert a protective effect by two mechanisms:

1. Beneficial effects on lipid pattern (Table 16.3). Oestrogen appears to induce favourable changes in lipid metabolism which probably account for about one-third of the reduction in cardiovascular mortality.
2. A direct effect on blood vessel wall physiology resulting in vasodilation. Oestrogen increases blood flow and, thereby, improves physiological function notably in the coronary and cerebral circulations. This is thought to be the major mechanism whereby oestrogen reduces cardiovascular risk.

Substantial benefits in reducing risk of cardiovascular disease would appear to result from the use of postmenopausal oestrogen. However, women who opt to take HRT are often a self-selected healthier group, generally at lower risk of cardiovascular disease. Moreover, most of the women involved in studies reporting a reduction in risk took oestrogen without additional progestogens. There is some current concern that progestogens may limit the protective effect of oestrogen particularly on lipids. Further epidemiological work is required to determine the true extent of the protective effect of oestrogen on cardiovascular disease.

TREATMENT

Treatment of menopausal symptoms with agents other than hormones is frequently recommended but gives largely disappointing results. Most studies on treatments for menopausal women demonstrate a marked placebo response.

Non-hormonal treatment

1. The antihypertensive agent Clonidine (50 μg b.d.) can be effective in the short-term management of vasomotor symptoms but longer-term studies have found the response to oestrogen significantly better.
2. The use of tranquillizers and antidepressants in women with climacteric problems is widespread but, in the absence of frank psychiatric disease, these drugs are probably best withheld until HRT has been tried.
3. Over-the-counter preparations such as vitamin B6 or oil of evening primrose are frequently tried by women but any beneficial effect may simply reflect a placebo response.
4. Some women find techniques such as relaxation or aromatherapy helpful and self-help groups or nurse-counselling sessions may assist women to cope better with their symptoms.

Oestrogen therapy

As the symptoms of the menopause are caused by oestrogen deficiency, the logical treatment is oestrogen replacement. Progestogen is added to preparations for women with an intact uterus to prevent the development of endometrial pathology (p. 396).

The oestrogens used in conventional HRT are described as 'natural' because they give rise to plasma oestrogens identical to those produced by the premenopausal ovary. Their pharmacological effect is achieved with plasma levels of oestradiol well within the physiological range. Natural oestrogens are far less potent than the synthetic oestrogens contained in combined oral contraceptive pills (COCs).

Oestrogen therapy is effective when administered by a variety of routes (Table 16.4) and generally causes few side-effects. Choice of

Table 16.4   Oestrogen administration

Oral
Transdermal patches
Subcutaneous implants
Vaginal delivery systems
Percutaneous (as creams and gels)
Sublingual or intranasal

how to take systemic HRT is largely a matter of patient preference, although for the majority of women, the cheaper, oral preparations will prove perfectly acceptable.

Oral oestrogens

Advantages

1. Cheap.
2. Convenient.
3. Well tolerated.
4. Easy to stop.

Disadvantages

1. 'First pass' through the liver – when oestrogen is taken orally, it has to pass through the portal circulation to the liver before reaching the systemic circulation and achieving the desired effect. During this 'first pass' through the liver, at least one-third is immediately metabolized to the weak oestrogen, oestrone, which is rapidly excreted. A higher dose of oral oestrogen has to be given compared to transdermal oestrogens to achieve the same therapeutic effect.
2. Occasional nausea and gastrointestinal upset.

The commonly used oral preparations are listed in Table 16.5.

Transdermal oestrogens

Transdermal delivery systems allow low-dose oestrogen therapy to be absorbed directly into the systemic circulation. Patches are designed to be changed twice weekly and should be placed on smooth, dry skin anywhere below the waist. Table 16.6 gives details of currently available transdermal patches.

Advantages

1. Highly acceptable to women.
2. Convenient, with application required only twice per week.
3. Avoid 'first pass' effect through the liver. Therefore, more 'physiological' and can be given in lower dosage. Less effect on hepatic synthesis of other products e.g. clotting factors and lipoproteins.
4. Combination patches with low-dose progestogen are also available, thus avoiding the need for any tablets to be taken orally.

Table 16.5 Oral HRT preparations

Proprietary name	Generic name	Dosages
Progynova	Oestradiol	1 mg, 2 mg
Climaval	Oestradiol	1 mg, 2 mg
Zumenon	Oestradiol (micronized)	2 mg
Premarin	Conjugated equine oestrogens	0.625 mg, 1.25 mg
Ovestin	Oestriol	1 mg
Harmogen	Oestrone	1.5 mg
Hormonin	Oestradiol/oestrone/oestriol	600 μg/1.4 mg/270 μg

Proprietary name	Type of oestrogen	Type of Progestogen
Prempak-C	Conjugated equine oestrogens 0.625 mg, 1.25 mg	Norgestrel 150 μg × 12 days
Nuvelle	Oestradiol 2 mg	Levonorgestrel 75 μg × 12 days
Climagest	Oestradiol 1 mg, 2 mg	Norethisterone 1 mg × 12 days
Trisequens	Oestradiol, oestrone (in varying doses)	Norethisterone 1 mg × 10 days
Cycloprogynova	Oestradiol 1 mg, 2 mg	Norethisterone 1 mg × 10 days
Menophase	Mestranol (in varying doses)	Norethisterone (in varying doses) × 13 days

Table 16.6 Transdermal patches

Proprietary name	Generic name	Release rate per 24 hours
Estraderm	Oestradiol	25 μg, 50 μg, 100 μg
Estracombi	Oestradiol + norethisterone	50 μg 250 μg (in 2nd half of cycle)
Evorel	Oestradiol	50 μg

Disadvantages

1. Expensive.
2. Allergic reactions affect around 10% of users and relate to the high alcohol content in the oestrogen-containing medium of the multi-layered patches. Newer patches are

single-layered units with oestrogen contained within the adhesive layer and are much less likely to cause skin sensitivity reactions.

Subcutaneous oestrogen implants

These consist of crystalline pellets of oestrogen which are inserted subcutaneously under local anaesthesia as a minor surgical procedure. The most common sites of insertion are the anterior abdominal wall or buttocks. The standard dose of implant is 50 mg which will be effective for around 6 months. Implants are now less widely used because of the increasing popularity of transdermal patches.

Advantages

1. Compliance is guaranteed.
2. Relatively higher serum oestradiol concentrations can be achieved with implants compared to other methods and this can be particularly beneficial in the treatment of women with very low bone densities, established osteoporosis or severe depression.
3. Oestrogen implants can be given simultaneously with testosterone implants when loss of libido is a particular problem.

Disadvantages

1. Insertion involves a minor surgical procedure.
2. Some women using implants experience the return of many of their menopausal symptoms while their circulating concentrations of oestradiol are very high (tachyphylaxis).

Vaginal oestrogen delivery systems

Local vaginal treatment with oestrogen is an effective way of improving atrophic change within the lower genital tract in women and consists of creams, pessaries, tablets and rings (Table 16.7).

Advantages

1. Can be used by women who do not wish to take systemic HRT or where contraindications exist to its use.
2. Vaginal preparations can be used in conjunction with systemic HRT if symptoms persist despite standard doses of HRT being used.

Table 16.7   Vaginal oestrogen preparations

Proprietary name	Generic name
Dienoestrol cream	Dienoestrol 0.01%
Ortho-gynest cream and pessaries	Oestriol 0.01%
Ovestin cream	Oestriol 0.01%
Vagifem tablets	Oestradiol 25 µg
Estring	Oestradiol 7.5 µg/24 hours

Disadvantages

1. Elderly women often find difficulty using creams and for some women they are unacceptably messy.
2. Most vaginal oestrogen preparations are only licensed for use over periods of 3–6 months because of the theoretical risk of endometrial cancer with prolonged use. If treatment is required for longer, the addition of cyclical oral progestogen is recommended for endometrial protection.

Other routes of oestrogen administration

Percutaneous creams and gels are widely used on the continent and will become available shortly in the UK. Oestrogen is also rapidly absorbed intranasally or sublingually although no commercially available products supply it by these routes.

Combined oestrogen–progestogen therapy

Use of unopposed oestrogen replacement in the United States led to a greatly increased incidence of endometrial cancer in the 1970s. The addition of progestogen regimens to oestrogen replacement will reduce this excess risk of endometrial cancer to below the risk for the general population (Gambrell 1986). The progestogen will bring about a regular withdrawal bleed and must be given:

1. In adequate dosage.
2. For an adequate number of days each cycle.

In the standard regimens, progestogens are added sequentially for around 10–12 days each month. The recommended daily

Table 16.8   Progestogens used in conventional HRT
and dosages required

Norethisterone acetate	1 mg
l-norgestrel	150 µg
Medroxyprogesterone acetate (Provera)	5–10 mg
Dydrogesterone (Duphaston)	10–20 mg

Each to be administered for 10–12 days each month.

dosages of different progestogens to oppose the effects of oestrogen are listed in Table 16.8. Calendar packs of combined oestrogen and progestogen regimens assist the woman in keeping to the correct sequence. Separate prescriptions of oestrogen and progestogen can also be given if a particular combination is not marketed. *There is no need to give women who have had a hysterectomy additional progestogen.*

HRT without bleeding

Continuous combined HRT

Continuous daily administration of both oestrogen and progestogen causes endometrial atrophy and thereby amenorrhoea. Women who are at least 1 year postmenopausal may find this regimen effective. Combined calendar packs are now available commercially. Separate prescription of oestrogen and progestogen can also be made. A regimen combining, for example, Premarin 0.625 mg and Duphaston 10 mg both daily is generally well tolerated, particularly by older women.

1. Spotting in the early months is very common before complete amenorrhoea is achieved.
2. As there is no cyclical effect with this regimen, women appear to tolerate the progestogen better with fewer side-effects.
3. Overall, the dose of progestogen given is greater than conventional therapy and this may adversely affect lipid levels.
4. There are no long-term safety data on this regimen.

Livial

The synthetic steroid tibolone (Livial) is a C-19 nortestosterone derivative which has weak oestrogenic, progestogenic and androgenic effects. Livial is a very popular product with patients because of the lack of regular withdrawal bleeding. It is a useful preparation when women experience heavy or painful withdrawal bleeds or marked cyclical symptoms with conventional HRT. Unfortunately, it is currently four times more expensive than the cheapest oral HRT.

1. It relieves acute menopausal symptoms.
2. It improves mood and libido.
3. It is not currently licensed for the prevention of osteoporosis but research does suggest it has a similar action to oestrogen in conservation of bone density.
4. The endometrium remains atrophic and, therefore, amenorrhoea occurs.
5. Its use should be restricted to women who are at least 1 year postmenopausal because irregular bleeding is common if given to perimenopausal women.
6. The long-term effects of Livial on the lipid profile have yet to be fully evaluated.

Contraindications to HRT

Absolute

The very few absolute contraindications to oestrogen therapy are listed in Table 16.9. Unfortunately, many contraindications to the combined oral contraceptive pill have been extrapolated to HRT use and are inappropriately listed on the data sheets of HRT preparations. Considerable effort is currently being made to alter data sheets to reflect recent knowledge on the contraindications to HRT.

Table 16.9   Absolute contraindications to HRT therapy

Unexplained vaginal bleeding
Pregnancy
Breast cancer (see p. 399)
Severe, active liver disease
Active thrombo-embolic disease

Relative

Among those commonly encountered are:

1. Hypertension – HRT can be used with caution and careful monitoring. An appropriate antihypertensive agent can be introduced, if necessary.
2. Previous episode of deep vein thrombosis or pulmonary embolism – this will require full evaluation and often referral to a haematology department for a pretreatment profile to exclude an underlying abnormality of fibrinolysis or coagulation.
3. Gallbladder disease – oestrogen can alter the composition of bile in a way that may predispose to gallstone formation. The non-oral routes of oestrogen delivery are probably preferable.
4. Fibroids – these may enlarge with HRT and cause bleeding problems. Hysterectomy or withdrawal of treatment may have to be considered.
5. Endometriosis – this may be reactivated by oestrogen postmenopausally but depends on the amount of residual disease present. Use of additional progestogen will reduce the risk of recurrence.
6. Previous myocardial infarction (MI) or cerebrovascular accident (CVA) – HRT can be given with careful monitoring after MI or CVA once 6 months have elapsed.
7. Cancer – HRT has no effect on the majority of cancers. Endometrial cancer was previously considered an absolute contraindication. Recent thinking is that women who have early stage disease and appear disease-free after treatment may take low dose HRT. Neither previous cervical nor ovarian cancer represents a contraindication to HRT. Breast cancer is still considered a complete contraindication by most specialists. Each woman should, however, be assessed individually and, for some, improving their quality of life with HRT may outweigh the small theoretical risk of reactivation of breast or endometrial cancer.
8. Otosclerosis – this progressive hearing disorder is frequently quoted as a contraindication to HRT use as it appears to worsen during pregnancy. If HRT is given, careful monitoring of hearing is recommended but in most cases there is no obvious deterioration of function.

Complications of HRT

Oestrogen causes few side-effects. Unfortunately, the addition of progestogen causes many troublesome side-effects. These are common and lead to many women discontinuing HRT after only a few months of therapy.

Side-effects of oestrogen

1. Nausea.
2. Breast tenderness.
3. Leg cramps.
4. Migraine.

Management

1. Reduce dose of oestrogen.
2. Change route of administration.
3. Try alternative oestrogen.

Side-effects of progestogen

1. Regular monthly withdrawal bleeds which may be heavy, prolonged or painful.
2. Premenstrual syndrome-type symptoms of irritability, depression, fluid retention and bloating.
3. Reversal of some beneficial effects of oestrogen on lipid levels, although this varies between the different progestogens.

Management

1. Reduce dose of progestogen to minimum recommended for endometrial protection.
2. Change progestogen to C-21 progestogen derivatives (dydrogesterone or medroxyprogesterone acetate) which are generally tolerated better but are not yet available in calendar packs.
3. Stopping the progestogen completely is not recommended, but some women opt to do this and then regular endometrial biopsies are mandatory. The increased risk of endometrial cancer continues for many years after the treatment has been stopped.
4. Use of the continuous-combined regimen or Livial (pp. 397, 398).
5. Endometrial resection or ablation.
6. Hysterectomy.

SPECIAL CONSIDERATIONS

Breast cancer

Currently 1 in 12 women in the UK will develop breast cancer. It is a disease universally dreaded by women, although it is still a much less common cause of death than cardiovascular disease. There is still no consensus on the increased risk involved in taking oestrogen postmenopausally.

Current epidemiological data suggest:

1. Up to 5 years of oestrogen use has never been shown to increase the risk of breast cancer.
2. Hormone replacement therapy for 10 years appears to increase the relative risk of breast cancer to a maximum of 1.3 (Jacobs & Loeffler 1992).
3. Women who develop breast cancer while taking HRT appear to have better survival rates, probably due to increased surveillance and earlier tumour detection.
4. The risk may be increased in the presence of a strong family history of breast cancer or a past history of benign breast disease.
5. There is no current consensus as to whether addition of progestogen confers any advantage or adds any additional risk in terms of development of breast cancer.

Compliance

Despite publicity of the well-established benefits of HRT, compliance remains relatively poor. Fear of cancer tends to discourage women from starting treatment and the withdrawal bleeds and cyclical progestogenic side-effects often cause women to stop treatment after only a brief trial. Women who are given adequate opportunity to discuss their fears and the risks and benefits of HRT often have a much higher compliance rate (McCleery & Gebbie 1994). Tolerance of preparations which induce amenorrhoea is often better than of those which cause withdrawal bleeding.

CLINICAL MANAGEMENT

Assessment of a woman prior to HRT

This can often be a lengthy consultation combining much information-giving with counselling. Use of standard menopause record cards can be helpful and a trained menopause-counselling nurse can do much of the basic information-giving.

History

1. Current symptoms attributable to the menopause; use of a symptom-rating questionnaire is often helpful.
2. Details of past gynaecological and obstetric history.
3. Past medical history; noting any contraindication to HRT use.
4. Family history; particularly breast cancer, ischaemic heart disease and stroke at a young age, osteoporosis.
5. Social history; employment, smoking, current relationship and any sexual problems.

Examination

1. BP.
2. Weight and height.
3. Breast examination.
4. Routine smear and pelvic examination; note degree of oestrogenization.

While breast and pelvic examinations are not absolutely essential, they are useful in screening for coincidental pathology (e.g. breast and ovarian malignancy) and also have medico-legal implications.

Investigations

In practice, investigations are often not necessary but may be indicated by the history or examination findings (Table 16.10). Mammography is not undertaken routinely prior to commencing HRT unless a woman has a first-degree relative with premenopausal breast cancer or a past history of benign breast disease, particularly the presence of atypia.

Table 16.10 Investigations occasionally indicated prior to HRT

Full blood count
Thyroid function tests
Hormone profile
Fibrinolysis/coagulation profile
Pelvic ultrasound scan
Endometrial biopsy and hysteroscopy
Bone density scan
Mammography
Lipid screen

In some younger women, particularly those who are still menstruating, it may not be clear whether symptoms are attributable to the menopause or not. A therapeutic trial of HRT for 3 months is often worthwhile and if there is no clear benefit in that time, an alternative diagnosis should be sought.

Monitoring

There is no scientific basis as to how often women should be followed-up or what exactly should be monitored. By convention, however, the first follow-up visit is usually after 3 months and, thereafter, visits can be 6-monthly or more frequently if problems arise.

History

1. Assess degree of symptom relief; oestrogen dose can be increased if necessary.
2. Note bleeding pattern.
3. Assess any side-effects.

Examination

1. BP and weight.
2. Annual breast examination.
3. Routine 3-yearly cervical smear.
4. Routine 3-yearly mammogram if within the age limits for screening.

Excess weight gain is frequently attributed to HRT use. Weight gain is a feature of increasing age and most studies show HRT users put on less weight overall than non-HRT users. Advice and support on dieting and exercise are frequently offered but rarely heeded.

Duration of use

There is no hard and fast rule as to how long HRT can be continued. For relief of acute menopausal symptoms, most women will require therapy for 3–5 years. To prevent osteoporosis in very elderly women, treatment would have to be continued for 10–15 years. The decision is an individual one and many women discontinue HRT without recourse to medical advice while others are extremely reluctant ever to stop.

CONTRACEPTION IN THE PERIMENOPAUSE

Over the years remarkably little attention has been paid by scientists and clinicians to fertility control in older women. It is obviously important that women are given the correct advice. If their fertility is underestimated they may have to cope with a late and unexpected addition to their family. Although most people believe that ovulation is less frequent in older women, it nevertheless continues to occur up to the menopause. The incidence of ovulation appears to be more closely related to the pattern of the menstrual cycle than to age alone. The quality of oocytes is almost certainly poorer in older women.

Frequency of intercourse declines with age in stable relationships. However, as divorce rates are ever increasing, coital frequency will inevitably increase as new relationships form.

Pregnancy in older women

Pregnancy above the age of 45 years increases the risks to both mother and fetus and may well be psychologically and socially catastrophic.

1. Maternal mortality rates sharply increase.
2. Perinatal mortality rates double compared with young mothers.
3. Chromosomal abnormalities increase in incidence, particularly Down's syndrome and, while screening and termination of pregnancy are an option, this presents moral and ethical dilemmas many older women could well do without.
4. Unwanted or unplanned pregnancies in this age group are often accompanied by a sense of shame or frustration and around 50% of these pregnancies will end in therapeutic abortion.

Contraceptive methods

As a rule of thumb, women are advised to continue contraception for one year after their last period if aged 50 years or above, and for two further years following their last period if below the age of 50 years. As fertility declines with age, most methods become almost 100% effective if used carefully and methods which would not be recommended for use in isolation by younger women become extremely acceptable and effective during the perimenopausal years.

Conventional HRT is not reliably contraceptive and if it is given to a woman who is still menstruating, a method of contraception should be recommended as well. Once HRT has been started, it becomes impossible to give an accurate indication of when contraception can safely be discontinued. If the woman is unwilling to discontinue HRT for a short period to assess her natural menstrual cycle and have her gonadotrophin levels measured, contraception can arbitrarily be continued until the age of 55. (The oldest recorded mother to give birth in the UK following a natural conception was 54 years old).

Combined oral contraception (COC)

The myth that all women should discontinue the COC at the age of 35 years must be exploded. *Selected, healthy, non-smoking women without risk factors can be prescribed low-dose combined preparations up to the age of 50 years provided they are carefully monitored.* The US Food and Drug Administration in 1989 confirmed that there is no upper age limit to COC use in healthy women.

Substantial benefits exist in taking COC in the later reproductive years and include:

1. Excellent cycle control.
2. A reduced incidence of most menstrual and gynaecological disorders with a greatly decreased admission rate to hospital for minor and major gynaecological operations.
3. Possible added protection against osteoporotic fractures in later life.
4. Relief of any early menopausal symptoms.
5. Protection against both endometrial and ovarian carcinoma.

However, these advantages have to be balanced against the possible disadvantages:

1. The prothrombotic tendency of synthetic oestrogens with a very small risk of serious arterial thrombosis.
2. An unknown effect on the risk of developing breast cancer.

Women with risk factors, particularly those who smoke cigarettes, should still discontinue COCs at the age of 35 years because of increased risk of serious arterial disease.

Progestogen-only contraception

The progestogen-only pill (POP)   This is an excellent and safe form of contraception for older women with almost no contraindications. It is virtually 100% effective in this age group with failure rates equivalent to that of COC use in women in their 20s.

Its biggest problem remains variable cycle control. Many older women become amenorrhoeic which causes them anxiety regarding possible pregnancy, despite the fact that it is an indication of high efficacy. Others experience excessive or irregular menstrual loss which can lead to gynaecological intervention.

Women who are amenorrhoeic on the POP may become confused as to their menopausal status. Measurement of FSH concentration remains a valid way of assessing this, as the POP does not exert a suppressive effect on gonadotrophins.

The POP can be given in conjunction with conventional HRT and appears to give effective contraception although no data exist on its use in this regimen.

Depo-Provera This shares some of the problems of POP use with amenorrhoea a common feature. Some women who are amenorrhoeic with Depo-Provera become hypo-oestrogenic and this has led to recent concerns regarding development of low bone mineral densities. At the present time, there is not sufficient evidence to allow this to affect clinical practice and any bone loss incurred would appear to be reversible. It may be wise to consider stopping Depo-Provera at 45 years if treatment has been prolonged, in order to allow time for reversal of bone loss before the menopause ensues.

Intrauterine devices

Pregnancy, expulsion, infection, perforation and ectopic pregnancy rates are all reduced in older IUD users. The criteria for insertion remain as for younger women, although careful account should be taken of the menstrual pattern prior to insertion in older women who may already have menorrhagia or dysfunctional bleeding. In this age group, copper devices remain effective far longer than the manufacturers' arbitrary 3 or 5 years, and any device inserted after a woman's 40th birthday can remain in situ, unchanged, until a year following the last menstrual period. IUDs should always be removed from postmenopausal women.

The levonorgestrel-releasing IUD will have important applications for older women with excessive menstrual loss and can be used in conjunction with systemic oestrogen as HRT, avoiding the need for systemic progestogen to be given.

Barrier methods

Generally speaking, barrier methods are not sufficiently 'user friendly' to be acceptable to older couples using them for the first time.

Condoms   These remain the most popular methods of contraception throughout the world, despite the fact that many doctors are loathe to recommend them because of a supposed high failure rate. They are widely used by older couples and are free from side-effects, although they may exacerbate erectile problems in older men.

Diaphragms   These are used more often by older than by younger women and for some the additional lubrication provided by the spermicide is advantageous in the presence of vaginal dryness.

The Today sponge / Delfen foam   These are successfully used by women at times of extremely low fertility such as the year following the last menstrual period or while taking hormone replacement therapy.

Natural family planning

As this relies on the ability to recognize signs of fertility, it is often difficult to use when cycles are irregular or anovulatory but can be appropriate if there are religious or ethical objections to other methods.

PROVISION OF SERVICES

Women naturally turn to their familiar providers of health services when they have menopausal problems. GPs, health visitors and practice nurses will provide most information and support for most women. Those who have been long-standing attenders at family planning and well woman clinics often turn there for advice regarding menopausal symptoms and fertility during their later years.

Most health authorities run a specialist menopause service where a local gynaecologist, or occasionally a psychiatrist, has a particular interest in problems associated with the menopause, thus providing a referral centre for patients with contraindications to HRT, or complex problems, or particular side-effects with its use. Most specialist clinics will have access to bone density screening and facilities such as vaginal ultrasound and hysteroscopy.

The development of trained menopause-counselling nurses has been very beneficial, providing a supportive role for women particularly those with contraindications to HRT.

Many women find self-help menopause support groups of benefit.

REFERENCES

Compston J E 1992 HRT and Osteoporosis. British Medical Bulletin 48: 309–44
Cummings S R, Black D, Rubin S M 1989 Lifetime risk of hip, Colles' or vertebral fracture and coronary heart disease among white postmenopausal women. Arch Intern Med 149: 2445–8.
Gambrell D R 1986 Prevention of endometrial cancer with progestogen. Maturitas 8: 159
Jacobs H S, Loeffler F E 1992 Postmenopausal hormone replacement therapy. British Medical Journal 305: 1403–1408
McCleery J M, Gebbie A E 1994 Compliance with hormone replacement therapy at a menopause clinic in a community setting. British Journal of Family Planning 20: 73–75
Stampfer M J, Colditz G A 1991 Estrogen replacement therapy and coronary heart disease: a quantitative assessment of the epidemiological evidence. Prev Med 20: 47–63.
Sullivan J, Van der Zwaag R, Hughes J et al 1990 Estrogen replacement and coronary artery disease: effect on survival in postmenopausal women. Arch Intern Med 150: 2557–62.

17. Contraceptives of the future

Paul Van Look

The need for new contraceptives

Improving existing methods
Male sterilization
  Valves and plugs
Female sterilization
  Cautery of the utero–tubal junction and the interstitial portion of the tube
  Occlusive plugs
  Chemical occlusion
Combined oral contraceptives
Progestogen-only pills
Implants
  Non-biodegradable implants
  Biodegradable implants
Injectable contraceptives
  Combined oestrogen–progestogen preparations
  Progestogen-only preparations
Intrauterine devices
Male condoms
  Male plastic condoms
Vaginal barrier methods
  Diaphragms
  Cervical caps
  Female condoms

  Vaginal sponges
  Chemical agents
Natural family planning
  Electronic devices
  Simple assay methods

The search for new methods
Contraception for men
  Hormonal methods
  Non-hormonal agents acting on sperm
GnRH analogues
  In female contraception
  In male contraception
Steroid hormone receptor antagonists
  Anti-androgens
  Anti-oestrogens
  Antiprogestogens
New delivery systems for steroid hormones
  Vaginal rings
  Transdermal systems
Antifertility vaccines
  Anti-hCG vaccines
  Antisperm vaccines
  Anti-ovum vaccines
  Other antifertility vaccines

THE NEED FOR NEW CONTRACEPTIVES

Over the last 3 decades there has been an impressive rise in the use of contraceptives all over the world. It has been estimated that, in 1990, up to 57% of all married women of reproductive age or their partners were using a method of contraception (Table 17.1). At that time, the prevalence of use of modern methods in both developed and developing regions was about the same, 49% and 48%, respectively. However, significant differences exist between the more developed and the less developed parts of the world in the types of fertility-regulating methods used. In the less developed regions, some 47% of women using contraception rely on female or male sterilization and another 25% use an intrauterine device (IUD) (Table 17.2). In contrast, in the more developed regions, use is

409

Table 17.1 Percentage of couples with wife in reproductive age using a contraceptive method

	World			More developed regions			Less developed regions		
	1983	1987	1990	1983	1987	1990	1983	1987	1990
All methods	51	53	57	70	71	72	45	48	53
Modern methods	42	44	49	46	47	49	40	44	48

Source: Khanna et al 1994.
Modern methods in this table include: female and male sterilization, oral pills, injectable methods, intrauterine devices, vaginal barrier methods (cervical cap, diaphragm), and the condom.

Table 17.2 Percentage distribution of current contraceptive users by type of method and year

	World		More developed regions		Less developed regions	
	1987	1990	1987	1990	1987	1990
Female sterilization	29	29	11	11	37	38
Male sterilization	8	9	6	6	9	9
Pill	14	14	20	22	11	11
Injectable	2	2	-	-	2	2
Intrauterine device	20	21	8	8	25	25
Condom	9	9	18	19	5	4
Vaginal barrier	1	2	3	3	1	1
Rhythm	7	5	13	11	4	4
Withdrawal	8	7	19	18	4	4
Others	2	2	2	3	2	2

Source: Khanna et al 1994.

more evenly spread amongst the different methods and a substantial proportion of users rely on the more traditional methods of withdrawal and periodic abstinence (rhythm or NFP methods).

The inadequacies of current methods of family planning underlie the high discontinuation rates seen with several contraceptive methods and they are probably responsible for the marked increase in the number of people, particularly women, undergoing sterilization at earlier and earlier ages.

It has been estimated that there are some 120 million women in developing countries who are not practising family planning despite wishing to avoid pregnancy. This applies particularly in Africa where the needs of less than one-third of all potential users are being met. But the most telling statistic by far of our inability to provide safe, effective, accessible, acceptable, and affordable methods of family planning is the fact that, worldwide, between 50 and 60 million unwanted pregnancies are terminated each year. Some 20 million of these abortions are induced under unsafe conditions and at least 70 000 women each year die as a result (World Health Organization 1994). The yearly number of unplanned pregnancies due to contraceptive failure has been estimated at between 8 and 30 million (Table 17.3).

Until the 1970s, contraceptive research was for the most part carried out in the private sector by large pharmaceutical companies, but at the present time only five major contraceptive manufacturers

Table 17.3 Typical first-year failure rates of various contraceptive methods

Method	Typical first-year failure rate (%)
Male sterilization	0.2
Female sterilization	0.4
Combined oral contraceptive	1-8
Progestogen-only pill	3-10
Norplant	0.4
Combined oestrogen/progestogen injectable	0.2
Progestogen-only injectable	0.4
Intrauterine device	3
Condom	12
Vaginal spermicide	21
Diaphragm, cervical cap, vaginal sponge	18-28
Natural family planning	20
Withdrawal	18

Source: World Health Organization.

(Leiras Pharmaceuticals, Organon International, Ortho Pharmaceuticals, Schering AG and Wyeth–Ayerst) remain involved. The reasons for this reduced involvement are cited as:

1. Product liability, coupled with the high cost of insurance to cover contraceptive development and introduction, particularly in the USA.
2. Stringent regulatory requirements for product approval, resulting in a long and expensive registration process and a concomitant decrease in patent protection.
3. A dearth of ideas for fundamentally new products.
4. A hostile political climate, particularly in the USA.
5. Competition from the public sector through the provision of free or low-priced contraceptives in developing countries.

More recently it has been suggested that there are two main reasons for the reduced involvement of industry in contraceptive research.

1. Pharmaceutical companies make most of their profit in developed countries where contraceptive use is already very high.
2. It is extremely expensive to develop new products – US$25–50 million over 3–7 years to adapt existing drugs to new delivery systems, and US$230 million to bring a new drug on to the market.

Fortunately a number of non-profit making, public sector agencies such as the World Health Organization, Population Council, and Family Health International, to name but three, have increased their efforts to improve existing methods and develop new ones.

The main research leads currently being pursued and which may ultimately result in new contraceptive products are, first, work aimed at improving existing methods and, secondly, development of new methods.

IMPROVING EXISTING METHODS

In recent years the improvement in several of the present methods of family planning (Table 17.3) includes the introduction of third-generation progestogens, new once-a-month injectables and the development of new progestogen-only injectables and implants. Further advances can be expected for some of these methods in the near future.

The worldwide increase in the incidence of STDs, particularly HIV infection, has stimulated renewed interest in barrier methods for both men and women and has increased investment in the search for vaginal agents with microbicidal and spermicidal activities.

Attempts are being made to develop simpler procedures for male and female sterilization in recognition of the fact that sterilization is the method of contraception used by the largest number of people in the world and that this is likely to remain so for the foreseeable future.

Male sterilization

Vasectomy is easier to perform and associated with fewer complications than female sterilization yet, worldwide, the number of men who have undergone vasectomy was estimated in 1990 to be about 30 million whereas there are estimated to be more than 140 million sterilized women. Behavioural research suggests that the necessity for a skin incision, and lack of certain reversibility limits its acceptability (Waites 1993). Two major technical improvements, *no-scalpel method of vasectomy* and the *percutaneous, non-surgical vas occlusion technique* have been developed to overcome these limitations (Ch. 8).

Valves and plugs

Various devices that are surgically inserted into the vas deferens to block sperm transport have also been tested but it has proved difficult to anchor them, and there have been problems with vas erosion and inflammatory reactions.

Female sterilization

Despite the large demand for female sterilization there have been surprisingly few technological developments during the last few decades in methods either of approach to the fallopian tube or of tubal occlusion. Attempts to overcome the disadvantages of transabdominal approaches to the tubes initially focused, during the 1970s, on procedures carried out through the anterior or posterior vaginal fornix, but these procedures have gradually been abandoned. Subsequent research has been directed at occluding the cornual portion of the tubes via the uterine cavity, but so far these attempts at transcervical sterilization have for the most part been unsuccessful. Procedures which have been investigated include those outlined below.

*Cautery of the utero–tubal junction and the interstitial portion
of the tube*

Failure rates are high and several interstitial or cornual ectopic pregnancies as well as thermal injury to bowel are reported.

More recent attempts to use laser coagulation of the tubal ostia have also proved to be unsuccessful.

Occlusive plugs

Materials that may either be pre-formed or formed-in-place are used.

The hydrogel plug or P-block   This is a pre-formed plug which is inserted through the hysteroscope into the lumen of the tube where it hydrates and swells to occlude the tube.

The Ovabloc   A formed-in-place occlusive plug made of silicone.

As in the male, it was hoped that these plugs would provide an effective and readily reversible method of tubal occlusion. However, rates of tubal occlusion and reversal are poor and insertion can be difficult.

Chemical occlusion

This is the method that holds the greatest promise but the ideal chemical i.e. one without toxic properties that will rapidly sclerose and occlude the tubal lumen and can be delivered in a reliable and simple manner to a defined segment of the tube, has yet to be realized.

The most often used tubal sclerosant has been quinacrine hydrochloride (Ch. 8). Recently, the long-term safety of quinacrine has been questioned.

Combined oral contraceptives

Much of the research aimed at producing new types of oral contraceptive pills (COC) has resulted in lower-dose, multiphasic and combiphasic preparations, and the development of new progestogens such as desogestrel, gestodene and norgestimate. Little work appears to have been done to date to find new oestrogens to replace ethinyloestradiol in COCs.

In an attempt to reduce the incidence of side-effects associated with oral pill use, a trial of vaginal insertion of the standard combined pills (50 µg ethinyloestradiol plus 250 µg levonorgestrel) showed that:

1. The incidence of side-effects was no different from that in the oral users.
2. Vaginal discharge was more common.
3. The 12-month gross discontinuation rate because of involuntary pregnancy was 3.25% compared to 1.03% in the oral group but this difference was not statistically significant (Coutinho et al 1993).
4. The adverse metabolic effects on lipids and lipoproteins appeared to be reduced, but this requires confirmation.

For women who are comfortable with the vaginal route of administration, vaginal rings that release both an oestrogen and a progestogen may provide a better alternative.

Progestogen-only pills

No major research is in progress in this area although it can be anticipated that progestogen-only pills (POPs) containing the newer progestogens will be introduced in the next few years. To achieve more consistent ovulation inhibition with POPs, concomitant administration of sulpiride or melatonin (Voordouw et al 1992) has been proposed but not yet evaluated.

Implants

The basic concept behind implants is that by maintaining a continuous sustained release of steroid hormone the contraceptive effect can be achieved with a much smaller daily dose than when the same steroid is given by the oral or intramuscular route. In addition, metabolic side-effects are reduced by avoiding the first pass through the liver.

To date, all implants release a progestogen and their main side-effects are menstrual disturbances and amenorrhoea, similar to other progestogen-only methods.

Norplant This levonorgestrel-releasing six-capsule system, was the first implant to reach the market (Ch. 4).

Research on second-generation implants is focusing on reducing the number of capsules, using steroids with better pharmacological profiles and biodegradable implants that do not require to be removed.

Contraceptive implants for men are also being investigated (p. 427).

Non-biodegradable implants

Norplant II A modification in design enables a two-implant system to release the same amount of levonorgestrel that is released from six Norplant capsules. Its performance proved similar to Norplant during the first 3 years of use. During year 4, plasma levels of levonorgestrel decreased and the pregnancy rate increased. In 1987 the implant was reformulated and results to date suggest that it may be effective for 5 years.

Norplant II may become available for routine use in about 3–4 years.

Sino-implant This is also a two-rod system. Each rod contains 75 mg of levonorgestrel. No data on the performance of this implant have yet been published outside China.

Implanon A single implant releasing 3-keto-desogestrel. In contrast to the other progestogen implants, Implanon has been designed to achieve plasma levels of 3-keto-desogestrel well above the threshold needed for ovulation inhibition. Ongoing studies indicate that plasma levels of the progestogen remain high enough to suppress ovulation for 3 years. No pregnancies have been reported in large clinical trials.

Implanon is likely to be available for routine use within the next 3–5 years.

Uniplant A single-capsule implant containing the progestogen nomegestrol acetate with an effective lifespan of 1 year.

Nestorone A single implant system that releases the progestogen ST 1435 (16-methylene-17-acetoxy-19 norprogesterone) designed to be effective for 2 years. This implant could be important for use in lactating women because, although small amounts of ST 1435 are secreted into breast milk and thus reach the breastfed infant, Nesterone is inactive by the oral route and would therefore have no biological effect.

The Nestorone implant is unlikely to become available for routine use within the next 5 years.

Biodegradable implants

Biodegradable implants have the potential advantage of not requiring removal, but the potential disadvantage of being difficult or impossible to remove some time after implantation. This would be important if side-effects necessitated removal, if the woman wished to regain her fertility before the end of the implant's lifespan, or if the tailing-down release of the remaining steroid after the end of the implant's lifespan was slow and prolonged, which could delay the return of fertility or increase the risk of an ectopic pregnancy.

Capronor   A single-capsule implant containing levonorgestrel. The capsules maintain their structural integrity even at 12 months and can be easily removed. No data are available as to the time required for the capsule to degrade completely.

Capronor 2 and Capronor 3   These are being developed with the aim of achieving a longer duration of effective release.

Norethisterone   Another form of biodegradable contraceptive implant that is under study consists of small pellets made of 90% norethisterone and 10% pure cholesterol and are expected to provide contraceptive protection for 12–18 months.

Injectable contraceptives

Injectable contraceptives have the advantage over subdermal implants in that they are easier to administer and do not require special training of providers. However, if the woman experiences side-effects she cannot discontinue use until the drug is depleted.

To overcome the problem of poor cycle control, research has been carried out to develop combined oestrogen–progestogen formulations (which are injected once a month) and other progestogens with better pharmacokinetic profiles.

Combined oestrogen–progestogen preparations

These are currently being used by approximately 2 million women (see Table 17.4).

The Chinese Injectable No. 1   This is used almost exclusively in China and neighbouring countries. The first injection is given on day 1–5 of the cycle with an additional injection 8–10 days later. Subsequent injections are given on day 10–12 after the onset of withdrawal bleeding, or 28 days after the previous injection if no bleeding occurs. In a recent WHO study the 12-month life-table contraceptive failure rate of this regimen was found to be 0.8%, whereas the failure rate was 6% when the preparation was used on a strict once-a-month schedule.

The second preparation is still used in Latin America even though the progestogen it contains was shown to cause breast abnormalities in beagle bitches.

Cyclofem (Cycloprovera) and Mesigyna   These have recently been approved as safe and effective products. The 1-year

Table 17.4   Once-a-month combined injectable preparations

Name	Progestogen	Dose	Oestrogen	Dose
Chinese Injectable No. 1	17α-Hydroxyprogesterone caproate	250 mg	Oestradiol valerate	5 mg
Topasel/Patector/ Perlutal (and various others)	Dihydroxyprogesterone acetophenide	150 mg	Oestradiol enanthate	10 mg
Cyclofem	Medroxyprogesterone acetate	25 mg	Oestradiol cypionate	5 mg
Mesigyna	Norethisterone enanthate	50 mg	Oestradiol valerate	5 mg

life-table pregnancy rates with these two preparations are less than 0.5% and discontinuation rates because of menstrual irregularity or amenorrhoea are generally less than half those seen with progestogen-only injectables such as DMPA or NET-EN.

Natural steroids   Research on aqueous suspensions of steroids has shown that, by controlling the range of crystal size, the release of the steroid from the injection site can be influenced. This approach using natural steroids could represent a new alternative in once-a-month injectable contraception and exploratory studies with a combination of 200 mg of progesterone plus 5 mg of 17β-oestradiol delivered as injectable microspheres are presently in progress.

Progestogen-only preparations

With the objective of developing compounds that would provide contraception at low doses for long periods, some 230 derivatives of levonorgestrel and norethisterone have been synthesized. One of these, levonorgestrel butanoate, is currently being developed further as a microcrystalline suspension with a duration of action of 3–4 months and possibly longer.

A microsphere preparation of norethisterone, expected to provide efficacy for 90 days with less than half the dose of the standard injectable formulation, and one of natural progesterone for breast-feeding mothers are at an early stage of clinical development.

Intrauterine devices

The most important reasons for discontinuing IUD use are pain, bleeding and expulsion. These side-effects are thought to be related to the relative size of the frame or shape of the device. A 'frameless' IUD should, in theory, minimize the problems and results from clinical trials are encouraging.

FlexiGard   This consists of six copper sleeves with a surface area of 330 mm² crimped onto nylon suture material (Ch. 5). A modified version for insertion immediately following delivery of the placenta appears to have a much reduced expulsion rate compared to conventional IUDs inserted postpartum.

Male condoms

Male latex condoms currently offer the best protection against STDs and HIV infection of any contraceptive. Unfortunately, they have a rather high contraceptive failure rate, probably due more to user failure than to failure from condom rupture. However, latex does deteriorate if exposed to excessive heat, light or humidity, and it is rapidly destroyed by oil-based lubricants such as Vaseline. Furthermore, men in many areas of the world, including regions such as sub-Saharan Africa where the prevalence of STDs and HIV is highest, dislike condoms mainly because of loss of penile sensitivity and interference with the spontaneity of intercourse.

Male plastic condoms

A range of plastic condoms currently under development could overcome many of these problems. The main advantages of plastic condoms are that they are loose-fitting apart from the region of attachment at the base of the penis, are stronger than latex condoms, do not deteriorate on storage, can be used with any type of lubricant and, being re-usable, are potentially also more 'environmentally-friendly' than the single-use latex condoms. They should come on the market within the next few years.

Vaginal barrier methods

The worldwide increase in STDs, including HIV/AIDS, and the growing awareness of the need to expand the contraceptive method mix, has led to a re-examination of the role of barrier methods for women. Greater resources are being devoted to finding new methods as well as to improving existing vaginal barrier methods.

Diaphragms

Research is being directed towards improving acceptability and effectiveness.

Diaphragm used continuously without spermicide The need to apply spermicide to the diaphragm and to insert it before intercourse and remove it later are all deterrents to its use (Ch. 6). In a recently reported retrospective study in Brazil, women who used the diaphragm with spermicide in the usual way had a significantly higher failure rate (9.8 pregnancies per 100 women at 12 months) than women who used it continuously without spermicide (2.8 per 100 women). Women in the latter group removed the diaphragm once a day for cleaning and during menses. Furthermore, there were significantly more discontinuations because of vaginal discharge and other medical reasons in the women using spermicide. Prospective randomized trials are required to confirm these findings.

Lea's shield   Made of flexible silicone rubber, this combines features of the diaphragm and of the cervical cap. It is concave like a diaphragm but thicker and slightly elongated, rather than round, to fit 'snugly' between the pubic bone and posterior fornix, which should reduce dislodgement during coitus. A flat, flexible tube, the 'flutter' valve, allows air to escape during placement so that a firm seal is obtained. The valve also allows the passage of cervical mucus and other upper genital tract secretions, thus reducing the risk of bacterial growth during long-term placement.

Long-acting, spermicide-releasing diaphragm   This device which is pH-sensitive releases only small amounts of spermicide at the normal vaginal pH, thus reducing the potential risk of vaginal irritation from continuous exposure to spermicide. When semen is deposited in the vagina at intercourse the pH rises above 6 and as a consequence up to 10 times as much spermicide is released. Clinical efficacy of this device has not yet been tested.

Cervical caps

A number of modifications have been made in the design of the cervical cap and in the materials used, to try to reduce the failure rate (Ch. 6).

Contracap   A 'personalized' device made from a mould of the woman's cervix, this had an unacceptably high failure rate and trials were stopped.

FemCap   This is made of silicone and shaped like a USA sailor's cap. It is claimed to fit the cervix better and to adapt more easily to changes in cervical shape and size during the menstrual cycle. Clinical experience is still limited.

'Diaphragm-tampon' device   This consists of two latex chambers surrounding each other. The inner chamber has a one-way valve which permits the passage of menstrual blood, cervical mucus and other secretions into the outer chamber which functions as a reservoir. It remains on the cervix by suction and is re-usable. The device was intended by its inventor to be used as a menstrual tampon or for the collection of cervical mucus in women using the Billings method or sympto-thermal method of natural family planning (Ch. 7). However, the design of the device might make it suitable as a barrier contraceptive, but clinical trial data to support this assumption are not available as yet.

Female condoms

Current research on the female condom is focusing on, inter alia, the device's acceptability and its contraceptive efficacy when used with or without spermicide (Ch. 6).

Vaginal sponges

The sponge has a lower efficacy and higher incidence of problems than other vaginal barriers.

Today sponge   See Chapter 6. Improvements in the sponge's performance will probably require a different material and a better spermicide as well as alterations in design to achieve better retention and coverage of the cervix. Little, if any, research towards attaining these goals appears to be in progress.

Chemical agents

Currently marketed spermicidal agents – foam, jelly, cream, suppository, film – inactivate spermatozoa by immobilizing them. The large doses of these substances required for contraceptive efficacy in vivo compared to in vitro, particularly if used repeatedly over prolonged periods, are thought to contribute to problems of vaginal irritation.

A variety of new chemical agents have been tested in recent years that immobilize sperm, interfere with sperm function through mechanisms other than spermicidal ones or harden cervical mucus so that sperm penetration is prevented. These compounds generally have antibacterial properties which could be considered an advantage in preventing STDs (Ch. 6). However, long-term use disturbs the normal vaginal flora and enhances the risk of vaginal infection and irritation.

A variety of other, sometimes ill-defined agents, including several plant products such as gossypol have been tried with little success.

As far as vaginal chemical contraception is concerned, we have made some progress since the days when women were advised to smear tar in the vagina or insert the pulp of pomegranates or elephant's dung, but a greater research effort is needed in this area if we are to control the spread of STDs.

Natural family planning

Successful use of a natural family planning method depends on correct identification of the fertile days of the cycle and, equally important, consistent abstinence from sexual intercourse on those days (Ch. 7). Better ways of identifying the beginning and the end of the fertile period should improve the performance of currently available methods and may widen the appeal not only of periodic abstinence by attracting the new, more 'technology-oriented' users but also users of barrier methods by limiting the need to use them to only a few days in each cycle.

Electronic devices

Devices such as the BabyComp, Cyclotest-D, Rite Time, Fertil-A-Chron and Bioself 110 have been developed for predicting the fertile and infertile days based on the basal body temperature (BBT) changes and on information, stored in the device, about previous cycle lengths. The most sophisticated device is The Rabbit (Rabbit Computer Company, Los Angeles, USA) which uses BBT measurements for up to 12 preceding cycles to predict the beginning of the fertile period and not simply the end. Although marketed in several countries, few of these devices have been rigorously tested for their accuracy in defining the fertile period and their effectiveness as a family planning aid. They are also very expensive.

In future, skin patches containing heat sensors may eliminate the need for thermometers.

Simple assay methods

Easy-to-use home tests for the measurement of hormones in urine are now available over-the-counter. They delineate the end of the fertile period through identification, in urine, of the luteinizing hormone (LH) peak (which is assumed to occur 3 days before the fertile period ends) or of the rise in pregnanediol glucuronide, the major metabolite of progesterone. Examples of such home kits are Ovutest, Clearplan-One Step (for LH) and the ProgestURINE RAMP test (for pregnanediol glucuronide).

Identification of the beginning of the fertile period, which requires detection of the pre-ovulatory rise in oestrogen, has been much more difficult to achieve but very recently, a 'Personal Contraceptive System' has been launched which is easy-to-use but requires a sophisticated reader with built-in programme to interpret the hormone changes. The usefulness and effectiveness of this system as a family planning aid still needs to be established; its (as yet unknown) cost may be a prohibitive factor.

Several other devices to identify the fertile period have been put on the market but almost always their reliability has not been adequately tested. The quantity and chemistry of mucus alters during the cycle. Disposable calibrated syringes have been developed to allow women to aspirate cervicovaginal fluid and record daily volumes. A miniature magnifying device has been designed to detect 'ferning' in saliva and tests to measure the content of various enzymes and proteins in saliva or mucus are being investigated. No doubt other such gadgets will appear in the coming years but it is very doubtful that a reliable, simple and affordable method for use in the home to identify the fertile days of the cycle will be available by the end of this decade.

THE SEARCH FOR NEW METHODS

Contraception for men

The development of reliable, reversible methods of contraception for oral or systemic use has proved to be much more difficult for men than for women. The process of spermatogenesis is poorly understood and suppressing the production of some 1000 spermatozoa per second is a much more formidable task than preventing the release of a single egg once a month.

In spite of inherent difficulties a contraceptive 'pill' for men based on systemically administered steroid hormones, which acts through inhibiting the secretion of LH and follicle stimulating hormone (FSH) by the pituitary gland, could be ready for more widespread testing by the end of the decade.

Hormonal methods

The ideal hormonal method of contraception for men should suppress sperm production while leaving testosterone secretion intact, thus rendering the man infertile but not impotent. To date, no hormonal approach has achieved this. It is also proving difficult to find a method which will completely inhibit sperm production (azoospermia) in the majority of men, which is cheap, effective within a short time of starting treatment, and rapidly reversible.

A trial of weekly injections of 200 mg testosterone enanthate (WHO 1990) resulted in azoospermia in 65% of 271 men after 6 months of treatment. After 12 months of relying on the method for contraception, only 1 pregnancy occurred (0.8 conceptions per 100 person years).

A second trial in which men who did not achieve azoospermia but whose sperm count fell to less than 3 million/ml (nearly 99% of subjects) resulted in a failure rate of 1.5 per 100 person years.

Research efforts are now concentrated on the development of long-acting methods, and regimens combining more potent androgens with either a progestogen (such as DMPA or desogestrel) or GnRH agonist or antagonist.

Non-hormonal agents acting on sperm

Affecting sperm production   A wide variety of chemical agents have been shown to suppress sperm production but most ultimately cause irreversible infertility.

Gossypol, a plant-derived product isolated initially from cotton seed, induces azoospermia or severe oligozoospermia in more than 90% of men. However, its use leads to irreversible infertility in 10–15% of men and is associated, in some cases, with potentially life-threatening hypokalaemia. Development of gossypol for male contraception has been discontinued by most investigators.

Physical agents such as irradiation and ultrasound also inhibit sperm production when used at certain doses but the application of such methods for contraception has not been pursued because of concerns about irreversibility and carcinogenesis.

Local, long-term application of a mild temperature increase (1–2°C), by bringing the testes closer to the inguinal canal, has possibilities. A polyester sling worn during waking hours has been employed for this purpose and led to azoospermia in all 14 men wearing the sling for 12 months. The inhibitory effect on sperm production was fully reversible within 6 months after stopping use of the sling.

Affecting sperm maturation   Drugs that affect sperm during storage in the epididymis would act quickly and, after withdrawal of the drug, normal spermatozoa would reappear rapidly in the semen. No compound has yet reached the stage of clinical efficacy testing in men because of toxicological concerns or insufficient efficacy in animal tests.

A traditional Chinese medicine containing extract of the plant *Tripterygium wilfordii* for treatment of psoriasis, rheumatoid arthritis, glomerulonephritis and other autoimmune diseases shows some promise. Work is under way to try and isolate the active principle(s) of this extract which is thought to act primarily at the level of the epididymis.

GnRH analogues

The discovery of GnRH, the hypothalamic peptide hormone that induces the pituitary gland to secrete FSH and LH, created great expectations of a novel form of contraception. Many hundreds of analogues – both agonists and antagonists – of GnRH have been synthesized, but the prospects of using these compounds in fertility regulation now look rather poor. They are expensive, short-acting, cannot be given orally and frequently cause local allergic reactions.

Vaccination against GnRH is summarized in the section on antifertility vaccines (pp. 432–433).

In female contraception

GnRH and its agonists normally stimulate the secretion of FSH and LH. Paradoxically, ovulation will be inhibited when agonists are given over long periods and in sufficiently high dose. If ovarian activity is completely suppressed, potentially deleterious effects on bone and on the cardiovascular system may occur (similar to changes in the postmenopausal state). The hypo-oestrogenism resulting from complete GnRH agonist-induced ovarian suppression would require replacement therapy with low-dose oestrogen and progestogen. Conversely, incomplete suppression of ovarian activity might result in long periods of unopposed oestrogen, increasing the risk of endometrial carcinoma.

The feasibility of keeping ovulation suppressed in the short term in breastfeeding women by giving the GnRH agonist, buserelin, by nasal spray has been demonstrated. Further development of this approach awaits cheaper agonists that can be more easily administered.

In male contraception

To date, pilot trials in humans and monkeys with combination regimens of GnRH agonists and androgens have not provided adequate suppression of spermatogenesis. Clinical research using implants is ongoing.

Steroid hormone receptor antagonists

Steroid hormone receptor antagonists bind with receptor sites to prevent the native steroid hormone from occupying the same

428 HANDBOOK OF FAMILY PLANNING

sites. They are often referred to as antihormones. Anti-androgens (e.g. cyproterone acetate in Dianette) and anti-oestrogens (e.g. clomiphene) have been in clinical use for some time but agents that block the receptor for progesterone were only discovered in the early 1980s.

Anti-androgens

Any effective anti-androgen e.g. cyproterone acetate is bound to have effects in the male on libido and potency which will require the concomitant use of exogenous androgens. These, in turn, would reduce the effectiveness of the anti-androgen and therefore, it seems unlikely that anti-androgens can be of use in male fertility control.

Anti-oestrogens

Many anti-oestrogens, including clomiphene, have proved inactive as contraceptive agents in the human.

A non-steroidal agent, centchroman, which has weak oestrogenic and potent anti-oestrogenic activities, is in use as a once-a-week pill in India only. Thought to exert its contraceptive action by preventing implantation, the compound is given in a dose of 30 mg twice a week for the first 3 months, followed thereafter by 30 mg once a week. A failure rate of 1.8 per HWY has been reported for this regimen.

Antiprogestogens

Because progesterone is essential for a range of reproductive functions, including the establishment and maintenance of pregnancy, antiprogestogens such as mifepristone offer considerable potential for the regulation of fertility (Van Look & von Hertzen 1995). The use of antiprogestogens, mifepristone in particular, for inducing abortion is described in Chapter 10. A summary of the current state of research in the other possible applications is given below.

Menstrual regulation The sequential combination regimen of mifepristone and a prostaglandin appears to be an effective method for menstrual regulation (induction of missed menses). In a recently completed trial by WHO, a total of 228 women with menstrual delay of up to 11 days were studied. Vaginal bleeding was induced in all of the 193 pregnant women and all but four of them had a complete abortion, giving a success rate of 98%. 35 women were not pregnant.

These results have brought closer the prospect of 'a menses inducer' comprising an antiprogestogen pill such as mifepristone followed, 36–48 hours later, by a prostaglandin tablet. The coming years should see this development reach fruition.

Once-a-month contraception   Antiprogestogens given during the luteal phase of the cycle have a profound effect on the endometrium and hence have been proposed for use as once-a-month contraceptives. Taken in the early luteal phase they could prevent implantation, while taken in the late luteal phase they could disrupt it.

Accurate timing of the antiprogestogen administration in the early luteal phase is essential. If the drug is taken too early, ovulation will be suppressed and menses will be delayed. If taken too late, endometrial bleeding may occur but an already implanting embryo may not be dislodged. Thus, the use of an antiprogestogen as a once-a-month contraceptive in the early luteal phase is not likely to be a practical method of family planning until such time that a simple and reliable method to detect ovulation has been discovered.

Trials of mifepristone as a *late* luteal, once-a-month contraceptive have been disappointing. Research is currently in progress to determine if monthly use of a combination of antiprogesterone with a prostaglandin is feasible.

Emergency contraception   Antiprogesterones may prove to be highly effective for emergency postcoital contraception (Ch. 9).

Once-a-week contraception   A small dose of antiprogesterone given once a week might disturb endometrial development without causing ovarian dysfunction. Alternatively, a higher dose of the compound might prevent ovulation. Unfortunately, in both approaches the endometrium is continually exposed to unopposed oestrogen and, therefore, to the potential risks of hyperplasia and cancer.

Daily use   Recent studies have shown that a very low daily dose of mifepristone (e.g. 1 mg or even less) does not upset ovarian cyclicity, yet profoundly disturbs endometrial development. This finding has led to the suggestion that antiprogestogens may represent a new generation of 'minipills'.

Cyclical use   An alternative contraceptive strategy would be to use a higher dose of mifepristone (e.g. 5–10 mg) in a sequential regimen with a progestogen. This regimen would allow development of a secretory endometrium and the occurrence of timely, well-controlled vaginal bleeding.

New delivery systems for steroid hormones

Non-oral routes of administering steroid hormones have several advantages.

1. The first pass through the liver is avoided which allows the use of lower doses of hormone and reduces metabolic side-effects.
2. It is possible to achieve steady hormone levels and avoid the peaks and troughs that are associated with the oral route of administration and which may be responsible for some of the side-effects.

The two new delivery systems discussed below – the hormone-releasing vaginal rings and transdermal systems – have major advantages in having contraceptive actions which can be easily reversed and are entirely under the control of the woman.

Vaginal rings

Most steroid hormones are absorbed efficiently through the vaginal epithelium and can be released from a vaginal ring made out of Silastic. Rings up to 75 mm in diameter usually stay in the vaginal fornix and fit around the cervix. To achieve release of the steroid at the desired dose and at a constant rate several designs are in use (Fig. 17.1). The release rate is a function of the surface area of the ring, the solubility of the steroid in the Silastic matrix, and the distance the steroid has to diffuse in order to reach the surface of the ring.

Combined oestrogen–progestogen rings   This type of ring is worn for 3 weeks and then removed for 1 week to allow withdrawal

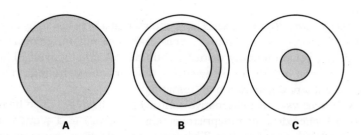

Fig. 17.1   Cross-sectional views of contraceptive rings in which the shaded areas are micronized steroid: **A**. Homogeneous ring; **B**. Shell ring; **C**. Core ring.

bleeding to occur. The '3-week-in/1-week-out' schedule is continued for the life-time of the ring.

Like combined oral contraceptive pills, vaginal rings releasing both oestrogen and progestogen are intended to inhibit ovulation with minimal disturbance of vaginal bleeding patterns. Examples of combined rings that are in development include one that releases 3-keto-desogestrel and ethinyloestradiol (Organon) and one that releases norethisterone acetate and ethinyloestradiol (Population Council).

Progestogen-only rings Depending on the amount of progestogen released, the ring acts either by inhibiting ovulation or in a manner similar to the POP. A ring that is intended to block ovulation would be used in a '3-week-in/1-week-out' schedule to ensure regular withdrawal bleeding. Rings that release a smaller dose of progestogen are worn continuously, although they can be removed for short periods if desired (e.g. for cleaning or during intercourse). Like the POP, the efficacy of rings that are worn continuously depends on a combination of effects, including thickening of cervical mucus, inhibition of ovulation and prevention of implantation. An example of a progestogen-only ring is the levonorgestrel ring with a daily release rate of 20 µg. This has recently been redesigned and is in the final phase of clinical testing prior to registration and marketing. Also under study is a ring delivering the progestogen ST 1435 (Nestorone), which is inactive when taken orally, and is intended for use by breastfeeding women in a '3 week-in/1 week-out' schedule.

Transdermal systems

The transdermal route of drug administration is an area of growing interest as can be seen by the increasing number of transdermal hormone replacement products. Drug delivery through the skin can be accomplished in two ways:

1. By an aerosol/aeropowder or a semisolid or liquid vehicle that contains the drug.
2. By a drug-delivery patch which ensures fairly constant release rates.

Transdermal delivery of contraceptive steroids is still in its infancy and currently focuses on the development of patches for the delivery of ethinyloestradiol plus levonorgestrel and of the progestogen ST 1435 (Nestorone).

Antifertility vaccines

The aim is to develop a vaccine – for either women or men – that will inhibit reproduction by immunological means and which is safe, effective, reversible, and free of endocrine and metabolic side-effects.

The first step in this development process is to identify a suitable, reproduction-specific molecule that can be used as an immunogen. A large number of reproduction-specific molecules exist but not all of them represent attractive options since their immunological removal or neutralization could result in endocrine or other side-effects. Molecules found in, or produced by, the sperm, egg and the peri-implantation embryo are the most appropriate targets.

Furthest advanced amongst the antifertility vaccines is the one directed against human chorionic gonadotrophin (hCG). Some work is also in progress on the development of vaccines for men against GnRH and FSH.

Anti-hCG vaccines

The main function of hCG, which is produced by the pre-implantation embryo within a few days of fertilization, appears to be the maintenance of the corpus luteum, thus ensuring the continued production of progesterone essential for successful implantation. Immunological inhibition of the production or function of hCG would lead to regression of the corpus luteum, followed by declining progesterone levels and the occurrence of menstrual bleeding.

One of the candidate vaccines being studied consists of an apparently unique part of the β-subunit of hCG (β-hCG-CTP) linked to an immunogenic carrier molecule such as tetanus or diphtheria toxoid and injected together with adjuvants that further enhance the immune response (Griffin 1991).

A Phase I study conducted by WHO with this vaccine preparation showed that it can induce a level of antibodies high enough to neutralize hCG for a period of some 6–12 months. To prolong the antifertility effect booster injections would need to be given.

An alternative approach is the use of the whole β-hCG subunit. In India, an anti-hCG vaccine is being tested that consists of the whole β-subunit coupled to the α-subunit of ovine LH. Studies conducted with this preparation have confirmed its antifertility effect.

In addition to lack of long-term safety data, one potentially major problem with anti-hCG vaccines is the individual variability in the antibody response. To detect those women who have responded poorly or not at all and to determine when the antifertility effect has worn off, it will probably be necessary to develop a simple, dipstick-type method for assessing the antibody level in blood following administration of the vaccine.

Antisperm vaccines

A small proportion (about 5%) of male and female patients attending infertility clinics appear to be infertile because they have antibodies against spermatozoa. Auto-antibodies are also found in a substantial percentage of vasectomized men and are thought to be responsible for the low pregnancy rate after vasectomy reversal even in men in whom the re-anastomosis procedure appears to have succeeded.

Since the presence of antisperm antibodies in either men or women seems to cause no ill effects other than infertility, the feasibility of developing a safe and effective antisperm vaccine appears very real. However, difficulty in finding an appropriate sperm antigen for use as the immunogen in the vaccine means that no antisperm vaccine is likely to become routinely available within the next 10–15 years.

Anti-ovum vaccines

Most of the research directed at developing an anti-ovum vaccine has focused on the zona pellucida (ZP), the outer layer of the ovum. One glycoprotein component, ZP3, is essential for fertilization. Active immunization of animals against ZP3 causes infertility. Unfortunately, the immunized animal eventually looses all the primordial follicles from its ovaries and experiences a premature, irreversible menopause. Research is currently under way to determine if this irreversible damage to the ovaries can be avoided.

Other antifertility vaccines

Pilot studies on the feasibility of immunizing men against GnRH have been initiated, but this approach would require hormone substitution therapy and could induce damage to the pituitary. Similar concerns have been voiced about vaccination of men against FSH, which is being tested in India, although no adverse physiological or behavioural effects have been observed in male monkeys actively immunized for periods of more than 10 years.

REFERENCES

Coutinho E M, Mascarenhas I, Mateo de Acosta O et al 1993 Comparative study on the efficacy, acceptability, and side effects of a contraceptive pill administered by the oral and the vaginal route: an international multicenter clinical trial. Clinical Pharmacology and Therapeutics 54: 540–545

Griffin P D 1991 The WHO Task Force on Vaccines for Fertility Regulation. Its formation, objectives and research activities. Human Reproduction 6: 166–172

Khanna J, Van Look P F A, Benagiano G 1994 Fertility regulation research: the challenges now and ahead. In: Khanna J, Van Look P F A and Griffin P D (eds) Challenges in reproductive health research. World Health Organization, Geneva, pp. 34–57

Van Look P F A, von Hertzen H 1995 Clinical uses of antiprogestogens. Human Reproduction Update 1: 19–34

Voordouw B C, Euser R, Verdonk R E et al 1992 Melatonin and melatonin–progestin combinations alter pituitary–ovarian function in women and can inhibit ovulation. Journal of Clinical Endocrinology and Metabolism 74: 108–117

Waites G M H 1993 Male fertility regulation: the challenges for the year 2000. British Medical Bulletin 49: 210–221

World Health Organization Task Force on Methods for the Regulation of Male Fertility 1990 Contraceptive efficacy of testosterone-induced azoospermia in normal men. Lancet 336: 955–959

World Health Organization 1994 Health, population and development (WHO Position Paper for the International Conference on Population and Development 1994, Cairo; document WHO/FHE/94.1). World Health Organization, Geneva

FURTHER READING

Drife J O, Baird D T (eds) 1993 Contraception. British Medical Bulletin 49: 1–258

Sitruk-Ware R, Bardin C W (eds) 1992 Contraception – Newer pharmacological agents, devices and delivery systems. Marcel Dekker, New York

Van Look P F A, Pérez-Palacios G (eds) 1994 Contraceptive research and development 1984 to 1994 – The road from Mexico City to Cairo and Beyond. Oxford University Press, Delhi

Abbreviations

AIDS	Acquired immune deficiency syndome
BBT	Basal body temperature
BIP	Basic infertile pattern
BMA	British Medical Association
BP	Blood pressure
BPAS	British Pregnancy Advisory Service
BSE	Breast self-examination
BTB	Breakthrough bleeding
CEP	Combined oestrogen-progestogen regimen
CFT	Complement fixation test
Ch.	Chapter
CIN	Cervical intraepithelial neoplasia
CMV	Cytomegalovirus
CNS	Central nervous system
COC	Combined oral contraception; combined oral contraceptive
CRC	Cancer Research Campaign
CVA	Cerebrovascular accident
CVS	Cardiovascular system
D & C	Dilatation and curettage
D & E	Dilatation and evacuation
DES	Diethylstilboestrol
DHSS	Department of Health and Social Security
DI	Donor insemination
DM	Diabetes mellitus
DMPA	Depot medroxyprogesterone acetate (Depo-Provera)
DNA	Desoxyribonucleic acid
DRCOG	Diploma of the Royal College of Obstetricians and Gynaecologists
EBV	Epstein Barr virus
ED	Every day
EE	Ethinyloestradiol

ELISA	Enzyme-linked immunoadsorbent assay
EU	European Union
FDS	Frequency–dysuria syndrome
FFPRHC	Faculty of Family Planning and Reproductive Health Care
FP	Family planning
FPA	Family Planning Association
FPC	Family planning clinic
FPIS	Family Planning Information Service
FR	Failure rate
FSH	Follicle stimulating hormone
GA	General anaesthesia
GIFT	Gamete intrafallopian transfer
GMC	General Medical Council
GMSC	General Medical Services Committee
GnRH	Gonadotrophin releasing hormone
GP	General practitioner
HAV	Hepatitis A virus
HBV	Hepatitis B virus
HDLC	High density lipoprotein/cholesterol
HEA	Health Education Authority
HFEA	Human Fertilisation and Embryology Authority
hCG	Human chorionic gonadotrophin
HIV	Human immunodeficiency virus
HPV	Human papilloma virus
HRT	Hormone replacement therapy
HSV	Herpes simplex virus
HWY	Hundred woman years
IMB	Intermenstrual bleeding
IUD	Intrauterine device
IVF	In vitro fertilization
JCC	Joint Committee on Contraception
JCTGP	Joint Committee on Training in General Practice
LA	Local anaesthesia
LAM	Lactational amenorrhoea method
LDLC	Low density lipoprotein/cholesterol
LH	Luteinizing hormone
LMP	Last menstrual period
MI	Myocardial infarction
MMR	Mumps, measles and rubella vaccine
MRCGP	Member of the Royal College of General Practitioners

MRCOG	Member of the Royal College of Obstetricians and Gynaecologists
MSSU	Mid-stream specimen of urine
NAFPD	National Association of Family Planning Doctors
NAFPN	National Association of Family Planning Nurses
NAOMI	National Association of Ovulation Method Instructors
NCCS	National Case Control Study
NCN	National Coordinating Network
NET-EN	Norethisterone enanthate
NFP	Natural family planning
NGU	Non-gonococcal urethritis
NHS	National Health Service
NSAID	Non-steroidal anti-inflammatory drug
NSU	Non-specific urethritis
NSV	No-scalpel vasectomy
OPCS	Office of Population Censuses and Surveys
PCB	Postcoital bleeding
PCC	Postcoital contraception
PCOS	Polycystic ovarian syndrome
PFI	Pill-free interval
PID	Pelvic inflammatory disease
PMB	Postmenopausal bleeding
PMS	Premenstrual syndrome
POP	Progestogen-only pill
PPNG	β-lactamase-(penicillinase) producing *Neisseria gonorrhoeae*
PREPP	Post-registration education and professional practice
RCGP	Royal College of General Practitioners
RCN	Royal College of Nursing
RCOG	Royal College of Obstetricians and Gynaecologists
RGN	Registered general nurse
RHC	Reproductive health care
RNA	Ribonucleic acid
SC	(referring to genes, Ch. 3 sickle cell disorders)
SLE	Systemic lupus erythematosis
Sp	Spotting
SPOD	Association to Aid the Sexual and Personal Relationships of People with a Disability
SS	(referring to genes, Ch. 3 sickle cell disorders)

STD	Sexually transmissible disease
TOP	Termination of pregnancy
TPFR	Total period fertility rate
TSH	Thyroid stimulating hormone
UK	United Kingdom
UTI	Urinary tract infection
VA	Vacuum aspiration
VIN	Vulvar intraepithelial neoplasia
WHO	World Health Organization
ZP	Zona pellucida

Useful addresses and helplines

ADDRESSES

Amarant Trust
Grant House
56–60 St John Street
London EC1M 4DT

Association for Voluntary Surgical Contraception
79 Madison Avenue
New York NY 10016
USA

Association to Aid the Sexual and Personal Relationships
of People with a Disability (SPOD)
286 Camden Road
London N7 0BJ

Breast Cancer Care
Kiln House
200 New Kings Road
London SW6 4NZ

British Association for Sexual and Marital Therapy
PO Box 62
Sheffield S10 3TS

British Association of Cancer United Patients (BACUP)
3 Bath Place, Rivington Street
London EC2A 3JR

British Heart Foundation
14 Fitzhardinge Street
London W1H 4DH

British Menopause Society
36 West Street
Marlow
Bucks SL7 2NB

British Pregnancy Advisory Service (BPAS)
Austy Manor
Wootton Wawen
Solihull
West Midlands B95 6BX

British Society for Clinical Cytology
The Quadrangle
West Mount Centre
Uxbridge Road
Hayes UB4 0HB

Brook Advisory Centre (Head Office)
153a East Street
London SE17 2SD

Cancer Research Campaign
10 Cambridge Terrace
London NW1 4JL

Faculty of Family Planning and Reproductive Health Care
Royal College of Obstetricians and Gynaecologists
27 Sussex Place
Regent's Park
London NW1 4RG

Family Planning Association[1]

Family Planning Association Head Office
27–35 Mortimer Street
London W1N 7RJ

Family Planning Association Northern Ireland
113 University Street
Belfast BT7 1HP

---

[1] The Family Planning Association bookshop 'Health Wise' has a large number of relevant books and leaflets.

Family Planning Association Northern Ireland
14 Magazine Street
Londonderry BT48 6HH

Family Planning Association Scotland
2 Claremont Terrace
Glasgow G3 7XR

Family Planning Association Wales
Grace Phillips House
4 Museum Place
Cardiff CF1 3BG

Greenhouse
Trevelyan Terrace
Bangor
Gwynedd LL57 1AX

Family Planning Nurses

FP Forum, RCN
Muriel Holroyd (Chair)
46 Balshagray Drive
Glasgow G11 7DA

National Association of FP Nurses
Vicky Padbury (Chair)
14 Belmont Road
Reigate
Surrey RH2 7EE

Scottish Society of FP Nurses
Jayne Nairn (Chair)
9 William Place
Scone
Perthshire PH2 6TF

Health Education Authority (HEA)
Hamilton House
Mabledon Place
London WC1H 9TX

Health Education Board for Scotland
Woodburn House
Canaan Lane
Edinburgh EH10 4SG

Health Promotion Agency for Northern Ireland
18 Ormeau Avenue
Belfast BT2 8HS

Health Promotion Wales
Ffynnon-las
Ty Glas Avenue
Llanishen
Cardiff CF4 5DZ

Institute of Psychosexual Medicine
11 Chandos Street
London W1M 9DE

International Planned Parenthood Federation
Regent's Park
London NW1 4NS

Irish Family Planning Association
36–37 Lower Ormond Quay
Dublin 1
Republic of Ireland

Joint Committee on Contraception
see Faculty of Family Planning and Reproductive Health Care

Marriage Counselling Scotland
Head Office
105 Hanover Street
Edinburgh EH2 1DJ

National Association of Family Planning Doctors
see Faculty of Family Planning and Reproductive Health Care

National Boards for Nursing, Midwifery and Health Visiting

   National Board for Nursing, Midwifery
      and Health Visiting, England
   Victory House
   170 Tottenham Court Road
   London W1N 0HA

National Board for Nursing, Midwifery
   and Health Visiting, Northern Ireland
RAC House
79 Chichester Street
Belfast BT1 4JE

National Board for Nursing, Midwifery
   and Health Visiting, Scotland
22 Queen Street
Edinburgh EH2 1JX

National Board for Nursing, Midwifery
   and Health Visiting, Wales
Pearl Assurance House
Greyfriars Road
Cardiff CF1 3JN

National Health Service Breast and Cervical Screening
Programme, National Coordination
Trent Regional Health Authority
Fulwood House
Old Fulwood Road
Sheffield S10 3TH

National Osteoporosis Society
PO Box 10
Radstock
Bath BA3 3YB

Natural Family Planning

   National Association of Family Planning Teachers
   Birmingham Maternity Hospital
   Queen Elizabeth Medical Centre
   Birmingham B15 2TG

   Natural Family Planning Centre
   Birmingham Maternity Hospital
   Queen Elizabeth Medical Centre
   Birmingham B15 2TG

   Natural Family Planning Service
   Catholic Marriage Advisory Council
   1 Blythe Mews, Blythe Road
   London W14 0NW

Northern Ireland and the Republic of Ireland
NAOMI/DOMAS
16 North Great George Street
Dublin 1
Republic of Ireland

Scottish Association for NFP
The Archdiocesan Offices
196 Clyde Street
Glasgow G1 4JY

Relate Marriage Guidance
Herbert Gray College
Little Church Street
Rugby
Warwickshire CV21 3AP

Royal College of General Practitioners
14 Princes Gate
London SW7 1PU

Royal College of Obstetricians and Gynaecologists[2]
27 Sussex Place
Regent's Park
London NW1 4RG

Women's Nation-wide Cancer Control Campaign
Suna House
128–130 Curtain Road
London EC2A 3AR

---

[2]The Royal College of Obstetricians and Gynaecologists has a comprehensive leaflet library for the lay person.

HELPLINES

Free

BACUP   0800 181199
Help for patients with cancer

Healthwise Heartline   0800 858585

Literature Line   0800 555777
Will send information by post

NHS Helpline   0800 665544
Information about diseases and self-help groups

Pay for

Breast Cancer Care Helpline   0171 867 1103

FPA Helpline   0171 636 7866
Monday to Thursday 9.00 a.m. to 5.00 p.m.
Friday 9.00 a.m. to 4.30 p.m.

Women's Nation-wide Cancer Control Campaign 0171 729 4688

Index

Abortion
  incomplete, 252–3, 379
  mental incapacity, 262
  recurrent spontaneous, 380
  therapeutic *see* Termination of
    pregnancy
Abortion Act (1967), 2, 241, 243–4,
    264
Acne, 371
  combined pill, 82–3
  progestogens, 111
Actinomycosis, pelvic, 138–9
Acyclovir (Zovirax), 319–20
Adenomyosis, 113–14
Adolescents
  choice of method, 25–8, 346–7
  combined pill, 26
  condoms, 26, 346–7
  confidentiality, 263–4
  progestogen-only contraception, 26,
    112
  services, 27–8
  sexuality, 345–7
  targets, 27
  uptake, 6
Age
  and choice of method, 25–8
  of consent, 260–61
  at first intercourse (coitarche), 24–5
  maternal, 22
  middle age, 349–50
  older women *see* Older women
Aggression, 343–4
AIDS *see* Human immunodeficiency
    virus
Alcohol
  health promotion, 296
  pregnancy, 378
Allergy
  combined pill, 55
  oestrogen patches, 394–5

Amenorrhoea, 370
  after stopping pill, 84
  causes, 370
  combined pill, 371
  Depo-Provera, 101
  injectable progestogen, 26, 29
  lactational, 198–9
  management, 370–71
  progestogen-only contraception, 110
Ampicillin, 309
Anal intercourse, 181, 324, 328
Anti-androgens, 428
Antibiotics, 63–6
Anti-epileptic drugs (anticonvulsants)
  combined pill, 64
  progesterone-only contraceptives,
    98, 115
Antifertility vaccines, 432–3
Anti-FSH vaccination, 433
Anti-hCG vaccines, 432–3
Anti-oestrogens, 428
Anti-ovum vaccines, 433
Antiprogesterones, 235, 428–9
Antisperm antibodies, 215, 220, 433
Antisperm vaccines, 433
Antithrombin-III, 53
Anxiety, reducing, 344
Arterial disease, 46, 48, 53–6
Arthritis, reactive, 310
Arthropod infestations, 334–5
Artificial insemination, 274
Aspirin, 368, 372
Association to Aid the Sexual and
    Personal Relationships of
    People with a Disability
    (SPOD), 17
Association of Sexual and Marital
    Therapists, 16–17
Atrophic vaginitis, 364, 369
Atrophy
  endometrial, 44

Atrophy (*contd*)
  urogenital, 388
Autoimmune system, 114
Azithromycin, 311
Azoospermia, 425–6

Bacterial infections, 303–13
Bacterial vaginosis, 137, 312–13
  diagnosis, 312–13
  prevalence, 302
  treatment, 313
Bacteroides spp., 312
Balanoposthitis, candidal, 315
Barrier methods, 147–81
  benefits, 181
  disability, 29
  history of, 147
  home-made, 168
  irregular lifestyle, 32
  perimenopause, 406–7
  postabortion, 255
  risks, 181
  see also Caps; Condoms; Diaphragm;
    Spermicides
Bartholin's cyst/abscess, 353, 364
Bartholinitis, 306
Basal body temperature method, 186–8
  effectiveness, 193
  electronic devices, 424
  intelligent thermometers, 195–6
Benign intracranial pressure, 73
Benzyl benzoate, 335
Billings method *see* Mucus method
Birth rates, 22
Bisphosphonates, 390
Bladder training, 377
Blood pressure, 55
  screening, 293
  see also Hypertension
Blood transfusion, 324
Bone density, 388
  screening, 390
Breakthrough bleeding, 42, 76,
    109–10
Breast cancer
  clinical examination, 291–2
  combined pill, 48, 79–81, 85
  Depo-Provera, 102
  hormone replacement therapy, 399,
    401
  mammography, 292
  management, 292
  progestogens, 97, 113
  screening, 290–92
  self-examination, 291, 298–9

Breastfeeding
  buserelin, 427
  combined pill, 33, 61, 200
  complementary contraception,
    199–201
  and fertility, 197–9
  HIV, 324, 329
  implants, 200, 417
  IUDs, 128, 200
  mucus method, 190–92
  Nestorene, 417
  progestogen-only contraception, 96,
    97, 98, 200
  sexual adjustment, 349
  vaginal rings, 431
Breasts
  cancer *see* Breast cancer
  clinical examination, 58, 291–2
  discomfort, 78–9
  progestogen-only contraception, 113
  self-examination, 291, 298–9
British Journal of Family Planning, 4,
    14
British Pregnancy Advisory Service, 5
Brook Advisory Centres, 3, 5, 12
Buserelin, 427

C-film, 159, 174, 175–6
Calcitonin, 390
Calcium supplements, 390
Calendar method, 183–4, 186
Cancer, 50
  breast *see* Breast cancer
  cervical *see* Cervical cancer
  endometrial *see* Endometrial cancer
  hormone replacement therapy, 399
  incidence, 281
  ovarian *see* Ovarian cancer
  pelvic, 281–90
  prostate, 216, 225–6
  sex-steroid dependent, 48
  testicular, 216, 226
Candidiasis (thrush), 72, 314–16
Canesten, 316
Capronor, 418
Caps, 148–66
  breastfeeding, 200
  cervical, 159–63, 422
  diaphragm *see* Diaphragm
  vault, 163–4
  vimule, 165–6
Carbaryl lotion, 334
Carbon dioxide laser, 208
Cardiovascular disease
  combined pill, 46, 53–6, 70–71

Cardiovascular disease (contd)
  postmenopausal, 390–91
  progestogen-only contraception, 113
  vasectomy, 215–16
Carpal tunnel syndrome, 81
Caruncle, 377
Catholic Marriage Advisory Council, 16
Centchroman, 428
Cerebral haemorrhage, 47
Cerebrovascular accident see Stroke
Cervagem (Gemeprost), 249, 250, 252, 254
Cervical cancer, 281–9
  cervical intraepithelial neoplasia (CIN), 283, 286, 321
  combined pill, 78
  Depo-Provera, 102
  diagnosis, 283
  human papillomavirus, 282, 302, 320–23
  incidence, 281–2
  mortality, 282
  national screening programme, 283–4
  prevention, 283–4
  risk factors, 282
  smear test see Cervical smear
  targets, 10, 289
  treatment, 287
Cervical cap, 159–63, 422
Cervical intraepithelial neoplasia (CIN), 283, 286, 321
Cervical palpation method, 192
Cervical smear, 58, 283–5
  abnormal, 286–7
  frequency, 287–9
  target payments, 10
Cervix
  cancer see Cervical cancer
  condylomatous lesions, 321–3
  ectropion (erosion), 365
  mucus see Mucus, cervical; Mucus method
  polyps, 365–6
  shock (vasovagal syncope), 131
Charges, 2
Chemical agents, 423
Childbirth
  and choice of method, 33
  family planning after, 197–201
  sexual adjustment, 348–9
  see also Pregnancy
Children
  AIDS, 326
  sexual abuse, 309, 321

Chinese injectable No-1 , 418
Chlamydia trachomatis infection, 246, 309–12
  diagnosis, 310–11
  treatment, 311–12
Chloasma
  combined pill, 82
  progestogen-only contraception, 115
Chlorhexidine, 179
Cholic acid, 179
Chorea, 73
Choriocarcinoma, 78
Ciprofloxacin, 309
Claim forms, 10
Climacteric see Perimenopause
Clindamycin, 313
Clitoromegaly, 372
Clomiphene, 428
Clonidine, 392
Clotrimazole (Canesten), 316
Clotting factors, 53, 54
Coagulations disorders, 97
Cohabitation, 23
Coitarche, 24–5
Coitus interfemora, 181
Coitus interruptus, 179–80
  sexual effects, 359
Coitus reservatus, 181
Collagen, 388
Combined oral contraceptive
  acne, 82–3
  adolescents, 26
  advantages, 51–2
  amenorrhoea/oligomenorrhoea, 371
  benign intracranial pressure, 73
  biphasic, 42, 61
  breaks in pill taking, 85
  breakthrough bleeding, 76
  breast cancer, 48, 79–81, 85
  breast discomfort, 78–9
  breastfeeding, 33, 61, 200
  cardiovascular system, 46, 53–6, 70–71
  carpal tunnel syndrome, 81
  central nervous system, 71–4
  cervical cancer, 78
  changing, 61
  chloasma, 82
  choice of pill, 58–9
  chorea, 73
  choriocarcinoma, 78
  complications, 69–83
  contraindications, 45–51
  cramps, 82
  Crohn's disease, 83
  depression, 71

Combined oral contraceptive (*contd*)
  diarrhoea, 63
  disabled people, 29
  disadvantages, 52–7
  drug interactions, 63–7
  drug-users, 31
  effectiveness, 44–5
  elective surgery, 69
  endometrial cancer, 85
  epilepsy, 66, 73
  everyday varieties, 60
  examination, 57–8
  eye problems, 74
  failure, 44–5
  fetal abnormalities, 84–5
  fibroids, 77
  follow-up, 67–8
  gall stones, 75
  gastrointestinal system, 74–5
  genital system, 76–8
  gynaecological conditions, 45
  headaches, 72–3
  hirsutism, 82–3
  history, 38
  HIV, 329
  hypertension, 70–71
  indications, 45
  infections, 83
  inflammations, 83
  instructions to patients, 59
  intercurrent disease, 49–51
  irregular lifestyle, 31
  jaundice, 75
  leg pains, 82
  libido, 71–2
  liver tumours, 75
  malignant melanoma, 48–9, 83
  melasma, 82
  metabolic effects, 52–3, 54
  migraine, 72–3
  missed pills, 61–3
  mode of action, 43–4
  monophasic, 42, 59–60
  morbidity, 86
  musculoskeletal system, 81–2
  myocardial infarction, 53, 56, 70
  nausea, 74, 233–4
  outcome of pregnancy, 84–5
  ovarian cancer, 51–2, 85
  patient history, 57
  perimenopause, 405
  photosensitivity, 82
  pigmentation, 82
  pill-free interval, 61–3
  postpartum, 33, 61
  preparations, 39–43

  prescribing, 44
  research, 415–16
  reversibility, 83–4
  risks/benefits, 85–8
  sexual effects, 356–8
  skin conditions, 82–3
  spotting, 76
  starting, 59–61
  stopping, indications, 68–9
  triphasic, 42–3, 61
  urinary system, 75
  vaginal administration, 416
  vaginal discharge, 77
  vomiting, 63, 74
  weight gain, 53, 74
  withdrawal bleeding, 44
  withdrawal bleeding, absent, 77
Combined oestrogen-progestogen
    (CEP) regimen, 230, 231,
    232
  side-effects, 233–4
Condoms, 169–72
  adolescents, 26, 346–7
  advantages, 170–71
  contraindications, 170
  disadvantages, 171
  effectiveness, 170
  female, 166–8, 423
  HIV, 21, 147, 169, 329
  indications, 170
  instructions for use, 171–2
  levels of use, 21
  perimenopause, 407
  plastic, 421
  postpartum, 33
  research, 420–21
  sexual effects, 358–9
  types, 169
Condylomata acuminata, 321–3
Confidentiality, 5, 263–4
  HIV, 273
Congenital malformations, 365
Consent, 260–63
  age of, 260–61
  AIDS testing, 273
  to medical treatment, 260
  mental incapacity, 261–3
  research subjects, 272
  to sex, 260
  sterilization, 269
Contact lenses, 74
Contracap, 422
Copper T380A, 128
Corpus luteum, 43, 184
Costs, and choice of method, 34–5
Co-trimoxazole (Septrin), 330–32

Counselling
  genetic, 378
  HIV infection, 328–9
  nurses, 16
  practice nurses, 9
  premenstrual syndrome, 373
  prepregnancy, 378
  sexual difficulties, 360–61
  sterilization, 32–3, 218–19
  termination of pregnancy, 244–5
  vasectomy, 214, 219
Cramps, 82
Crohn's disease, 83
Cu-Fix, 121
Culture see Religion/culture
Cyclizine, 234
Cyclofem (Cycloprovera), 418–20
Cycloprovera, 418–20
Cyproterone acetate, 83, 371, 428
Cystic fibrosis, 66
Cystitis, 75
Cytomegalovirus, 334

Danazol, 234
Dapsone, 332
Deep venous thrombosis see
      Thromboembolism
Delfen foam, 407
Depo-Provera (depot
      medroxyprogesterone acetate;
      DMPA), 92
  administration, 106–7
  amenorrhoea, 101
  animal toxicology, 102
  breast cancer, 102
  cervical cancer, 102
  contraindications, 97
  controversial aspects, 101–3
  delayed return of fertility, 112,
      116
  effectiveness, 94
  endometrial cancer, 98, 102
  fetal abnormalities, 103
  follow-up, 109
  GP home visits, 8
  informed consent, 103
  libido, loss of, 100
  license, 95
  osteoporosis, 103
  ovarian cancer, 102
  perimenopause, 406
  weight gain, 111
Depression, 49, 71
Desogestrel, 39, 415
Developing countries, 409–12

Diabetes mellitus
  candidiasis, 315
  combined pill, 51
  IUDs, 128
  progestogen-only contraception, 99,
      115
Dianette, 83, 371
Diaphragm, 148–59
  adolescents, 26
  advantages, 151
  C-film, 159
  contraindications, 151
  disadvantages, 151–2
  effectiveness, 150
  fitting, 152–6
  follow-up, 159
  HIV, 329
  indications, 151
  instructions for use, 158–9
  introducer, 158
  levels of use, 22
  long-acting spermicide-releasing,
      422
  mode of action, 150
  patient teaching, 156–8
  perimenopause, 407
  removal, 156
  research, 421–2
  sexual effects, 358
  spermicides, 150, 158–9
  used continuously without
      spermicide, 421–2
Diaphragm-tampon device, 422
Diarrhoea, 63
Diathermy, 205, 212
Diazepam, 66
Didanosine, 332
Diethylstilboestrol, 365
Dilapan rods, 250
Diploma of the Royal College of
      Obstetrics and Gynaecology
      (DRCOG), 14–15
Disability, 28–30, 261–3
Divorce, 23
DMPA see Depo-Provera
Dominance, 343
Donor insemination, 274
Doxycycline, 311
Drug users
  barrier methods, 32
  combined pill, 31
  HIV, 324
  IUDs, 32
Duphaston, 374
Dydrogesterone, 400
Dysmenorrhoea, 372–3

Dyspareunia, 353–4, 375
    menopausal, 388
Dysuria, 377–8

Ectopic pregnancy
    female sterilization, 211
    IUDs, 126, 140, 268
    progestogen-only pill, 94
Ectropion, 365
Ejaculation
    failure, 355
    lack of control, 347–8
    premature, 354
    retrograde, 355
Embryo research, 274
Emergency contraception, 8, 13
    adolescents, 27
    antiprogesterones, 235
    availability, 237–9
    contraindications, 232–3
    danazol, 234
    effectiveness, 231–2
    examination, 235–6
    fetal abnormalities, 236
    follow-up, 237
    indications, 232
    information, 236–7, 239, 240
    IUDs, 8, 230–34
    levonorgestrel, 230, 234
    litigation, 267–8
    methods, 230–31
    mode of action, 231
    patient history, 235
    side-effects, 233–4
Endocervical brush smear, 285
Endocrinology, 43
Endometrial cancer, 52
    combined pill, 85
    Depo-Provera, 98, 102
    hormone replacement therapy, 396,
        399
    progestogen-only contraception,
        109–10, 113–14
    screening, 290
Endometriosis
    hormone replacement therapy, 399
    progestogen-only contraception,
        113–14
Endometrium
    atrophic, 44
    biopsy, 367, 369
    cancer see Endometrial cancer
    IUDs, 124
    progestogen, 93
    proliferation, 43

Enovid, 38
Enzyme-inducing drugs
    combined pill, 63, 66
    progestogen-only contraception, 98
Epididymitis, 310
Epididymo-orchitis, 306
Epilepsy
    combined pill, 66, 73
    IUD insertion, 131
    progestogen-only contraception,
        115
Epstein Barr virus, 333–4
Erectile dysfunction, 354–5
    condoms, 359
Erythromycin stearate, 311
Ethics, 259–77
Ethinyloestradiol, 39, 42, 431
    emergency contraception, 230
Ethnic background see Religion/culture
Ethynodiol diacetate, 39, 92
Etidronate, 390
Evening primrose oil, 374, 392
Exercise, 296
Eye problems, 74

Faculty of Family Planning and
        Reproductive Health Care, 3, 4,
        13–14, 15, 17
Failure rates, 412
Fallopian tubes
    occlusion see Tubal occlusion
    plugs, 415
Falope ring, 207
Family Planning Association, 3
    multidisciplinary seminars, 16
Family planning clinics, 1-2, 5,
        11–12
Family structures, 23
Female condom, 166–8, 423
Female sterilization, 203–11
    complications, 210–11
    counselling, 219
    ectopic pregnancy, 211
    effectiveness, 219
    examination, 208–9
    follow-up, 210
    laparoscopy, 204–5, 222
    litigation, 269
    menstrual disturbance, 210–11
    minilaparotomy, 205
    occlusive plugs, 415
    postoperative advice, 209, 222
    preoperative advice, 209
    reversibility, 219–20
    techniques, 205–8

Female sterilization (*contd*)
  technological developments, 414–15
  utero-tubal junction cautery, 415
  see also Sterilization
FemCap, 422
Femidom, 167
Femulen, 93
Fertile period, identifying, 423–5
Fertility, 341
  awareness, 183
  and breastfeeding, 197–9
  perimenopause, 404
  see also Infertility
Fetal abnormalities
  combined pill, 84–5
  Depo-Provera, 103
  emergency contraception, 236
  NET-EN, 96
  progestogen-only contraception, 116
  rubella, 293
  termination of pregnancy, 251
Fetal tissue, use for research/
    treatment, 275
Fibrinolysis, 53
Fibroids
  combined pill, 77
  hormone replacement therapy, 399
  IUDs, 127
Filshie clip, 207
FlexiGard (GyneFix), 121, 420
Fluconazole, 316
Fluoxetine hydrocholoride, 354, 374
Folate supplements, 378
Follicle stimulating hormone, 43, 371,
    384, 385
  anti-FSH vaccination, 433
Fourex, 169
Fractures, 389
Frequency dysuria syndrome (urethral
    syndrome), 377
Fungal infection, 314–16

Gallbladder disease
  combined pill, 75
  hormone replacement therapy, 399
Gamete intrafallopian transfer
    (GIFT), 274
Gamma benzene hexachloride, 335
Gamolenic acid, 374
Gardnerella vaginalis, 312, 313
Gastrointestinal system, 74–5
Gemeprost, 249, 250, 252, 254
Gender
  identity, 342
  selection, 275

General practice
  contraceptive list, 7, 15
  family planning clinic, 8
  fundholding, 4
  home visits, 8
  IUDs, 7
  oral contraceptive pill, 7
  policies, 7
  remuneration, 10
  research, 10
  services, 6–10
  shared care, 9
  training, 10, 15
  vasectomy, 7
Genetic counselling, 378
Genital herpes *see* Herpes simplex
    virus
Genital tract
  combined pill, 76–8
  progestogen-only contraception,
    113–14
Genital warts (human papilloma
    virus), 282, 302, 320–23
Genitourinary medicine clinics, 302–3
Gestodene, 39, 42, 415
GnRH analogues, 427
Gonorrhoea, 303–9
  diagnosis, 307
  pelvic inflammatory disease, 306
  penicillinase producing strains
    (PPNG), 303, 308
  pharyngeal, 306, 309
  prepubertal girls, 306
  prevalence, 302, 303
  rectal, 306
  treatment, 307–9
  urethral, 303–6, 307
Gossypol, 423, 426
Gracial, 42, 82
Gramicidin, 179
Gynaecological problems, 45, 363–81
GyneFix, 121, 420

Headaches, 72–3
  see also Migraine
Health promotion, 295–7
Health of the Nation, 4
Hepatitis
  A, B, C, D viruses, 332–3
  progestogen-only contraception, 114
Herpes simplex virus, 316–20
  clinical features, 318–19
  diagnosis, 319
  treatment, 319–20
High-density lipoproteins, 39, 49, 99

Hirsutism, 82–3, 371–2
History of family planning, 1–4
Hormonal contraception
    combined *see* Combined oral
        contraceptive
    emergency *see* Emergency
        contraception
    litigation, 266–7
    for men, 425–6
    non-oral routes, 430–31
    postabortion, 254–5
    prescribing, 266
    sexual effects, 356–8
Hormone replacement therapy (HRT),
    384
    assessment, 401–3
    breast cancer, 399, 401
    combined oestrogen-progestogen,
        396–7
    compliance, 401
    complications, 400
    contraindications, 398–9
    duration of use, 403
    endometrial cancer, 396, 399
    monitoring, 403
    oestrogen, 392–6
    without bleeding, 397–8
Hospitals, 12–13
Hostility, 343–4
Hot flushes, 386
Hulka-Clemens clip, 207
Human chorionic gonadotrophin, 43,
    252
    anti-hCG vaccines, 432–3
Human Fertilisation and Embryology
    Acts, 271, 274, 275
Human immunodeficiency virus
    (HIV), 323–32
    breastfeeding, 324, 329
    clinical features, 324–6
    combined pill, 329
    condoms, 21, 147, 169, 329
    confidentiality, 273
    contraception, 329–30
    counselling, 328–9
    course of infection, 326
    diagnosis, 326–8
    diaphragm, 329
    drug users, 324
    epidemiology, 324
    ethical aspects, 272–3
    follow-up/treatment, 330–32
    injectable progestogens, 32
    IUDs, 29, 32, 329–30
    pregnancy, 324, 328–9
    prevalence, 302

    random testing, 273
    secondary neoplasms/infectious
        diseases, 325
    spermicides, 174, 179, 329
Human papilloma virus, 282, 302,
    320–23
Hydatidform mole, 113–14
Hydrogel plug (P-block), 415
Hyperprolactinaemia, 49, 371
Hypertension
    combined pill, 70–71
    hormone replacement therapy, 399
    progestogen-only contraception, 97,
        99, 113
    see also Blood pressure
Hypnotics, 65

Immunity, 55
Immunization *see* Vaccination
Implanon, 417
Implants, oestrogen, 395
Implants, progestogen
    advantages/disadvantages, 101
    biodegradable, 417–18
    breastfeeding, 200, 417
    insertion, 107–8
    non-biodegradable, 417
    removal, 108
    research, 416–18
    see also Norplant
Implants, testosterone, 395
In vitro fertilization, 274
Incontinence, urinary, 376–7
Infertility, 274–5
    investigations, 380–81
    pelvic inflammatory disease, 138
    postabortion, 253
    see also Fertility
Inhibin, 385
Injectable progestogens
    administration, 106–7
    adolescents, 26
    advantages/disadvantages, 100–101
    amenorrhoea, 110
    breastfeeding, 200
    coagulation disorders, 97
    combined oestrogen-progestogen,
        418–20
    consent, 267
    disability, 29
    effectiveness, 94
    HIV, 32, 329
    irregular lifestyle, 31–2
    levels of use, 22
    natural steroids, 420

Injectable progestogens (*contd*)
  postpartum, 33
  progestogen-only, 420
  research, 418–20
  see also Depo-Provera;
      Medroxyprogesterone acetate;
      Norethisterone enanthate
      (Noristerat; NET-EN)
Institute of Psychosexual Medicine, 16
Insulin, 39, 51
Intermenstrual bleeding, 367–8
Internal market, 4
Intimacy, 342
Intrauterine devices (IUDs), 119–44
  abnormal bleeding, 134–6
  adolescents, 26
  advantages, 101, 125
  breastfeeding, 128, 200
  choice, 128–9
  complications, 134–40
  contraindications, 126–8
  copper-bearing, 120
  disability, 29
  disadvantages, 101, 125–6
  drug-users, 32
  duration of action, 125
  ectopic pregnancy, 126, 140, 268
  effectiveness, 124–5
  emergency contraception, 8,
      230–234
  endometrium, 124
  epilepsy, 131
  examination, 128
  expulsion, 142
  failure rates, 124–5
  fibroids, 127
  flexible, 121
  follow-up, 133
  historical aspects, 119–20
  HIV, 29, 32, 329–30
  indications, 126
  inert (non-medicated), 120
  insertion, 129–32
  instructions to patients, 132–3
  intercurrent therapy, 133
  intrauterine pregnancy, 139–40
  irregular lifestyle, 32
  item of service fee, 13
  levels of use, 22
  levonorgestrel-releasing *see*
      Levonorgestrel-releasing IUDs
  litigation, 268
  lost threads/devices, 140–44
  medicated, 123–4
  menorrhagia, 127
  mode of action, 124

  pain, 136
  patient history, 128
  pelvic inflammatory disease, 29, 126,
      127, 137–9
  perforation, 131
  perimenopause, 406
  postabortion, 255
  postpartum, 33, 420
  removal, 133–4
  research, 420
  reversibility, 125
  safety, 125
  sexual effects, 358
  termination of pregnancy, 129–30
  training, 15
  vaginal discharge, 137
Irritable bowel syndrome, 374
Ischaemic heart disease, 295

Jaundice, 75
Joint Committee on Contraception, 3

3–Keto-desogestrel, 92, 417, 431

Lactation *see* Breastfeeding
Lactational amenorrhoea method,
    198–9
Lamicel rods, 250
Laparoscopy, 204–5, 222
Lea's shield, 422
Learning disability, 28–30
Leg pains, 82
Legal aspects, 259–77
  termination of pregnancy, 243–4,
      264–5
Levonorgestrel, 39, 82, 92
  acne, 111
  emergency contraception, 230, 234
Levonorgestrel butanoate, 420
Levonorgestrel-releasing IUDs, 92,
    123–4
  breastfeeding, 200
  effectiveness, 95, 125
  follow-up, 109
  perimenopause, 406
Libido, loss of, 351–2, 355–6
  combined pill, 71–2
  Depo-Provera, 100
Lice, 334
Lichen sclerosis, 364
Lifestyle, 25–6, 31–3
Lipid disorders, 46
Lippes Loop, 120

Litigation, 265–71
Liver
  combined oral contraceptive, 47–8,
    52–3, 54, 75
  oestrogen metabolism, 393
  progestogen-only contraception, 96,
    97, 114
Livial, 398, 400
Loestrin-20, 42
Low-density lipoproteins, 39, 99
Lubricants, oil-based, 166, 171–2
Luteinizing hormone, 43, 184, 371,
    384
  home testing kits, 196, 424

Malabsorption, 49
Malathion, 334
Male contraceptives, 425–6
Malignant melanoma, 48–9, 83
Mammography, 292
Marriage, 23, 347–8
Marvelon, 66, 82
Medical defence organizations, 271
Medical ethics, 259–77
Medical research see Research
Medroxyprogesterone acetate, 92, 400
  depot (DMPA) see Depo-Provera
Mefenamic acid, 368, 372, 374
Melasma, 82
Melatonin, 416
Menopause, 383–407
  cardiovascular disease, 390–91
  consequences of ovarian failure,
    385–91
  diagnosis, 385
  endocrine changes, 384–5
  hot flushes, 386
  night sweats, 386
  palpitations , 386
  provision of services, 407
  psychological symptoms, 387
  sexuality, 350
  treatment, 391–400
Menorrhagia, 367, 368
  IUDs, 127
Menstrual cycle
  endocrinology, 43
  hormones, 184–6
  manipulation, 67
Menstrual disturbance, 366–8
  antiprogestogens, 428–9
  female sterilization, 210–11
  irregularity, 367, 368
  perimenopause, 385
Mental incapacity, 28–30, 261–3

Mercilon, 66
Mesigyna, 418–20
Mestranol, 39
Method of contraception, choice,
    19–36
  adolescents, 25–8, 346–7
  and age, 25–8
  childbirth, 33
  and cost, 34–5
  current trends, 20–22
  and disability, 28–30
  lifestyle, 25–6, 31–3
  provider's influence, 33–4
  religion/culture, 30–31
  sexual behaviour, 24–5
  social trends, 22–4
Metronidazole, 311, 313, 314
Micronor, 93
Microval, 93
Middle age, 349–50
Midwives, 16
Mifepristone (RU, 486)
  fertility regulation, 428–9
  termination of pregnancy, 235,
    248–9, 250, 251–2
Migraine
  combined pill, 72–3
  menstrual, 373
  progestogen-only contraception,
    115
Minerals, 55
Minilaparotomy, 205
Miscarriage see Abortion
Missed pills, 62
Mobiluncus spp., 313
Molluscum contagiosum virus, 333
Mothers
  age of, 22
  single, 23
Mucus, cervical, 44, 93
  Spinnbarkeit, 190
Mucus method, 189–92
  research initiatives, 196
Multiload, 124
Multiple index method, 192–3
Musculoskeletal system, 81–2
Mycoplasma genitalium, 309
Myocardial infarction
  combined pill, 53, 56, 70
  hormone replacement therapy, 399
  progestogen-only contraception, 113
Myomas, 113–14

National Association of Family
    Planning Doctors, 4

National Association of Family
    Planning Nurses, 4, 14
National Association of Ovulation
    Method Instructors, 16
National Birth Control Council, 3
National Health Service Act (1946), 1
National Health Service (Family
    Planning) Act (1967), 2
National Health Service Indemnity
    Scheme, 271
National Health Service
    reorganisation, 4, 17
National Health Service
    Reorganisation Act (1973), 2-3
Natural family planning, 16, 183–201
    advantages, 194
    calendar method, 9, 183–4, 186
    after childbirth, 197–201
    disadvantages, 194–5
    effectiveness, 193–4
    future prospects, 195–6
    hormone measurements, 196
    levels of use, 22
    methods, 186–93
    perimenopause, 407
    research, 423–5
    scientific basis, 184–6
    sexual effects, 359
    training, 195
Nausea, 74, 233–4
Neogest, 93
Nestorone, 417, 431
NET-EN see Norethisterone enanthate
Night sweats, 386
Non-specific urethritis, 309–12
Nonoxynol-9 , 172, 174, 176, 329
Norethisterone, 39, 82, 92, 368
Norethisterone acetate, 39, 431
Norethisterone enanthate (NET-EN),
    92
    acne, 111
    administration, 106–7
    contraindications, 96
    effectiveness, 94
    fetal abnormalities, 96
    follow-up, 109
    implants, 418
    license, 95
    microsphere preparation, 420
    weight gain, 111
Norgestimate, 39, 415
Norgeston, 93
Noriday, 93
Norplant, 92
    adolescents, 26
    breakthrough bleeding, 110

    effectiveness, 94
    follow-up, 109
    insertion, 107–8
    irregular lifestyle, 32
    levels of use, 22
    removal, 108
    remuneration, 10
    see also Implants, progestogen
Norplant-II , 417
19–Nortestosterone, 39
Novagard, 128–9
Nova-T, 124, 128–9
Nurses
    counselling, 16
    extended role, 16
    family planning clinics, 11
    practice nurses, 9
    training, 15–16
Nystatin, 316

Occlusive pessaries see Caps
Oestrogen, 39, 43, 184
    cardioprotection, 390–91
    deficiency, menopausal, 385–91
    emergency contraception, 230
    hormone replacement therapy,
        392–6
    implants, 395
    oral, 393
    osteoporosis prevention, 389
    percutaneous creams/gels, 396
    side-effects, 400
    subcutaneous implants, 395
    transdermal (patches), 393–5
    vaginal delivery systems, 395–6
    vaginal preparations, 364
Oestrone, 384
Older women
    method, choice, 28
    pregnancy, 404
    see also Menopause; Perimenopause
Oligomenorrhoea, 370
    causes, 370
    management, 370–71
Once-a-month contraception, 429
Once-a-week contraception, 429
Oral contraception
    combined see Combined oral
        contraceptive
    levels of use, 21
    progestogen-only see Progestogen-
        only pill
Oral sex, 181
Organon, 431
Orgasm, 341–2

Orgasmic dysfunction, 352
Ortho-Gyne-T380S, 120
Osteoporosis, 388–90
  Depo-Provera, 103
Otosclerosis, 399
Ovabloc, 415
Ovarian cancer
  combined pill, 51–2, 85
  Depo-Provera, 102
  family history, 289
  screening, 289–90
Ovarian cysts, 97, 366
  progestogen-only contraception, 111
Ovaries
  cancer see Ovarian cancer
  failure see Menopause
  progestogen, 93
Ovran, 66
  emergency contraception, 230
Ovulation, 43, 184
  breakthrough, 61–3
  method see Mucus method
Ovum donation, 274
Oxytetracycline, 311

P-block, 415
Pair-bonding, 342
Palpitations, 386
Pelvic actinomycosis, 138–9
Pelvic disease
  cancer screening, 281–90
  non-malignant, 290
Pelvic examination, 290
Pelvic floor exercises, 377
Pelvic inflammatory disease
  chlamydial infection, 310
  gonorrhoea, 306
  infertility risk, 138
  IUDs, 29, 126, 127, 137–9
Pelvic masses, 366
Pelvic pain, 374–5
Pentamidine esithionate, 332
Peptostreptococcus spp., 312
Perforation, 131
Perihepatitis, 310
Perimenopause (climacteric), 384
  contraception, 404–7
  endocrine changes, 385
  see also Older women
Persistent generalized
    lymphadenopathy, 325
Pessaries, occlusive see Caps
Pharmacies, 13
Photosensitivity, 82
Phthiriasis, 334

Pigmentation, 82
Pleasure, 341–2
Pneumocystis carinii pneumonia, 330,
  332
Polycystic ovarian syndrome, 83,
  370–71
Polyps, cervical, 365–6
Postcoital bleeding, 367–8
Postcoital contraception see Emergency
    contraception
Postgraduate training, 14–15
Postmenopausal bleeding, 368–9
Potassium citrate, 378
Practice nurses, 9
Prednisolone, 66
Pregnancy
  alcohol, 378
  bleeding in early, 379–80
  combined pill, 84–5
  cytomegalovirus, 334
  ectopic see Ectopic pregnancy
  genital herpes, 320
  HIV, 324, 328–9
  IUD in place, 139–40
  older women, 404
  prepregnancy counselling, 378
  risk, 229–30
  sexual adjustment, 348
  smoking, 378
  video display terminals, 296
  see also Childbirth
Pregnanediol glucoronide estimation,
  424
Premenstrual syndrome, 373–4
Prentif cavity-rim cap, 160
Prescribing, 5
  GP versus clinic, 33–4
  hormonal contraception, 266
  oral contraceptive pill, 44
Privacy, 5
Private practitioners, 13
Proctitis, 310
Professional bodies, 13–14
Progestasert, 123
Progesterone, 43
Progestogen ST-1435 (Nestorone),
  417, 431
Progestogen-only contraception,
  91–117
  adolescents, 112
  advantages, 98–9
  amenorrhoea, 110
  breakthrough bleeding, 109–10
  breastfeeding, 96, 97, 98, 200
  cardiovascular system, 113
  chloasma, 115

Progestogen-only contraception (*contd*)
  coagulation factors, 99
  compliance, 99
  contraindications, 96–7
  disadvantages, 99–100
  drug interactions, 98–9, 115–16
  effectiveness, 94–5
  endometrial cancer, 109–10, 113–14
  endometriosis, 113–14
  epilepsy, 115
  examination, 104
  fetal abnormalities, 116
  follow-up, 109
  future fertility/pregnancy, 116
  genital tract, 113–14
  hypertension, 97, 99, 113
  implants *see* Implants, progestogen;
      Norplant
  indications, 95–6
  indications for stopping, 116–17
  menstrual changes, 99–100
  metabolic effects, 99
  method, choice, 104
  migraine, 115
  mode of action, 93
  oral *see* Progestogen-only pills
  ovarian follicular cysts, 100
  overdosage, 99
  patient history, 104
  post-treatment menstrual
      disturbance, 110
  side effects, 109–12
  surgery, 99
  tolerance, 99
Progestogen-only pills
  administration, 105–6
  adolescents, 26
  advantages/disadvantages, 100
  breastfeeding, 200
  compliance, 99
  ectopic pregnancy, 94
  effectiveness, 94
  failure rates, 94
  follow-up, 109
  HIV, 329
  perimenopause, 405–6
  postcoital contraception, 106
  research, 416
  sexual effects, 356–8
  transferring to combined pill, 106
  types, 93
Progestogens, 39–42
  breast cancer, 97, 113
  hormone replacement therapy, 396–7
  implants *see* Implants, progestogen;
      Norplant

injectable *see* Injectable
    progestogens
  irregular bleeding, 368
  mode of action, 93
  oral *see* Progestogen-only pills
  side-effects, 400
Prolactin-secreting pituitary tumours,
    356
Propanalol, 179
Prostaglandin synthetase inhibitors,
    368, 372
Prostaglandins, 249, 250, 252, 254
Prostate cancer, 216, 225–6
Prostitution, 345
Protectaid sponge, 176, 179
Protozoal infestation, 313–14
Psychological symptoms, menopausal,
    387
Psychosexual medicine, 16–17
Pulmonary embolism, 53
Purchaser/provider split, 4
Pyridoxine (vitamin B_6), 71, 374, 392

Quinacrine hydrochloride, 208, 415

Rabbit, 424
Rape, 343–4
Record keeping, 270
Reiter's disease, 310
Rejection, 343
Religion/culture
  choice of method, 30–31
  coitarche, 25
  and sexuality, 341
Remuneration, 10
Research, 10, 271–2, 412–13
  embryos, 274
  ethical principles, 277
  mucus method, 196
  use of fetal tissue, 275
Resuscitation, 131–2
Rhythm (calendar) method, 183–4, 186
Rifampicin
  combined pill, 66
  progesterone-only contraceptives,
      98, 115
Risk taking, 344
Royal College of General Practitioners,
    3
Royal College of Nursing, 14
Royal College of Obstetricians and
    Gynaecologists, 3, 14–15
RU-486 *see* Mifepristone
Rubella screening, 293–4

Sacral radiculitis, 318
Safer Sex campaign, 147, 169
Scabies, 334–5
Screening, 279–99
  antenatal, 378
  blood pressure, 293
  bone density, 390
  breast cancer, 290–92
  cervical cancer *see* Cervical smear
  endometrial cancer, 290
  human papilloma virus, 323
  ovarian cancer, 289–90
  pelvic disease, 281–90
  rubella, 293–4
  tests, 280
Self-esteem, 343
Septrin, 330–32
Serotonin uptake inhibitors, 374
Services, 5–13
  adolescents, 27–8
  cost-effectiveness, 35
  future of, 17
  guidelines, 4
Sex
  education, 27–8
  functions of, 340–45
  selection, 275
Sexual abuse, 309, 321
Sexual assault, 343–4
Sexual aversion, 352
Sexual difficulties, 350–56
  female problems, 351–4
  helping with, 360–61
  male problems, 354–6
Sexuality, 339–61
Sexually transmissible diseases,
    301–37
  clinics, 302–3
  examination, female patient, 303,
    336–7
  IUDs, 127
  prevalence, 302
Sickle cell disease
  combined pill, 50–51
  progestogen-only contraception, 115
Sino-implant, 417
Skin
  combined pill, 82–3
  menopausal changes, 388
  patches, 431
  progestogen-only contraception, 115
Smoking
  cervical cancer, 282
  combined pill, 56
  health promotion, 295–6
  pregnancy, 378

progestogen-only contraception,
    95–6
  targets, 295
Social class, 23, 24
Sodium fluoride, 390
Sperm granulomas, 215, 225
Sperm production, suppressing, 425–6
Spermicides, 172–9
  adolescents, 27
  advantages, 175
  and condoms, 171
  breastfeeding, 200
  chlorhexidine, 179
  cholic acid, 179
  contraindications, 174
  with diaphragm, 150, 158–9
  disadvantages, 175
  effectiveness, 174
  gramicidin, 179
  HIV, 329
  indications, 174
  instructions to patients, 175–6
  mode of action, 174
  propanalol, 179
  research, 423
SPOD, 17
Sponges, 176–9
  adolescents, 27
  effectiveness, 177
  perimenopause, 407
  Protectaid, 176, 179
  research, 423
  Today *see* Today sponge
Sterilization, 203–227
  adolescents, 27
  advantages, 217, 220
  breastfeeding, 201
  consent, 269
  contraindications, 217
  cost, 35
  counselling, 32–3, 218–19
  disability, 29–30
  disadvantages, 217–18
  effectiveness, 219
  fees, 13
  female *see* Female sterilization
  history of, 2
  indications, 216
  irregular lifestyle, 32–3
  laparoscopic, 204–5
  learning disability, 30
  litigation, 269
  male *see* Vasectomy
  mental incapacity, 262–3
  postpartum, 33
  rates, 21

Sterilization (*contd*)
  regret, 217
  reversibility, 5, 219–20
  risks, 220
  services, 5
  sexual effects, 360
  and social class, 23
Steroid hormone receptor antagonists,
    427–9
Stress incontinence, 376–7
Stroke
  combined pill, 53, 56, 73
  hormone replacement therapy, 399
  progestogen-only contraception, 113
Subarachnoid haemorrhage, 53
Subdermal implants *see* Implants
Sulpiride, 416
Surgery
  combined pill, 69
  progesterone-only contraceptives,
    99
Surrogacy, 274–5
Sympto-thermal method, 192
Syphilis, 309

Targets, 4
  adolescents, 27
  cervical cancer, 10, 289
  smoking, 295
TCu-380 , 125
Teenagers *see* Adolescents
Teratogenesis *see* Fetal abnormalities
Termination of pregnancy, 241–58
  Abortion Act (1967), 2, 241, 243–4,
    264
  abortion rate, 241–2
  assessment, 245–6
  availability, 23–4
  combined pill, 61
  complications, 252–3
  conscientious objection, 264–5
  counselling, 244–5
  dilatation and evacuation, 251
  dilation of cervix, 250
  early first trimester, 247–50
  fetal abnormalities, 251
  follow-up, 254–5
  incomplete abortion, 252–3
  information for patients, 257–8
  IUD insertion, 129–30
  late first trimester, 250
  legal aspects, 243–4, 264–5
  litigation, 270
  medical abortion, 248–50, 251–2,
    257–8

  menstrual extraction technique,
    247–8
  mid-trimester, 250–52
  mifepristone, 235, 248–9, 250, 251–2
  pelvic infection, 246, 253
  private sector, 13
  prophylactic antibiotics, 246
  prostaglandins, 249, 250, 252, 254
  psychiatric disease, 253
  referral, 246
  regret, 253
  rhesus isoimmunisation, 246
  services, 5
  subsequent pregnancies, 253
  techniques, 246–52
  vacuum aspiration, 247–8, 250, 257
Testes, temperature modification, 426
Testicular cancer, 216, 226
Testosterone, 352, 360
  implants, 395
  injections, 425–6
Tetracyclines, 63–6
Therapeutic abortion *see* Termination
    of pregnancy
Thermometers *see* Basal body
    temperature method
Thromboembolism
  combined pill, 29, 39, 47, 53–6
  hormone replacement therapy, 399
  oestrogens, 39
  postpartum sterilization, 33
Thrombophilias, congenital, 53
Thrush, 72, 314–16
Tibolone (Livial), 398, 400
Today sponge, 176–7
  improvements, 423
  perimenopause, 407
Total period fertility rate, 22
Toxic shock syndrome
  diaphragm, 152
  sponges, 178
Toxoplasma gondii, 330, 332
Training, 14–17, 195
Tranquillisers, 65
Transdermal systems, 431
Triadene, 42
Trials, randomized controlled, 272
Trichomoniasis, 313–14
  prevalence, 302
Tricycle regimen, 67
Tri-Minulet, 42
Tripterygium wilfordii, 426
Tubal occlusion
  breastfeeding, 201
  chemical, 208, 415
  clips, 207

Tubal occlusion (*contd*)
  diathermy, 205
  Falope ring, 207
  laser, 208
  non-surgical, 208, 415

Undergraduate training, 14
Uniplant, 417
Uptake, 6
Ureaplasma urealyticum, 309
Urethral prolapse, 377
Urethral syndrome, 377
Urethritis, non-specific/non-
      gonococcal, 309–12
Urinary system disorders, 375–8
  combined pill, 75
  diaphragm, 152
  incontinence, 376–7
  menopausal, 388
  urgency/frequency, 376
Urine testing, 293
Urogenital atrophy, 388

Vaccination
  antifertility, 432–3
  hepatitis A, 332
  hepatitis B, 333
  measles/rubella, 293–4
Vaginal adenosis, 365
Vaginal discharge, 77
  investigation, 303, 304–5
  IUDs, 137
Vaginal rings, 88, 95, 416, 430–31
  advantages/disadvantages, 101
  breastfeeding, 431
  combined oestrogen-progestogen,
      430–31
  insertion, 108
  progestogen-only, 431
  removal, 108–9
  replacement, 108
Vaginal wall cysts, 364–5
Vaginismus, 348, 352–3
Vaginitis, atrophic, 364, 369
Vaginosis, bacterial *see* Bacterial
      vaginosis
Valvular heart disease
  combined pill, 47
  IUDs, 127
Vas deferens valves/plugs, 414
Vasectomy, 211–16
  assessment, 213
  breastfeeding, 201
  cancer, 216, 225–6
  cardiovascular disease, 215–16

complications, 215–16, 224–6
  counselling, 214, 219
  effectiveness, 219, 223–4
  examination, 213
  failure, 215
  follow-up, 214
  information for patients, 223–7
  late recanalization, 215
  litigation, 269
  no-scalpel, 212–13, 414
  non-surgical, 213, 414
  open-ended, 213
  percutaneous non-surgical vas
      occlusion technique, 213, 414
  perioperative advice, 214, 226–7
  prostate cancer, 216, 225–6
  reversibility, 220, 226
  services, 5
  technical improvements, 414
  techniques, 211–13
  testicular cancer, 216, 226
  timing, 214
  see also Sterilization
Vasovagal syncope (cervical shock),
      131
Vault cap, 163–4
Venous disease, 53
Video display terminals, 296
Vimule, 165–6
Viral infections, 316–34
Virilism, 372
Visual disturbance, 74
Vitamin B_6, 71, 392, 374
Vitamins, 55
Vomiting, 63, 74, 233–4
Vulval intraepithelial neoplasia (VIN),
      320–21
Vulvovaginitis
  candidal, 315
  prepubertal girls, 306, 309

Warfarin, 67
Weight, screening, 292–3
Weight gain
  combined pill, 53, 74
  Depo-Provera, 111
  hormone replacement therapy, 403
  injectable progestogens, 111
  progestogen-only contraceptives,
      100

Zalcitabine, 332
Zidovudine, 332
  pregnancy, 324
Zovirax, 319–20